Occupational Therapy: Advanced Concepts and Techniques

Occupational Therapy: Advanced Concepts and Techniques

Edited by Abraham Miller

STATES
ACADEMIC PRESS
www.statesacademicpress.com

States Academic Press,
109 South 5th Street,
Brooklyn, NY 11249, USA

Visit us on the World Wide Web at:
www.statesacademicpress.com

ISBN: 978-1-63989-391-1

Cataloging-in-Publication Data

Occupational therapy : advanced concepts and techniques / edited by Abraham Miller.
p. cm.
Includes bibliographical references and index.
ISBN 978-1-63989-391-1
1. Occupational therapy. 2. Occupational therapy--Technological innovations.
3. Medical rehabilitation. I. Miller, Abraham.
RC487 .O23 2022
616.891 65--dc23

Table of Contents

Preface

Every book is a source of knowledge and this one is no exception. The idea that led to the conceptualization of this book was the fact that the world is advancing rapidly; which makes it crucial to document the progress in every field. I am aware that a lot of data is already available, yet, there is a lot more to learn. Hence, I accepted the responsibility of editing this book and contributing my knowledge to the community.

The branch of health care which assists people who suffer from sensory, physical or cognitive issues is termed as occupational therapy. The challenges related to emotional and social needs are addressed within this field. People who suffer from sensory processing disorders, birth defects, autism, cancer and developmental delays are assisted in a variety of ways such as visual perception, sensory-processing problems and fine motor skills. It involves tailoring the therapy for each person's individual needs. The strengths and challenges are analyzed in order to design a schedule of activities and exercises. This book traces the progress of clinical research on occupational therapy, and highlights some of its key concepts and applications. It elucidates new techniques and their applications in a multidisciplinary manner. The book will help the readers in keeping pace with the rapid changes in this field.

While editing this book, I had multiple visions for it. Then I finally narrowed down to make every chapter a sole standing text explaining a particular topic, so that they can be used independently. However, the umbrella subject sinews them into a common theme. This makes the book a unique platform of knowledge.

I would like to give the major credit of this book to the experts from every corner of the world, who took the time to share their expertise with us. Also, I owe the completion of this book to the never-ending support of my family, who supported me throughout the project.

Editor

1

Yoga for Anxiety Management in the Workplace

S. Doria, F. Irtelli, R. Sanlorenzo and F. Durbano

Abstract

Anxiety is a potential cause of serious influence in a person's daily life. This chapter is focused specifically on the effects of the work environment factors in disease development and progression. Working environments are places of significant sources of stress: they put us in connection with our duties and expectations (often not coincide with reality) and with a "forced socialization." Especially forced socialization is to be considered a main source of stress in work places, inducing negative outcomes in work and social relationships. The psychosocial risks of work places can so be defined according to design, organization and management of work as well as to social and environmental contexts that may lead to damage of physical, social and psychological domains. Stress can then be defined as a pattern of emotional, cognitive, behavioral, and physiological reactions to adverse and noxious aspects perceived as the contents of the working environment. Thanks to the beginning of psychosocial research on the working environment, the impact of some aspects of the work environment on health has become an object of study, as the interventions to mitigate it. Yoga, meditation, and mantra techniques, as described in this work (presenting others' experiences and two of own current projects, used in a hospital workplace to control the condition of occupational stress but also in a clinical sample), showed the potential in considerably reducing anxiety and mood symptoms.

Keywords: anxiety, yoga, work, environmental factors, stress, coping and vulnerability, prevention

1. Introduction

This perspective is deep-rooted in the history of medicine. From this perspective, George Engel introduced the term "biopsychosocial approach" as a privileged model for decoding and comprehending in many ways health and stress as existential processes, and to articulate forms of care and of taking responsibility [1]. The biopsychosocial model is based on the paradigm of complexity, in sharp contrast with classical biomedical reductionism, as well as the hierarchy of the sciences. It adopts the perspective of the General Systems Theory developed by Von Bertalanffy, which considers a set of events interrelated as a system with specific properties and functions depending on the level at which it is located with respect to a larger system. The systems theory in fact claims that all levels of an organization are interrelated to each other, so that changing one affects the other, mitigating the dichotomy between holism and reductionism [1]. The model refers to three basic principles: free dialogue, relationship, and humility. In other words, it aims at looking at the person as a "whole" genetic element (bio), the subject of discussion and decision (psycho), as well as a historical, cultural, and familiar subject (social). The axioms of the model are inclusiveness (understanding of diversity) and nonexclusiveness (putting aside what is regarded as their competence), the answers to which are total and global whatever the point of entry into the system (the biological now, psychological time, social hour). The centrality of this model has been confirmed and validated by almost uncountable literature marking the transition to a person-centered medicine [2] and it is now of widespread knowledge that biopsychosocial screening, rather than a compartmentalized approach, can help plan a more effective treatment and help an early and useful stress management. Human beings tend to form themselves through the development of groupal complex systems affecting the three main areas explored in the biopsychosocial model. Therefore, one must bear in mind that every action must always consider the construction of or refunding the mind–body integration. A person's discomfort cannot be considered only in terms of somatic or psychic discomfort, because any discomfort brings the indissoluble unity of consciousness of the self. This should be emphasized because not everyone knows how to use this knowledge in the care of the person as a whole.

2. Work, a question of balance and psychosocial aspects

Workplace can be assumed as a model of a complex system involving biological, psychological, and social aspects, so we have to rely on a biopsychosocial approach to deal effectively with any issue concerning individuals and teams. These three dimensions are interlinked, in fact effective management of health and safety in the workplace is important and recommended to individuals and society alike. This approach is particularly important and relevant in times of economic uncertainty when it is essential for companies to maintain high productivity levels despite the decreasing number of resources and when mistakes and accidents are most likely to occur [3]. The psychosocial risks should be taken in to account when designing, organizing, managing, and evaluating the social and environmental contexts that may lead to damages of the "physical, social, and psychological health." In the '60s, psychosocial research in the work environment highlighted the impact of some aspects of the workplace on health. Today we have strong evidence of how the work-related stress exposes the individual to danger, inefficiency, and error: stress increases the production of cortisol, damages the hippocampus, and causes damage to memory and cognitive skills (which can be reduced by up to 60%) [4].

But what is stress? In the '50s Selye introduced the term stress in everyday language and such term began to take on the meaning which it still retains, also in the field of psychology. Stress, a term that means "pressure," derives from the field of engineering; it is used to refer to any force that is applied to a body in order to test its durability under stress. Over time, this term was progressively used to refer more specifically to "a state of non-specific stress of living matter, which is manifested by morphological transformations tangible in various organs, particularly in the endocrine glands that are under the control of the pituitary" [5,6]. Originally the syndrome "just being sick" covered the stereotypical response of an organism to a wide range of physical, biological, or chemical agents. Selye was the first to use the term stress to describe a range of physical and psychological responses to adverse conditions or influences [7]. Stress occurs when we have to respond to a stimulus from the external world: this response consists of a behavioral adaptation and the activation of biological systems (psycho-neuro-endocrine) in such a way to prevent potential negative consequences and, where it is not possible to solve the situation, possibly develop forms of adaptation. The first important consideration relates to the fact that stress is the result of a process of human adaptation to the environment. There are some specific mechanisms that underlie the identification of a response to stress: a) a dynamic stimulus-response reaction, b) the required adjustment in order to respond appropriately and effectively to the stimulus, c) the high energy (mental and physical) needed to achieve this adaptation effort. In addition to the "active" and "passive" reaction, characterized by inhibition, recent studies have demonstrated the existence of ways of reacting with a great intersubject variability. We filter the stressor by attributing different and personal meanings and values to it depending on a wide range of constitutional and experiential factors, and also on the context. When exposed to stressful situations, the individual puts in place strategies that modify or attempt to modify his/her environment. These strategies are strictly individual and are linked to the personal characteristics of the subject and their historical experience. The term stress stands for stressful event (or stressor), a term that describes the stimulus factor that causes the reaction. Stressors can be major factors (the loss of work), minor factors (small facts of everyday life, or hassles), acute factors (accidents) and chronic factors (a very competitive business environment) [8]. The stress effect is potentially pathogenic when the conditions from which it is derived are chronic or recur with some frequency. Selye also distinguished between eustress (or good stress) and distress (bad stress); such terms were originally included in the broader definition of stress but were immediately indicated as distinct from one another. Selye stated that stress is an inevitable consequence of living, but that distress appears when the requests to which the person is exposed (both in the psychological and physiological dimensions) overtake the capacity and energy that the person has or believes to have to maintain the homeostasis. The stimulus demand can, therefore, have a more or less acceptable meaning [7,9]. Holmes and Rahe, in the construction of the "Social Readjustment Rating Scale [10]," discovered that each stress can be classified into distress and eustress, where the first is caused by a response considered disproportionate in size, while the eustress is caused by a response considered acceptable, which creates a moderate level of tension enabling to successfully address the perceived challenge. This is, however, only one aspect of Eustress. The concept of an optimal level of stress derives from the studies of Yerkes and Dodson Law that explained how stress is beneficial for increasing the performance until it is moderate, after surpassing a certain level of stress the performance will deteriorate according to a inverted "U" diagram—see Figure 1 [11,12].

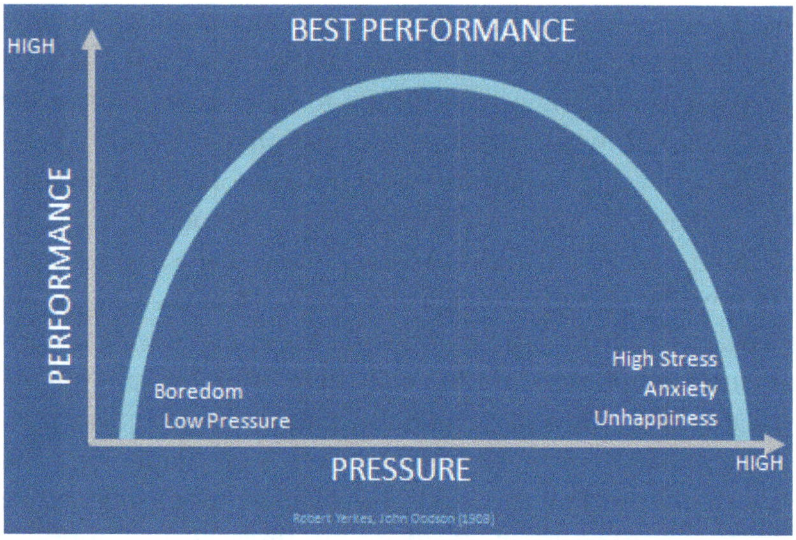

Figure 1. The stress–performance relationship according to Yerkes and Dodson [12] modified.

In order to clarify the connection between the theory of Yerkes and Dodson and Seyle's work, it has to be clear that the effect of any stimulus depends on how each individual interprets it and chooses to react to it. It is the individual that determines whether the stressor will generate eustress or distress. The eustress is the primary result of a positive perception of the stressor, while the distress is the result of a negative perception. The classification depends on how the stressor is perceived by the individual, on which kind of value is assigned to it. Selye suggested that learning how to respond to stressful stimuli with positive emotions, such as hope, maximizes eustress and minimizes the distress, whereas responding with negative emotions, such as despair, greatly increases the distress [9]. In the perception of stressor, and when assigning of its meaning, a key characteristic of the individual is involved: the locus of control (or self-efficacy); people with an internal locus of control (believing they can control and master all external situations) tend to perceive and to respond to stressors quite differently with respect to people with an external locus of control (believing they cannot at all control and master all external situations) [13]. Self-efficacy is the belief of being able to control the environmental challenges by deploying an adaptive action, and, according to the social cognitive theory, strongly influences the effectiveness of self-perceived behaviors being positively associated with adaptation [13]. In fact, it is positively related to an active strategy and negatively to a passive reaction [14]. In the aforementioned works, Selye introduced the notion of "general adaptation syndrome" to describe the way in which the body copes with stressful events; he distinguished three phases that follow this order: 1) alarm phase: it is activated by the autonomic nervous system in the occasion of intense stressful events; 2) resistance stage: the body reacts to stress and, if the stress is intense, there are transient events such as the enlargement of the adrenal glands, gastrointestinal ulcers, etc.; 3) exhaustion stage: if the stressor persists or if the body is not able to put in place appropriate responses, the body undergoes irreversible responses, which can include death. The distress, specifically, is characterized by a stage of alarm, a stage of resistance, and a stage of functional exhaustion. R.S. Lazarus has integrated Selye's model with the purely cognitive aspects related to the subjective perception of specific stressors, creating a more complex model [15,16]. In his model, the same event, as already mentioned, may have different meanings in different subjects, and it is unquestionable that when confronted with stressful factors different people react in different ways with quite different outcomes. The ideal response requires strategies which are active but also multiple, flexible, and tailored to the specific factors or stressful events in action. The stress response is then modulated in two ways by the psychological characteristics of the individual: in the process of perception and processing of the stressors, and in coping with these factors.

3. Workplace and anxiety

Working environments put us in connection with our duties and expectations (which often do not coincide with the reality of the context) and with a "forced socialization." This is a clear model of stress defined as a psychosocial phenomenon; therefore, specific interventions have to be based on the identification of stressors and their original context. Over time, this has led to the identification of two areas of research: 1) study of stress measures, scales, and 2) tools for assessing the effects of stress on individuals. We must remember that the measured stress level may not be strictly related to the work environment and that subjective aspects play a decisive role in the type of reaction. Being subjective, this measure allows us to identify the sources of stress that have occurred in causing discomfort and to certify its effects only [4]. If the stressful events are easily identified, it is much more difficult to predict the subjective reactions to them. In fact, as already stated, the individual response to stress depends on constitutional and experiential factors. There are also particular types of stress and forms of anxiety (i.e., stress response) that could be directly related to the workplace, like "stress in social situations." This is a particular stress that arises from forced participation in social situations perceived as anxiety provoking. People affected by stress in social situations are very upset when forced to interact in social gatherings, tend to avoid public speaking, show anxiety in group settings and invent excuses to avoid encounters with people they do not know; furthermore, those who exceed in this stress often feel uncomfortable when talking with "superior" people of the opposite sex and/or with whom they have never spoken before. Therefore, the resulting stress involves a state that may evolve from an acute condition (where the mind/body is enabled to effectively react to external events that must be addressed and solved) to a chronic condition in which stress remains constant and generates harmful effects on the physiological functions with repercussions on the ability of interpersonal adaptation. Another kind of anxiety that could characterize a person is also "social concern": it is closely related to the activation and the consequent negative emotional condition of tension that occurs in situations in which the subject feels under observation. Individuals with high levels of social concern are very uncomfortable when thinking someone is looking at him, as he often fears negative evaluations by others. Feeling apprehensive about someone becoming aware of their shortcomings, or not approving what they do, is a cause of great anxiety for these individuals, especially when the feared opinion comes from their superiors. People with high social concerns usually see their image as is potentially perceived by others, and believe that physical appearance is very important to establish positive and functional relationships with others. This induces a dysfunctional groping to inspire confidence at all costs, with the negative and unwanted pitfall to behave ridiculously. These elements can originate a condition defined mismatch [17-19]. Concerns about the image perceived by others can lead to the complete avoidance of any potentially stressful situations and, consequently, to a state of interpersonal closure and loss of motivation to affiliate to others [15,20]. In this context, it is very important to prevent negative stress, distress, which occurs when the situation needs an effort to adapt to it that exceeds our perceived ability to achieve it. Since the '60s, there has been a growing awareness on the unavoidable essence of stress as a human condition while coping skills and resources make the difference in the outcomes of the adaptation process [16,21]. The features involved in the modulation of the stress response strategies are called coping skills, and the whole process of reaction and coping of stress is referred to as "coping" [15,16]. Studies on the so-called "good copers" clearly show that these people persistently believe that they will be able to cope with the stress: they are practical and directly address the issues straightforward; on the contrary, "bad copers" are characterized by disappointment and pessimism [22,23]. There are quite recurrent types of coping, which is why we talk about "styles" of coping. They are crucial in the success to achieve personal goals [24-27]. The most common coping styles can be summarized as follows:

1. **Combat**: this style is characterized by the challenge of defeating the stress: the person sees the situation of stress like a challenge, has an optimistic view of the future, and believes that it is possible to exercise control over the stress. This kind of person reveals a coping style aimed at direct confrontation [27]. Therefore, those who adopt this strategy have a so-called internal locus of control, they want to know as much as possible about their own condition, their source of stress and the context and actively change their lifestyle in order to preserve their health; this strategy can be defined as an active, positive coping, because it represents a tendency to actively confront and cope with stress and protects from anxiety. The optimism that characterizes this style of coping has beneficial effects on the health, well-being, and the quality of life of those who adopt it. Recent research confirmed these assumptions [27]. The combative coping mediates these effects positively, while fatalism, anxious worries, and despair mediate these effects negatively. However, it is not enough to be optimistic, if you do not take a combative style of coping. The combative style induces lower levels of anxiety and demoralization, empowers individuals in finding answers for discussion and gives them the feeling they are able to control events, at least partially: "I see this stress as a challenge," "I am determined to overcome it," "I am very optimistic;" combative people adopt more flexible and differentiated cognitive and

behavioral strategies, such as "I am actively trying to improve my health," which promote a more positive view of the events. As a result, and as mentioned above, this style is associated with lower psychological morbidity and a greater sense of personal control [27].

2. **Avoidance-disclaimer**: this strategy is very complex, it is generally characterized by the tendency to not directly address any issues related with stress, and is associated to the use of the refusal defense mechanism (to avoid seeing the unpleasant aspects of reality); it is very common, often plays a really useful role in protecting from anxiety. However, if taken to the extreme and used as the only form of defense, it can cause problems. It has been divided into denial of adaptation and maladaptive avoidance; the first can be defined as a natural method of emotional self-protection, which has positive effects on health, so it was also called "healthy denial" by Druss in 1988 [28]. The maladaptive avoidance, instead, splits up into more extreme forms of denial that can lead to poor cooperation and cause strong anxiety when it is no longer effective as defense mechanism. A high level of avoidance, used as the only coping strategy, can also lead to an unrealistic perception of self-efficacy.

3. **Fatalism**: it is a strategy characterized by an attitude of fatalistic resignation and passive acceptance of the stress. People who adopt this strategy recognize the gravity of the situation and believe they have little control over events. Therefore, they accept what fate ordained with resignation as if that was their destiny. Therefore, we must point out that the tendency to perceive external events as related to fate is typical of those who have an external locus of control, a place of external control, which causes poor adaptation to the stress.

4. **Anxious preoccupation**: it is a strategy characterized by constant feelings, the feelings of danger, stress, and high level of anxiety. Stress assumes a central position in person's existence. It is negatively related to social and emotional functioning. Those who adopt this style of coping are continuously searching for reassurance, demand for visits, or otherwise escape from the context because it is too distressing. It is positively related to coping style despair [27].

5. **Despair**: it is characterized by feelings of loss and the oppression; it is related to high levels of anxiety, poor cognitive strategies, and the belief of having little control over events. In fact, there is a correspondence between despair and demoralization, which leads to affective symptoms of existential distress, cognitive tendency to pessimism, sense of personal failure, lack of motivation to deal with the event, feelings of social isolation and alienation [24-27].

3.1. Burn out, source of stress in workplaces

The '**burn out**' syndrome is a stress-related phenomenon, even if distinct from it. It happens particularly to people working in the social sector and in the helping professions. Burn out consists in a progressive loss of motivation, idealism, objectives and the meaning associated with them, a decreased perception of social utility of one's own work. The "burn out" condition does not coincide with stress but it induces stress in a work environment when the balance between the following three important factors is lost: a) required level of performance, b) control over one's own work, c) reward and gratification. In order not to get into a condition of stress, the worker has to perceive these three factors as balanced. With regard to the analysis of occupational stress the cognitive aspects are very highlighted, assuming that an event can have very different effects on each individual. To better understand the development of burn out it is useful to introduce also the concepts of "work stress" and "work strain." "Work stress" is an objectively measurable occupational stress (an acceptable level of overtime); "work strain" is defined as the particular emotional and mental reverb of the same condition or activity on different people (e.g., the effects of demotivation on a single person in relation to his/her actual potential professionalism or his/her culture) [4]. Only in certain circumstances can an experience of stress turn into a real illness. Since the autonomic nervous system and the neuroendocrine system mediate the body's response to stress, as a result of prolonged and repeated stress a normal physiological response can turn into a meaningful damage to health, especially affecting the cardiovascular, endocrine, gastrointestinal, and immune systems [4]. When the need to tackle stress is over, the chemical responses previously activated should terminate. But when the physiological reaction to stress is not able to recover, the areas assigned to the production of adrenaline and cortisol continue their secretion, creating chronic stress, this in turn leads in particular to systemic alterations that in turn cause physical and psychological problems, such as behavioral and emotional symptoms like recurring irritability, poor concentration, decreased performance, tearfulness, changes in appetite, loss of self-esteem, sleep disorders, cardiovascular disorders, tendency to hyperglycemia, headache, and poor functioning of the immune system [4].

3.2. The importance of stress prevention in working organization

The high psychological and social costs that a person has to pay as a result of negative experiences (stress) at the workplace is becoming an increasing problem not only for the workers or the management, but also for organizations. For this reason, organizations are gearing up (e.g., by promoting yoga courses for employees). In the past, it was noted that the reduction in efficiency due to work stress probably has comparable effects to those caused by the strikes on the economic front [4].

Potentially stressful factors at work involve the relationship with work environment and work content (material factors), the role people play in the organization (organizational factors), and interpersonal relationships (psychosocial factors). Referring to the role that a person plays in the organization we can talk about role-stress when there is a discrepancy between the actual role and the role to that the worker wishes to reach in the organization (this phenomenon is called inconsistency of position).

The classical three levels of prevention are:

1. **Primary prevention**, the purpose of which is to decrease the incidence of the arising of the negative phenomenon, it consists in an attempt to prevent the development of a discomfort in a population at risk.

2. **Secondary prevention**, which tends to reduce the prevalence of morbidity through the curtailment of the period, the spread of the stress.

3. **Tertiary prevention**, which tends to mitigate the effects of negative factors on those affected.

The timing of the intervention with the onset of pathological symptoms is, therefore, the discriminating factor between these three levels. The earlier the preventive intervention takes place, the more efficacy it has in preventing potential damages generated by work processes and environment. Developing trainings aimed at improving stress management can help to reduce stress through greater mastery of the work process, strengthening self-esteem, and developing a higher sense of self-efficacy, but also improving motivation and mood. In the process of designing the work flow it is essential to take in to account not only ergonomic principles, but also the need to develop proper systems of performance evaluation, based on known criteria (preferably shared), on a transparent communication and on constructive feedback from the management. Such evaluation system will concretely reduce stress and increase the sense of control and involvement, facilitating the employees in the assignment of meaning to their activities and contribute to self-esteem [4].

3.3. Mental disorders in the EU, the importance of an early intervention

It is estimated that a third of the European population suffers from mental disorders [29]. Psychiatric disorders are the prominent cost of disability-adjusted life years worldwide [30]. Anxiety is one of the most common psychiatric disorders affecting adults and young adults [29,31-36]. Anxiety disorders have the potential to cause serious interference with a person's daily life, work, and career [29,37]. It is also known that all pharmacological treatments with benzodiazepines can cause troublesome side effects, including anterograde memory impairment, sedation, and the risk of dependence; therefore, they are not recommended for long-term use [38]. Furthermore, response to these treatments tends to be highly variable, ranging from 40% to 70% [39-42]. These limits in terms of efficacy and tolerability often result in poor patient adherence to medication and, thus, long-term remission is often difficult to achieve [43]. On average, only a third of patients achieve remission within a year of follow-up, while patients who do achieve an initial response often relapse [44].

Can we, therefore, intervene before the appearance of a psychiatric disorder? Here stands the importance of primary prevention, which is finalized to prevent pathogenesis preserving the subject from the risk of taking pathogenic behaviors. The literature has largely emphasized that improving "coping style" to stress, and all the problems related to it, may prevent and decrease anxiety and its consequences on working processes (and on social functioning as a whole). In this perspective yoga can be a very effective and promising approach.

3.4. Yoga: A biopsychosocial approach to health

Why should organizations promote yoga and not a generic physical activity for their employees? What is the difference between generic physical activity benefits and yoga benefits? The difference in benefits has been shown in a fairly recent study made by Bonura: both fitness and yoga lead to an improvement of psychological health, although the changes obtained with yoga were generally higher and more durable [45].

Yoga has shown greater enhancement in psychological health than the simple physical exercise, substantiated by the decrease of anger, anxiety, and depression, and increased global wellness, positive overall effects, and feeling of an increase of self-efficacy. Clance and coworkers (1980) concluded that yoga is an effective method to improve the image of the body and, consequently, the self-image [46].

We need to point out that yoga is a time-tested, *ante litteram*, biopsychosocial approach to life: it includes health in the body, peace in the mind, and helps to develop good relationships and harmony in the society; moreover, the body-mind-spirit unity is a key feature of the yogic approach to health and happiness. Yoga techniques range from yoga postures (asanas) and purification techniques (kriyas), more focused on body health, to breathing techniques, cognitive strategies, and meditation for clarity of mind and emotional balance (pranayama, gyana, and dyana), to ethical codes of conduct aimed to establish harmony in the society (yama and nyama). The yoga approach to life is very reliable with the general system theory and to the work of Nicolis and Prigogyne [47] on dissipative systems: life is seen as a flow of energy where the individual (subsystems) is part of the whole (the bigger system) and is striving to keep its harmony (sattva) utilizing energy from nature to implement proper actions and assuming a proactive attitude toward events. The imbalances of the system can be of two types: excess of tamas (inertia) like in depression and misunderstandings or excess of rajas (activity) like in anxiety, and all yoga techniques are aimed at recreating balance (sattva) at physical, psychological and social level. Often yoga is seen as an intangible and philosophical practice that is not suitable for the modern world of competitions and the fast pace that characterizes the work environment. This misunderstanding is due to a lack of knowledge and a cultural bias; in fact Patanjali (a prominent character in the yogic tradition that systematized the discipline in his "yoga sutras" (400 BC)) defines yoga as "skill in action" [48] The usefulness of yoga postures and breathing techniques for general health, stress management and anxiety is easy to understand and to demonstrate and there is a growing body of studies showing evidences in this direction [49,50]. But yoga can also provide cognitive tools to approach stressors in a healthy way. In fact yoga promotes a proactive approach to events and challenges, encouraging the apprentice to develop a keen self-awareness and to take responsibility for how he perceives events and people and for how he responds to events and people's behavior. When properly understood and followed this "practice" leads to a balanced and constructive combative attitude toward stressors. Yoga can be helpful for the development of an effective strategy for reducing tension, through short and simple exercises that are easy to replicate autonomously. In particular, for the constant attention paid to the body–mind relationship, yoga seems to be particularly influential on the activities related to the sympathetic system and, therefore, on the typical symptoms of anxiety: accelerated heartbeat, palpitations, tremors, sweating, increased blood pressure, dry mouth, avoidance behaviors, restlessness, etc. [51]. Yoga can also stabilize mental activity and enhance brain function and resilience to stress [52-54]. Yoga and breathing techniques can also favor a regular nasal breathing, with better lung expandability. Some yogic exercises of relaxation and cleansing of the nasal passages are also very effective in the prevention of sinusitis and rhinitis, and the resulting pharyngitis, laryngitis, and tracheitis [55]. Specific exercises can procure greater elasticity in the muscles needed for breathing, which is important because respiratory deficits are due in large part to the lack of movement secondary to a sedentary lifestyle. Yoga breathing techniques can also prevent excessive tachycardia and hypertensive crises related to anxiety, because of their help in regularizing breathing. Finally, it is also known that stress and sleep disorders, such as insomnia and frequent interruption of sleep, can be fought with specific breathing techniques associated with sequences of dynamic yogic exercises [56]. Yoga can be also considered one of the strategies to cope with pathological conditions that have already taken place (secondary prevention), like Generalized Anxiety Disorder. Today there is enough evidence to consider yoga to be a beneficial, low-risk, low-cost integration to the treatment of stress and anxiety [57-60]. The antidepressant efficacy is also important as demonstrated by quite numerous studies [61-66]. Yoga could be considered a complementary therapy to classical psychological and psychiatric approaches, because many traditional yogic exercises have a therapeutic value. For these reasons today more and more doctors and psychologists recommend yoga as a relaxation technique.

3.5. Yoga and work organization

There are many evidences supporting the hypothesis that the introduction of yoga and meditation in the workplace at a large scale will benefit both the single workers and the performance of teams and organizations. We think that can be useful to analyze the "access barriers" that yoga shows for organizations and also to highlight cases where these barriers have been surpassed:

1. **Language and cultural bias**: yoga is perceived by many managers and decision takers in the corporate and institutional world as unpractical, philosophical, esoteric, religious, and anyway as something that concerns personal life and personal choices. To overcome such preconceptions the yoga teachers need to develop the skill to present yoga and conduct yoga classes with a secular language, introducing scientific evidences of the benefits of yoga. It is a huge cultural experiment that offers very interesting horizons of integration of eastern and western culture.

2. **Budget allocation**: in the middle of the shrinking of budgets, HR departments struggle to give priority to initiative that do not seem very concrete and with short term results. Again to overcome this problem it is necessary to show scientific results both in terms of health prevention and health strategies (and also the reduction of lost working hours) but also in terms of increased personal and team performance.

Some successful initiatives highlighted the potential of introducing yoga and meditation in working organizations, suggesting how to overcome the aforementioned barriers.

The Project Response has been supported and funded by the EU Commission's Directorate General (DG) Research to develop knowledge and understanding on the degree of alignment between companies and their stakeholders about what Corporate Social Responsibility (CSR) entails. The main objective was to study CSR at the level of individual manager's behavior, assessing the relative effectiveness of diverse training interventions on the development of social consciousness in managers. It was conducted from 2004 to 2007 by a multidisciplinary team of academic researchers from a consortium of leading business schools in Europe (INSEAD, France; Copenhagen Business School, Denmark; Università Commerciale Luigi Bocconi, Italy; Leon Kozminski Academy of Entrepreneurship and Management, Poland) and a training consultancy (Impact, Austria). Part of the study was aimed to evaluate, on 93 managers, the impact on their CSR behaviors after following stress management and meditation programs. In the words of Maurizio Zollo, leading the research team, "meditation and relaxation techniques seem to enable managers to break free from patterns of decision making driven by short term outcomes, self interest and reliance on safe solutions to embrace more proactive and innovative approaches to social and environmental challenges" [67]. One might even posit that the strain placed on managers in the workplace leads to short-term time horizons, narrow self-interests and familiar approaches to problem solving. This would, thus, prevent sound decision-making based on search for creative solutions to unstructured problems, on caring and trusting attitudes and on long-term views of the implications of one's decisions on broader audiences internal and external to the company [67].

Mindfulness Based Stress Reduction: the roots of this method are in the Tibetan Buddhist tradition. Mindfulness Based Training was conceived in a hospital setting and developed by Jon Kabat-Zinn at the University of Massachusetts Medical Center, it uses a combination of mindfulness meditation, body awareness, and yoga to help people become more mindful. His specific secular and scientific approach to yoga and meditation coupled with the effectiveness are the base of the wide success of the program in corporations and organizations worldwide [68-70].

TLEX Program: TLEX program is another positive example of how to overcome the barriers expressed in points 1 and 2. The origin of this set of programs is the Sudarshan Kriya Yoga (SKY), a complete yoga method created by Sri Sri Ravi Shankar in 1982. The TLEX program started form the personal experience of some entrepreneurs and managers that experienced SKY and, seeing the potential of introducing such techniques and cognitive strategies in their working environment, requested Sri Sri Ravi Shankar to tailor specific programs for their employees and managers. Starting as a very innovative service, TLEX is now offered in corporations and organizations worldwide [71,72].

4. Two studies focused on yoga and health — The Milan "Fatebenefratelli e Oftalmico" Hospital experience

The promising results of the scientific research, embracing both the neurophysiologic approach and the management approach, the "commercial" success of programs based on yoga and meditation, and positive case histories (like the program conducted at Fatebenefratelli Hospital in Milan, Italy) show the important impact that yoga training has on individual workers and organizations in general. We are still in the initial phase; much more has to be done.

Here we describe two studies regarding yoga and health.

In the first study we applied a particular yogic protocol called SKY (which stands for Sudarshan Kriya Yoga) as a treatment for patients affected by Generalized Anxiety Disorder and depression.

In the second study that we present, yoga, meditation and mantras have been used to deal with work-related stress for employees of a hospital.

4.1. SKY for anxiety disorders

A sample of patients (n=69) diagnosed and treated for anxiety and depression disorders was included in an experimental treatment with SKY techniques [73]. The adult participants (from 25 to 64 years old) were consenting persons with primary diagnosis of DSM-IV-TR Mood (n=18), anxiety disorders (n=39), or mixed condition (n=12) [74]. All patients signed informed consent for participation in the study. The sample was divided in two groups:

Group 1 undergoing pharmacological treatment, SKY treatment and participating to self-help group weekly; Group 1 subjects had a minimum of six months of stable condition due to standard pharmacological treatment with appropriate dose of antidepressant and/or anxiolytic.

Group 2 was not treated with psychiatric medication for at least six months prior to the study. This group received only SKY treatment and participated to self-help group weekly. These subjects were characterized by poor response and/or inadequate adherence to pharmacological treatment, had at least six months of participation to self-help groups and stable conditions.

The procedure of SKY was documented previously [62,63,74,75]. SKY was taught by trained, certified facilitators. The experimental group participated in an intense SKY workshop consisting of 10 sessions in two weeks followed by weekly SKY follow-up classes for six months. Each session lasted approximately two hours.

Assessments were done by a psychologist, uninvolved in treatment, in a quiet ambulatory environment. The severity of anxiety was assessed using Hamilton Rating Scale for Anxiety (HRSA) [76] and Zung Self-Rating Anxiety Scale Inventory (ZASI) [77]. The severity of depression was assessed using Hamilton Rating Scale for Depression (HRSD) [78] and Zung Self-Rating Depression Scale Inventory (ZDSI) [79]. The global symptom situation of patients was also assessed using Symptom Checklist-90 Revised (SCL-90-R) [80].

One of the aims of the study was to verify if SKY was an efficacious adjunctive treatment in pharmacological resistant, anxious-depressive subjects. Other objectives are related to neurophysiological evidences of the effects of SKY on the autonomic nervous system; the data are currently in evaluation for a specific publication.

Table 1 shows the results on anxiety severity assessment both with a subjective and an objective measure (ZASI and HRSA, respectively). Statistical analysis is in press [73], but some results are summarized in Table 1. All the tests measuring anxiety showed a significant improvement, which reaches statistical significance. The Global Score Index of SCL–90–R also showed a marked improvement from the baseline onward, the main effect of medication consumption over GSI scores being not significant.

Statistical analyses have shown that SKY therapy significantly reduces the levels of anxiety as measured by different scales.

SKY seemed to promote a meaningful remission of anxiety symptoms in the outpatients but the study should be replicated on a larger clinical sample for a more in-depth analysis of the efficacy of SKY Protocol and a longer follow-up is needed to evaluate the response maintenance.

Scale	Group	T0	T1	T2	T3	P
Hamilton	Medicine n=30	16,9	12,9	8,8	11,4	P <0.001
	No Medicine n=25	16,6	8,9	8,5	7,6	P <0.001
Zung	Medicine n=30	44,4	36,7	36,6	35,3	p <0.001
	No Medicine n=25	43,3	34,2	32,6	31,8	p <0.001
Scl-90	Medicine n=30	1,27	0,86	0,79	0,78	p <0.001
General Symptoms Index	No Medicine n=25	1,21	0,75	0,71	0,56	p <0.001

In the table the mean scores are reported. Statistical analysis was conducted by ANOVA (see text for details)

T0 (before SKY treatment), T1 (after 15 days of SKY training), T2 (after 3 months), T3 (after 6 months).

Table 1. The improvement of Anxiety level

4.2. Yoga, meditation, and mantras to deal with work-related stress for employees of a hospital

This project took place at the Fatebenefratelli and Ophthalmic Hospital in Milan since 2012, and it is currently ongoing as a quality project of the hospital.

This intervention includes five lessons, two hours weekly; every lesson is structured as follows: 30 minutes for relaxation, breathing, and full asanas (yoga postures to promote lengthening of column and muscles); 60 minutes for asana specifications; and 30 minutes for meditation with mantra listening.

The experimental sample is composed mainly by females (n=90) and to a lesser extent by males (n=10), the mean age being 47.51 yrs (sd=8.3).

The work-related stress measure utilized was the Perceived Stress Scale (PSS) [81]; this self-assessed questionnaire measures the perception of stress (degree to which situations in the life of the subject are evaluated as stressful). This is one of the tools most frequently used for evaluating work-related stress. To evaluate the stress response, the GHQ-12 - General Health Questionnaire [82] was chosen: the questionnaire consists of 12 items, it assesses the degree to which a person experiences the presence of stress symptoms. It can signal a situation of distress and in particular depression, anxiety, somatic symptoms and dysfunction at the social level. It can also discriminate between well-being conditions (scores below 5) and the presence of symptoms of psychological distress (scores greater than or equal to 5). Finally, Profile of Mood

States (POMS) [83] was utilized. This questionnaire evaluates six factors, each of which identifies a particular state of mood: tension-anxiety, depression, aggressiveness-anger, vigor-activity, tiredness-indolence, and confusion-bewilderment.

The results of the pilot study on 100 workers attending the treatment program are summarized by the following Tables 2, 3, and 4.

PSS **(N=100)**	**Mean (sd)**
before	18.55 (5.089)
after	14.87 (4.923)
Anova: F(1,99) = 63.990, p=.000	

Table 2. Descriptive statistics for Perceived Stress Scale (PSS). Average score of the sample before and after the treatment.

GHQ **(N=100)**	**Mean (sd)**
before	2.55 (2.749)
after	1.01 (1.664)
Anova: F(1,99) = 46.615, p=.000	

Table 3. Descriptive statistics for General Health Questionnaire Scale (GHQ): Average score of the sample before and after the treatment

POMS-T **(N=100)**	**Mean (sd)**
before	11.33 (5.853)
after	6.77 (5.272)
Anova: F(1,99) = 76.112, p=.000	

Table 4. Descriptive statistics for POMS-Tension and Anxiety Scale: Average score of the sample before and after the treatment.

For the Scale for the Perceived Stress (PPS) there is a significant decrease in the average score of the sample, from 18.55 to 14.87; for General Health Questionnaire (GHQ) there is a significant decrease in the average score of the sample, from 2,55 to 1,01; and for POMS, in particular, in the subscale tension and anxiety, there is also a significant improvement; finally, there is a clear and significant reduction in the percentage of subjects who experience a condition of distress (from 21% to 8%).

5. Conclusion

In the light of the benefits and the effectiveness showed in preventing and treating anxiety symptoms, yoga and meditation protocols would reasonably be helpful if proposed in organizations and to the general public health system. This person-centred approach generates a prevention culture and a significant costs reduction among all three levels of prevention mentioned earlier.

Workplace being a main place of high level and high intensity interactions, the intervention models presented could be positive examples of an institutional response to stress issue. Another positive outcome is the creation of a widespread culture of efficacious prevention of stress responses without the induction of secondary costs due to medication side effects, medication costs, lost days of work (as the traditional approaches induce instead) and with evident benefits on work efficacy and work–life balance. Moreover, these interventions do not generate a stigmatizing response in the whole system, being "not psychiatric" even if deeply rooted in psychic life and equilibrium. Yoga is focused on empowerment and self-efficacy, acting on body level to effect mind–body system, and it promotes a central role of the worker/patient in pursuing health and balance in daily life.

Probably it will be necessary to tailor the interventions to the different settings, target groups, and patients. The experience of programs like Mindfulness Based Stress Reduction Program, the project at Hospital Fatebenefratelli, and the TLEX Program can be examples to follow confirming that when yoga and meditation programs are presented in a proper way and adequately sponsored by an organization's leaders, not only is the participation of employees and managers assured, but they also show encouraging results.

More work has to be done in this direction to identify the most effective approaches and to differentiate the interventions based on the target population and the nature of the challenges that the context proposes. Yoga is, however, a new low-risk, without side effects, way to improve health and quality of life [84].

Author details

S. Doria, F. Irtelli*, R. Sanlorenzo and F. Durbano

*Address all correspondence to: dott.ssaflorianairtelli@gmail.com

Department of Psychiatry and Neuroscience, "Fatebenefratelli e Oftalmico" Hospital, Milano, Italy

References

[1] Engel G. The Need for a New Medical Model: A Challenge for Biomedicine. Science; 1977, 196:129-136.

[2] Engel G. How Much Longer Must Medicine's Science Be Bound by a Seventeenth Century World View? Psychother Psychosom. 1992; 57:3-16.

[3] EU-OSHA European Agency for Safety and Health at Work [internet]; 2014. Available from: http://osha.europa.eu; or https://www.healthy-workplaces.eu/en

[4] Ferrari G. Manuale di valutazione dello stress e dei rischi psicosociali [Manual for evaluation of stress and psychosocial risks]. Edizioni Ferrari Sinibaldi, Italy, 2010.

[5] Selye H. A Syndrome Produced by Different Nocuous Agents. Nature, 1936; 138: 32.

[6] Selye H. History of the Stress Concept. In: Goldberger L and Bretznitz S (Eds.), Handbook of Stress: Theoretical and Clinical Aspects. 2nd Ed. New York: The Free Press, 1993.

[7] Selye H. From Dream to Discovery: On Being a Scientist. Ayer Co Pub; New edition, 1975.

[8] Sanavio E, Cornoldi C. Psicologia Clinica [Clinical Psychology] Il Mulino, Bologna, Italy, 2001.

[9] Selye H. Stress without Distress. New York: Harper & Row, 1974.

[10] Holmes T.H, Rahe R.H. The Social Readjustment Rating Scale. J Psychosom Res. 1967; 11: 213-218.

[11] Benson H, Allen RL. How Much Stress is Too Much. Harvard Business Review, 1980; 58(5): 86-92. Available from: https://hbr.org/1980/09/how-much-stress-is-too-much

[12] Yerkes RM, Dodson JD. The Relation of Strength of Stimulus to Rapidity of Habit-Formation. J. Comp. Neurol. Psychol. 1908; 18: 459-482. doi: 10.1002/cne.920180503.

[13] Bandura A. Self-efficacy: The Exercise of Control. New York: Freeman, 1997.

[14] Luszczynska A, Scholz U, Swarzer R. The General Self-efficacy Scale: Multicultural Validation Studies. J Psychol, 2005; 139(5): 439-457.

[15] Lazarus RS. Psychological Stress and the Coping Process. New York: Mc Graw-Hill, 1966.

[16] Lazarus RS, Folkman S. Stress Appraisal and Coping. New York: Springer,1984.

[17] Clarck JV, Arkowitz H. Social Anxiety and Self-evaluation of Interpersonal Performance. Psychological Reports, 1975; 36: 211-221.

[18] Buss AH. Self Consciousness and Social Anxiety. San Francisco: Freeman, 1980.

[19] Villone Betocchi G, Asprea AM. Ansia, Ansia Sociale e Ansia da Esame nella Prospettiva Cognitiva. Arch psicol Neurol psichiatr. 1994; LV(1-2): 326-338.

[20] Bellack M, Hersen AS. (Eds.) Research and Practice in Social Skills Training. New York: Plenum Press, 1979.

[21] Lazarus RS. Coping Theory and Research: Past, Present and Future. Psychosom Med. 1993; 55: 234-247.

[22] Weisman A. Worden JW. Coping and Vulnerability: A Research Report. Boston. MA: Massachusetts General Hospital, 1977.

[23] Folkman S. Positive Psychological States and Coping with Severe Stress. Soc Sci Med. 1997; 45(8): 1207-1221.

[24] Scheirer MF, Carver CS. Optimism, Coping and Health: Assessment and mplications of eneralized Outcome Expectancies on Health. Health Psychology. 1985; 4(3): 219-247.

[25] Scheirer IH, Carver CS. Distinguishing Optimism From Neuroticism (and trait Anxiety, self-mastery, and self-esteem): A Reevaluation of the Life Orientation Test. J Pers Soc Psychol. 1994; 67(6): 1063-1078.

[26] Grassi L, Buda P, Cavana L, Annunziata M, Torta R, Varetto A. Styles of Coping with Cancer: The Italian version of the MINI-MAC Scale. Psycho-Oncol. 2005; 14: 115–124.

[27] Schou I, Ekberg O, Ruland CM. The Mediating Role of Appraisal and Coping in the Relationship between Optimism-Pessimism and Quality of Life. Psycho-Oncol. 2005; 14: 718-727.

[28] Druss RG, Douglas CJ. Adaptive Responses to Illness and Disability. Healthy Denial. Gen Hosp Psychiat. 1988; 10: 163-168.

[29] Wittchen HU, Jacobi F. Size and Burden of Mental Disorders in Europe: A Critical Review and Appraisal of 27 Studies. Eur. Neuropsychopharmacol. 2005; 15: 357–367.

[30] Balasubramaniam M, Telles S, Doraiswamy M. Yoga on Our Minds: A Systematic Review of Yoga for Neuropsychiatric Disorders. 2012; 3: 117.

[31] Da Silva TL, Ravindran LN, Ravindran AV. Yoga in the Treatment of Mood and Anxiety Disorders: A Review. Asian J Psychiat. 2009; 2(1): 6-16.

[32] Alonso J, Angermeyer MC, Bernert S, Bruffaerts R, Brugha TS, Bryson H, et al. Prevalence of Mental Disorders in Europe: Results from the European Study of the Epidemiology of Mental Disorders (ESEMeD) Project. Acta Psychiat Scand. 2004; 109(420): 21–27.

[33] Cassano P, Fava M. Depression and Public Health: An Overview. J Psychosom Res. 2002; 53: 849-857.

[34] Wittchen HU, Lieb R, Schuster P, Oldehinkel AJ. When Is Onset? Investigations into Early Developmental Stages of Anxiety and Depressive Disorders. In: Rapaport JL

(Ed.), Childhood Onset of "adult" Psychopathology, Clinical and Research Advances. American Psychiatric Press, Washington, pp 259–302, 1999.

[35] Wittchen HU, Kessler RC, Beesdo K, Krause P, Höfler M, Hoyer J. Generalized Anxiety and Depression in Primary Care: Prevalence, Recognition and Management. J Clin Psychiatry. 2002; 63 Suppl 8: 24-34.

[36] Wittchen HU, Jacobi F, Rehm J, Gustavsson A, Svensson M, Jönsson B. et al. The Size and Burden of Mental Disorders and Other Disorders of the Brain in Europe. Eur Neuropsychopharmacol. 2010; 121(9): 655–679.

[37] Wittchen HU. Generalized Anxiety Disorder: Prevalence Burden and Cost to Society. Depress Anxiety. 2002; 16(4): 162-171.

[38] Michelini S, Cassano GB, Frare F, Perugi G. Long-term Use of Benzodiazepines: Tolerance, Dependence and Clinical Problems in Anxiety and Mood Disorders. Pharmacopsychiatry. 1996; 29: 127-134.

[39] Rickels K, Downing R, Schweizer E, Hassman H. Antidepressants for the Treatment of Generalized Anxiety Disorder. A Placebo-controlled Comparison of Imipramine, Trazodone, and Diazepam. Arch Gen Psychiatry. 1993; 50: 884-895.

[40] Gelenberg AJ, Lydiard RB, Rudolph RL, Aguiar L, Haskins JT, Salinas E. Efficacy of Venlafaxine Extended-release Capsules in Non-depressed Outpatients with Generalized Anxiety Disorder: A 6-month Randomized Controlled Trial. JAMA. 2000; 283: 3082-3088.

[41] Pollack MH, Zaninelli R, Goddard A, McCafferty JP, Bellew KM, Burnham DB, et al. Paroxetine in the Treatment of Generalized Anxiety Disorder: Results of a Placebo-Controlled, Flexible-Dosage Trial. J Clin Psychiatry. 2001; 62: 350-357.

[42] Baldwin DS, Nair RV. Escitalopram in the Treatment of Generalized Anxiety Disorder. Expert Rev Neurother. 2005; 5: 443-449.

[43] Katzman MA, Vermani M, Jacobs L, Marcus M, Kong B, Lessard S, et al. Quetiapine as an Adjunctive Pharmacotherapy for the Treatment of Non-remitting Generalized Anxiety Disorder: A Flexible-Dose, Open-label Pilot Trial. J Anxiety Disord. 2008; 22: 1480-1486.

[44] Andrews G, Slade TC, Issakidis SC. Deconstructing Current Comorbidity: Data from the Australian National Survey of Mental Health and Well-being. Br J Psychiat. 2002; 181(4): 306-314.

[45] Bonura KB. The Impact of Yoga on Psychological Health in Older Adults. Florida State University. Electronic Theses, Treatises and Dissertations. Paper 3549, 2007. Available from: http://diginole.lib.fsu.edu/cgi/viewcontent.cgi?article=2537&context=etd

[46] Clance P, Mitchel M, Engelman S. Body Cathexis in Children as a Function of Awareness Training and Yoga. J Clin Child Psychol. 1980; 9: 82-85.

[47] Nicolis G, Prigogine I. Self-Organization in Nonequilibrium Systems: From Dissipative Structures to Order through Fluctuations. NY: Wiley, 1977.

[48] Woods JH. The Yoga-System of Patañjali. Cambridge, MA: Harvard University Press, 1914.

[49] Brown RP, Gerbarg PL. Sudarshan Kriya Yogic Breathing in the Treatment of Stress, Anxiety, and Depression. Part II-Clinical Applications and Guidelines. J Altern Complement Med. 2005; 11(4): 711-717.

[50] Ravindran AV, Lam RW, Filteau MJ, Lespérance F, Kennedy SH, Parikh SV, Patten SB. Canadian Network for Mood and Anxiety Treatments (CANMAT) Clinical Guidelines for the Management of Major Depressive Disorder in Adults. V. Complementary and Alternative Medicine Treatments. 1. J Affect Disord. 2009; 117 Suppl 1: S54-64.

[51] Michalsen A. Die Komplementärmedizin und der «menschliche Faktor». Forsch Komplementmedizin Innere Medizin V und Integrative Medizin, Kliniken Essen-Mitte, Deutschland 2006; 13(2): 68-69.

[52] Agte VV, Chiplonkar SA. Sudarshan Kriya Yoga for Improving Antioxidant Status and Reducing Anxiety in Adults. Alternative and Complementary Therapies, 2008, 14(2): 96-100. Available from: http://online.liebertpub.com/doi/pdfplus/10.1089/act.2008.14204

[53] Meti BL, Desiraju T. Study of Changes in BEG and Autonomic Parameters After 4 Months of Initiation and Practice of Pranayama. Indian J Physiol Pharmacol. 1984; 28: 34.

[54] Meti BL, Raju TR. Auditory Middle Latency Evoked Potentials in Kriya Yoga. Health Administrator. 1993; 4: 56-58.

[55] Iyengar BKS. Light on Pranayama: The Yogic Art of Breathing. New York: Crossroads Publishing, 1997.

[56] Sarris J, Byrne GJ. A Systematic Review of Insomnia and Complementary Medicine Sleep Medicine Reviews. 2011April; 15(2): 99–106.

[57] Gilbert C. Yoga and Breathing Journal of Bodywork and Movement Therapies, Elsevier, 1999.

[58] Gupta N, Khera S, Vempati RP, Sharma R, Bijlani RL. Effect of Yoga Based Lifestyle Intervention on State and Trait Anxiety. Indian J Physiol Pharmacol. 2006; 50(1): 41-47.

[59] Brown RP, Gerbarg PL. Sudarshan Kriya Yogic Breathing in the Treatment of Stress, Anxiety, and Depression. Part II-Clinical Applications and Guidelines. J. Altern. Complement. Med. 2005b ;11(4): 711-717.

[60] Zope SA, Zope RA. Sudarshan Kriya Yoga: Breathing for Health. Int J Yoga. 2013; 6(1): 4-10.

[61] Naga Venkatesha Murthy PJ, Janakiramaiah N, Gangadhar BN, Subbakrishna DK. P300 Amplitude and Antidepressant Response to Sudarshan Kriya Yoga (SKY). J Affect Disorders. 1998; 50(1): 45-48.

[62] Janakiramaiah N, Gangadhar BN, Naga Venkatesha Murthy PJ, Harish MG, Subbakrishna DK, Vedamurthachar A. Therapeutic Efficacy of Sudarshan Kriya Yoga (SKY) in Dysthymic Disorder. NIMHANS J. 1998; 17: 21–28.

[63] Janakiramaiah N, Gangadhar BN, Naga Venkatesha Murthy PJ, Harish MG, Subbakrishna DK, Vedamurthachar A. Antidepressant Efficacy of Sudarshan Kriya Yoga (SKY) in Melancholia: A Randomized Comparison with Electroconvulsive Therapy (ECT) and Imipramine. J Affect Disord. 2000; 57: 255–259.

[64] Rohini V, Pandey RS, Janakiramaiah N, Gangadhar BN, Vedamarthachar A. Comparative Study of Full and Partial Sudarshana Kriya Yoga (SKY) in Major Depressive Disorder. NIMHANS J. 2000; 18(1-2): 53-57.

[65] Vedamurthachar A, Janakiramaiah N, Hegde JM, Shetty TK, Subbakrishna DK, Sureshbabu SV, Gangadhar BN. Antidepressant Efficacy and Hormonal Effects of Sudarshana Kriya Yoga (SKY) in Alcohol Dependent Individuals. J Affect Disorders. 2006; 94(1-3): 249-253.

[66] Gangadhar BN, Janakiramaiah N, Sudarshan B, Shety KT. Stress-Related Biochemical Effects of Sudarshan Kriya Yoga in Depressed Patients Study #6. Presented at the Conference on Biological Psychiatry. New York: UN NGO Mental Health Committee, 2000.

[67] European Commission's Directorate General [internet]; 2014. Available from: http://www.insead.edu/media_relations/press_release/docs/RESPONSE-Executive-Briefing.pdf

[68] Bazarko D, Rebecca AC, Azocar F, Jo Kreitzer M. The Impact of an Innovative Mindfulness-Based Stress Reduction Program on the Health and Well-Being of Nurses Employed in a Corporate Setting. J Workplace Behav Health. 2013; 28(2):107-133.

[69] University of Massachussetts Medical School; 2014. Available from: http://www.umassmed.edu/cfm/stress-reduction/workplace-programs/

[70] Awareness and Relaxation Training (ART); 2014. Available from: http://www.mindfulnessprograms.com/corporate-program.php

[71] Sri Sri Ravi Shankar, [interneet]; 2014. Available from: http://srisriravishankar.org/entry/tlex-transformational-leadership-for-excellence/

[72] Sri Sri Ravi Shankar; [internet]; 2014. Available from: www.tlexinstitute.com

[73] Doria S, Sanlorenzo R, Irtelli F, Mencacci C. Anti-anxiety Efficacy of Sudarshan Kriya Yoga in General Anxiety Disorder: A multicomponent, Yoga Based, Breath Intervention Program for Patients Suffering from Generalized Anxiety Disorder with or without Comorbidities. J Affect Disorders (2015 in press).

[74] American Psychiatric Association, 1994. Diagnostic and Statistical Manual of Mental Disorders, 4th ed. American Psychiatric Association, Washington, DC.

[75] Yoga Research Group. Treating Depression with Sudarshan Kriya Yoga: A Demonstration Video Cassette. Department of Health Education, National Institute of Mental Health and Neurosciences, Bangalore (1995).

[76] Hamilton M. The Assessment of Anxiety States by Rating. Br J Med Psychol. 1959; 32(1): 50–55.

[77] Zung WWK. A Rating Instrument for Anxiety Disorders. Psychosomatics. 1971; 12(6): 371–379.

[78] Hamilton M. A Rating Scale for Depression. J Neurol Neurosurg Psychiatry. 1960; 23: 56–62.

[79] Zung WWK. A Self-Rating Depression Scale. Arch Gen Psychiatry. 1965; 12(1): 63-70.

[80] Derogatis LR: SCL-90-R, Administration, Scoring and Procedures Manual-II for the R(evised) Version and Other Instruments of the Psychopathology Rating Scale Series. Townson: Clinical Psychometric Research; 1992 [italian version: Emanuele Preti, Antonio Prunas, Irene Sarno e Fabio Madeddu, OS Editions, Florence, Italy, 2011.

[81] Cohen S, Kamarck T, Mermelstein R. A Global Measure of Perceived Stress, J Health Soc Behavior. 1983; 24: 385-396.

[82] Goldberg DP, Gater R, Sartorius N, Ustun TB, Piccinelli M, Gureje O, Rutter C. The Validity of Two Versions of the GHQ in the WHO Study of Mental Illness in General Health Care Psychol Med. 1997; 27(1):191-197.

[83] Spielberger CD. Review of Profile of Mood States. Professional Psychol. 1972; 3(4): 387-388.

[84] Balasubramaniam M, Telles S, Doraiswamy PM. Yoga on Our Minds: A Systematic Review of Yoga for Neuropsychiatric Disorders. Front Psychiatry. 2013; 25(3): 117(1-16). Available from: http://journal.frontiersin.org/Journal/10.3389/fpsyt.2012.00117/full

2

Safety Measures for Handlers/Workers against Herbicide Intoxication Risk

Joaquim G. Machado-Neto

Abstract

With the use of herbicides, there is a certain risk of intoxication to directly exposed workers, which depends on several factors. Risk factors can be grouped in the toxicity of herbicides and exposure provided by the specific working conditions. From the assessment of the risk of intoxication, working conditions can be classified as safe or unsafe. The safety of working conditions is based on the chronic toxicity of the pesticide and the absorbable amount of dermal and respiratory exposure. Safety can be determined by calculation of the margin of safety calculation (MOS). If the value of MOS ≥1, the working condition is classified as safe, but if the MOS <1, the condition and work is classified as unsafe. For working conditions classified as unsafe, workers should adopt safety measures to become safe. Safety measures at work are grouped into preventive and protection. The preventive safety measures are grouped into the selection of workers/personnel: psychological meas-ures; administrative: legislation, standards, and procedures; and hygiene, cleaning, main-tenance, and safety of the environment. The protection safety measures are grouped into collectives and individual. The Brazilian labor law mandates the use of preventive measures and protection, according to the pesticide manufacturers' recommendations on the labels.

Keywords: Pesticides, herbicides, occupational exposure, risk of intoxication, measure

1. Introduction

The convention 012 (C012) of the International Labour Organization (ILO) on the Compensation for Work Accidents (Agriculture), 1921, became internationally effective on 02.26.1923. Convention 012 extends the benefit of the laws to agricultural workers and regulates mandatory indemnification of victims of work accidents [4].

Work accidents occur due to the existence of risks in the working environment. Work risk is any possibility that some element or condition in a given process can cause damage or be destructive to the physical and/or psychological health of the worker. The risk outcome can be an accident, illness or suffering, or exposition to environmental pollution.

The ILO Convention 184 on safety and health in agriculture, 2001, states that member states should define, implement, and revise a coherent national policy on agriculture safety and health periodically. The purpose is to prevent accidents and health injury related to or as a consequence of work and to eliminate, mitigate, or control the risks in the agricultural working environment [9].

In Brazil, the NR 31 approved in 2005, and amended in 2011 and 2013, is still in force [6]. It is related to safety and health in agriculture, livestock, forestry, and aquaculture, meeting the obligations of signatory member countries of the ILO Convention 184.

Pesticides are chemical compounds used to control organisms harmful to crops. Pesticides are carefully selected to intoxicate the target organisms. Toxicity is the ability to cause harm and death of the target organisms [21]. However, nontarget organisms that come into direct contact with pesticides can be intoxicated, especially if they have the points of the toxic action. Therefore, working with pesticides poses a chemical poisoning risk to exposed workers [1].

The overall Brazilian legislation on health safety (NR 9) in the workplace provides that companies must implement the environmental risk prevention program (ERPP). The ERPP consists of the following steps: anticipation, recognition, quantitative assessment, and control of risks according to specific action levels [7].

This chapter informs the reader about the safety procedures required while working with pesticides. It aims at motivating the worker to make a habit of preventing herbicide poisoning. Moreover, it also serves to motivate the businessmen to implement safety measures in the working environment, to keep the risks at acceptable levels, while increasing business productivity and competitiveness.

2. Risk of intoxication with herbicides

The risk of worker intoxication with pesticides, especially herbicides, depends on several elements that can be grouped into two major factors: the toxicity of the handled herbicides and the exposure under the specific working conditions [1]. Therefore, the safety and health management during work with herbicides should be addressed using the steps set out by the industrial hygiene and the ERPP [7]. The steps are the ability to anticipate, identify, recognize, evaluate, and control the risks in the workplace.

2.1. Anticipation and identification of the intoxication risks associated with herbicides

A safety and health management plan for workers exposed to herbicides must anticipate and identify potential risks and health hazards before a given production process is implemented or modified, or new risk agents are introduced in the workplace.

The risks can be anticipated during the planning phase of the productive activity such as acquiring new equipment and/or materials (including pesticides), determining the work process, and preventive maintenance plans.

The identification of pesticide poisoning risks starts with the specific agricultural production system. The production systems can be organic, when the use of synthetic toxic products is not allowed, or conventional, when the use of new agricultural technologies is allowed, including the use of pesticides. Therefore, the risk of occupational intoxication with pesticides exists only in conventional farming systems.

The use of pesticides in conventional crops depends on a wide variety of interrelated factors that can be grouped according to the direct relation to the crop, crop environment, and target organisms.

During the planning of an agricultural crop, the professional must be able to predict the occurrence of harmful organisms and control methods. The pesticides recommended for chemical control are legally required to inform the formulation registered in the Ministry of Agriculture, Livestock and Supply, MAPA, in the package leaflet [10].

2.2. Recognizing the intoxication risks of pesticides

In this step, the work environment is observed and carefully analyzed to identify the agents and their potential risks. The priority assessment and control of the risk involved must be established. Risk analysis should answer the following questions: What? Where? andHow? A deep knowledge of the products involved in the process, working methods, process flow, and facilities layout is necessary to answer these questions [27].

It is necessary to analyze the information contained in the package leaflet regarding the product, the environment and protection of human health to recognize the poisoning risks of pesticides [10]. The leaflet also contains information about application methods and calibration settings of the application equipment. The handler is exposed to the product by drift, that is, the portion of the product that does not reach the target and drifts away. The extent of drift and exposure depends on several factors, predominantly the type of application and the equipment used. Therefore, the type of formulation is an important information contained in the leaflet regarding the handler's safety since it determines the type of application equipment to be used. The leaflet must also contain mandatory information on poisoning, acute and chronic toxicity of pesticides, the first aid procedures should an intoxication occur, and preventive measures to protect handlers.

The identification of the working conditions and the job are critical to determining the risk of poisoning with pesticides. Handler exposure is determined by the working conditions while working conditions are identified by the activities performed. The legislation on pesticide working safety (NR 31) defines workers in direct exposure as those handling pesticides, additives, and related products in any of the stages of storage, transportation, packaging opening, pesticides preparation and application, disposal and decontamination of equipment, and clothing [6].

Thus, it is necessary to identify homogeneous work groups (HWG). The HWG consists of workers performing the same activity and exposed to the same risks. Therefore, safety measures will be similar for all workers of the same HWG since the working conditions are the same [14]. The exposure assessment for any worker of the HWG is representative of the exposure of all workers of the group [29].

2.3. Quantitative assessment of pesticide poisoning risks

The procedure to perform risk assessment of intoxication with pesticides has been established in a document of the American National Academy of Sciences (USA) in 1983 as a four-step process [33]. The four steps are outlined in the diagram shown in Figure 1 [18].

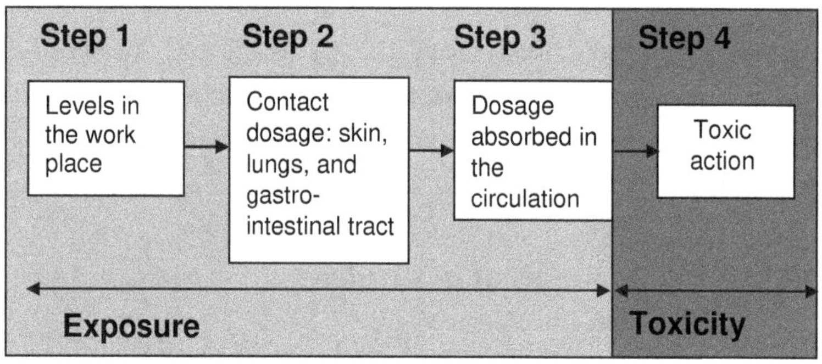

Figure 1. The steps of the intoxication risk assessment when working with pesticides [18].

Occupational exposure to pesticides is influenced by the type of work or activity performed, the way it is conducted, and the product formulation [20]. Toxicity is an intrinsic property of pesticides that is determined following national regulations, even before they are placed on the market.

2.3.1. Occupational exposure to pesticides

The worker's exposure to pesticides can be real or potential. The actual exposure refers to the absolute amount of pesticide that comes into contact with the body during a determined working period and is readily available to be absorbed via dermal, respiratory, or oral routes [1].

Potential exposure refers to the amount of the pesticide that could be absorbed via dermal, respiratory, and oral routes if the worker had not worn personal protective equipment during the operation [32].

The potential exposure results from the interaction of the dominant risk factors in specific working conditions. It has been determined that during the application of herbicides in field conditions, 99% or more of total exposure occurs via dermal and only 1% or less, via respiratory [35, 34, 26].

Therefore, knowledge about pesticide exposure and the relative importance of each pathway to the total exposure is essential to select the most effective, comfortable, economical, and applicable safety measures given the specific conditions.

2.3.1.1. Exposure routes

The potential routes of exposure to pesticides in the workplace are dermal and, to a lesser extent, respiratory. The relative importance of each exposure route is directly related to the specific working conditions or determinants of exposure. To tractor operators spraying eleven pesticides in a citrus orchard using a turbo type sprayer, 99.7–99.9% of the total exposure occurs via dermal, and only 0.1–0.3%, via respiratory route, on average [35]. This finding is greatly important for adopting safety procedures, especially regarding personal protective equipment (PPE).

The predominance of the dermal exposure under field conditions is explained by the spray droplets or mist, which drifts away towards the handler reaching the skin. The lower respiratory exposure is explained by the low contamination of the air that the handler breathes. The low contamination of breathable air is due to the fantastic dispersion of the spray droplets in the atmospheric air. Wolfe et al. reported that it is due to the distance between the tractor driver and the nozzles of the spray jet, the area with the greatest concentration of drops [35].

The potential reach of the bloodstream and the absorption of pesticides on the exposure routes should be also considered. After contact, the first entry stage of the toxic compound is absorption by the body. The absorption of a pesticide that reaches the lungs via respiratory route is fast and complete [16]. On the contrary, the absorption of herbicides via the dermal route is slower, partly because the skin is a natural, efficient barrier.

Respiratory exposure

Respiratory exposure consists of exposure to spray droplets containing the toxic compounds and possible toxic vapors present in the air that the worker breathes. The drops are particles suspended in the air, called liquid aerosols. Liquid aerosols are liquid particles produced by mechanical disruption of liquid, called mist [28]. The pesticide spraying is a mist of water droplets. The aerosols are classified by the diameter (Ø), as shown in Table 1 [27].

Type of particulate	Size (μm)
Sedimentable	10 < Ø < 150
Inhalable	Ø < 10
Breathable	Ø < 5
Visible	Ø > 40

Table 1. Classification of aerosols according to the type and size of particulates, for respiratory exposure [27].

The inhaled and breathable particles are the most harmful. Inhalable particles are usually deposited in the respiratory tract. However, the breathable particles enter the upper and lower respiratory tracts, reaching the lungs and the pulmonary alveoli. In the alveoli, the toxic compounds permeate the cellular membranes reaching the bloodstream and the toxic action site in the body.

The droplet size is one of the most important parameters of pesticide application technology. The spray droplets typically have a mean volume diameter (MVD) in the range of sedimentable and visible particulates (Table 1), or higher, from 100 to 300 μm. The droplet size can be one of the factors that explain lower respiratory exposure under certain field conditions [35, 34, 26].

Dermal exposure

The skin consists of the outermost and innermost layers, the epidermis and dermis, respectively. The dermis consists of connective tissue, blood vessels, nerves, hair follicles, sebaceous, and sweat glands. Direct contact with the external environment occurs through the follicles and the dermal glands. Thus, chemicals can be absorbed mainly by the epidermal cells and hair follicles.

The absorption speed of chemicals into the skin is mainly limited by the continuous stratum corneum. The fat-soluble substances penetrate through the lipids existing between the keratin filaments by passive diffusion. The rate of absorption of oily substances is indirectly proportional to their viscosity and volatility. For polar substances of low molecular weight, the absorption occurs through the outer surface of the keratin filament, the hydrated extract. The transepidermal absorption is the most frequent due to the high number of epidermal cells, although not very easy for toxicants.

The transfollicular absorption is less significant than the transepidermal. Some chemicals can penetrate the hair follicles and quickly reach the dermis. Penetration is easier for chemicals because they do not need to go through the stratum corneum. Fat-soluble or water-soluble, ionized or nonionized, gas or vapor, and acidic or basic substances can penetrate the follicles. The penetration of toxic compounds in the skin depends on its absorption pharmacokinetic model [25] and can vary from 0.8% to 6.0% [19] up to 80% [11].

2.3.2. Quantification of dermal and respiratory exposures

The whole-body method is the most suitable for assessing dermal exposure. In this method, the worker dresses in a cotton coverall, according to the protocol VBC 82.1 [36]. This method evaluates the potential and actual dermal exposures directly on the coverall used by the worker over the safety equipment, under normal working conditions for a certain evaluation period (Figure 2A and B).

The coveralls are long-sleeved with a hood made of white denim material. They are used to quantify the dermal exposures of the head + neck, trunk (back and front), arms, and legs (back and front). Cotton gloves are used to quantify the dermal exposure of the hands. The face and feet exposure is evaluated using Carefree™ female sanitary napkins that are attached to the semidisposable facial masks and rubber boots [22, 23].

Respiratory exposure is evaluated using personal continuous air flow pumps (Figure 2A and B) with specific respirator filters, cartridges, or cassettes for collecting particulates, gasses, and vapors [27].

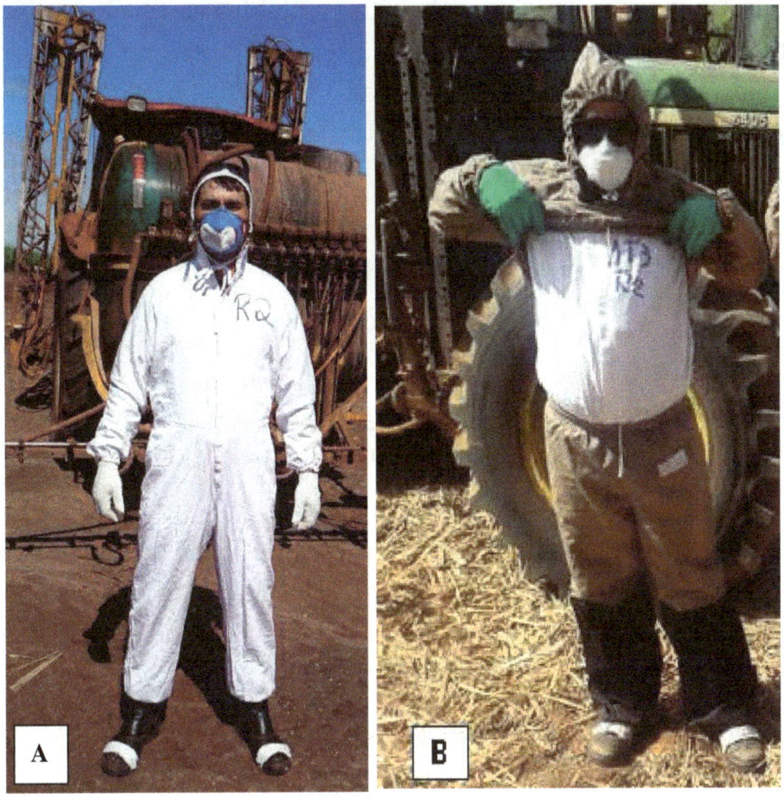

Figure 2. Workers applying pesticide in the field during assessment of potential dermal exposure: A—quantified in coverall and unprotected, exposure real: B—quantified in coverall worn under the personal protective equipment during the evaluation period, according VBC 82.1 [36].

2.4. Controlling the risk of intoxication with pesticides

Safety, health, and environment management is regulated by a specific labor legislation for pesticides, the regulatory standard no. 31, known as NR 31 [6]. The NR 31 prioritizes implementation of safety measures to eliminate the risks by replacing or adjusting the production processes, machines, and equipment; by adopting collective protective measures to control the risk at the source; and by introducing personal protection. Safety procedures should be implemented based on risk assessment and risk acceptability criteria. Working conditions can be classified as safe or unsafe according to the adopted risk acceptability criterion. The acceptability criterion of poisoning risk with pesticides is based on toxicity and handler exposure determined by working conditions.

Safety evaluation is fundamental to classify working conditions and select the appropriate safety procedures needed to reduce the risk of poisoning to acceptable levels.

2.4.1. Acceptability criterion of intoxication risk with pesticides

The acceptability criterion of pesticide risk is based on the no observable effect level (NOEL) in mg/day/kg body weight. The NOEL is determined by assessment tests of the chronic toxicity of pesticides using mice in laboratory conditions. The studies follow international standard procedures.

The acceptability criterion of poisoning risk with pesticides can be quantified by calculating the margin of safety (MOS) proposed by Severn [30] and adapted by Machado-Neto [23]. MOS is determined dividing the safe dose (calculated by multiplying the NOEL value and the worker body weight) by the absorbable quantity of exposure (AQE) via the dermal and respiratory tract, under working conditions:

$$MOS = \frac{NOEL \text{ x } W}{AQE \text{ X } SF}$$

where NOEL is the no observed effect level (mg/kg/day); W is the mean body weight of the worker, considered to be 70 kg; AQE is the absorbable quantity of exposure (mg/day); and SF is the safety factor.

AQE via the dermal route is determined for each molecule in the dermal exposure studies with laboratory animals or human skin tissue grown in the laboratory. For molecules wherin dermal absorption has been determined, it is considered to be 10% of the evaluated dermal exposure for each working condition, according to Byers et al. [13].

The AQE in the respiratory tract can be considered as 100% of respiratory exposure evaluated for each working condition [23].

The SF, which multiplies AQE, is used to compensate for the extrapolation of the NOEL results obtained in laboratory animals, to humans [12]. The used safety factor may be 10 [12], to compensate for interspecies extrapolation, or 100; 10 for interspecies times 10 for intraspecies extrapolation.

The MOS is calculated for the activities and daily exposure times according to working conditions. For formulations with two or more active ingredients, the commercial product safety rating is based on the smallest value among the MOS calculated for the active ingredients.

The risk acceptability criterion depends on the toxicity of the pesticide, while the intensity of risk depends directly on the intensity of worker exposure to pesticides.

The working condition is classified as safe if MOS ≥ 1; exposure as tolerable and intoxication risk as acceptable.

The working condition is classified as unsafe if MOS <1; exposure as intolerable and intoxication risk as unacceptable.

2.4.2. Control action level of intoxication risk

According to NR 9, the action level is a value above which preventive measures should be initiated to minimize the likelihood that exposures to environmental agents exceed the exposure limits [7].

For pesticides, the action level to implement the risk control measures is when the working condition is classified as unsafe (MOS <1). For unsafe conditions, preventive and protective measures should be intensified enough to make the working conditions safe (MOS ≥ 1). The preventive safety and protection measures should control toxicity and/or exposure to make unsafe working conditions safe.

3. Safety measures while working with pesticides

Controlling the intoxication risk with safety measures is a key step to planning health and safety management while working with pesticides. The specific labor legislation for pesticides, the NR 31 [6], states that the rural employer or similar should conduct risk assessments to ensure the safety and health of workers. Based on the results, the employer must adopt preventive and protection procedures to ensure that all activities, workplaces, machinery, equipment, tools, and processes are safe and in compliance with health and safety standards. The legislation also determines the prioritization of measures to prevent accidents and occupational diseases [6].

3.1. Preventive safety measures

The preventive safety measures may be applied early in the planning of agricultural activities, during the previously described steps of anticipation, identification, and recognition of the risks. Preventive safety measures target the risk factors and can be divided into two groups, to eliminate and to reduce poisoning risk. Preventive measures aim to ensure a safe work environment and maintain workers skilled and motivated and in good health conditions.

Most safety measures determined in the specific legislation to work with pesticides, NR 31, are preventive [6]. The administrative measures are highlighted among the preventive safety measures determined in the legislation on safety and health at work. Administrative preventive measures are adequate policies and procedures to the specific working conditions.

In the planning of agricultural activities with the use of pesticides, prevention measures will act on risk factors, to reduce the toxicity of the pesticide and/or exposure caused to the workers by the working conditions.

3.1.1. Selection of workers/personnel

The personnel selection process is critical to prevent the occurrence of accidents. To work with risky activities, employees must have a physical and psychological profile suitable to the working conditions.

Every worker acquires personal characteristics that form the personality resulting from physical and mental growth over the years in the work environment in which he/she lived. The personality traits can be strong and striking, positive and negative, displaying strengths and weaknesses as irresponsibility, stubbornness, irritability, etc. [3].

The worker's personality, whether positive or not, is carried into the working environment and can cause unsafe acts or unsafe working conditions. Due to negative traits, the worker can act unsafely ignoring safety rules and make mistakes when performing his or her work that may result in work accidents. Unsafe acts are the way workers expose themselves, consciously or unconsciously, to accident risks (e.g., using machines without a license or permission, not using the required PPE, etc. [3]).

Therefore, the selection process should take into account the physical and psychological profile of the employee required to work in risky activities. Thus, the occurrence of accidents can be prevented. Once selected properly, the worker must be trained to perform especially risky activities.

3.1.2. Psychological measures

When the worker interacts in the workplace as a whole (physical or abstract space), he/she is influenced positively or negatively, thus changing his or her physical, mental, and social state. On the other hand, it is natural that the worker brings his or her personal problems to the workplace [2]. Therefore, it is impossible to pretend that all is well when, in fact, the worker is experiencing personal problems. The only one able to understand and evaluate the anguish of losing a loved one, the disappointment of a treacherous love, among others is the person itself. These factors are, for the most part, largely responsible for the increase in the indices that measure delays, work absences, illnesses, and accidents [2].

In working activities, there is a personal unsafety factor when the employee works grudgingly, under abnormal physical conditions (illness, physical, or mental disability), without experience, knowledge, and proper training. Due to personal unsafety factors, the worker may cause accidents and/or occupational illnesses that result from negligence, recklessness, or malpractice [2].

Companies must implement measures that value the worker, by enabling professional growth and personal development to control the human factor effects on the risk of poisoning with pesticides. Such actions elevate the workers' self-esteem and improve performance and commitment, thus making the working environment more pleasant. There are other positive actions such as dynamics between employees, awards campaigns, and the willingness to hear suggestions to improve the workplace.

The work environment should be a harmonious and welcoming place for all to engage in their activities with satisfaction and enthusiasm. The standards and rules set by the company are also important to promote good communication. The basic behavioral rules that are desirable in the workplace are as follows: mutual respect, call people by name, be calm, participate actively in the activities that are delegated to you, be willing to help others, do not judge people, and do the best you can. Dialogue is always important to avoid conflicts, to respect people differences, and to avoid intrigues, gossip, and side conversations.

Companies, more than ever, are looking for professionals who can work in groups, be proactive, and capable of leading. The website of a Brazilian company recruiting employees states, "For all opportunities, Eldorado Brazil seeks professionals with good communication and interpersonal skills and 'owner' attitude" [17].

3.1.3. *Administrative: Legislation, standards, and procedures*

The companies should implement security measures to meet specific labor laws and local regulations to prevent workplace accidents. The preventive security administrative measures are mandatorily applied at all stages, starting at the registration of pesticides up to before labor legislation. The legal commercialization of pesticides in the country is regulated by the legislation on pesticide registration, Decree Law no. 4074 [10].

According to the Decree Law no. 4074 [10], pesticides can only be produced, handled, imported, exported, commercialized, and used in national territory after being registered with the appropriate federal agency. They are required to meet the guidelines and requirements of federal agencies responsible for the sectors of agriculture, health, and environment.

The Ministry of Agriculture, Livestock and Supply (MAPA) is the federal agency responsible for registering pesticides. The Ministry of Health (MS) is responsible for evaluating and classifying toxicologically the pesticides; performing preliminary toxicological evaluation of pesticides, technical products, premixes, and the like, used for research and experimentation; and establishing the reentry interval in a treated environment, among others, as set out in Decree Law no. 4074 [10].

The main administrative preventive measure prohibits the registration of pesticides that can cause harm. The Decree Law no. 4074 [10] prohibits pesticide registration for which there are no available methods for disabling its components in Brazil. There is no antidote or effective treatment.

The teratogenic and carcinogenic compounds present enough evidence as such from observations in humans or studies in experimental animals.

The mutagenic compounds might induce mutations observed in at least two tests, one for detecting genetic mutations, performed using even metabolic activation and the other to detect chromosomal mutations.

Some compounds cause hormonal disorders and harm the reproductive system. They are more dangerous to humans than animals based on tests, according to updated technical and scientific criteria, and some compounds harm the environment.

Tests, trials, and studies about mutagenesis, carcinogenesis, and teratogenesis, conducted in at least two animal species should be performed according to criteria accepted by national or international technical and scientific institutions.

The legislation on working with pesticides (NR 31) requires a management plan regarding health, environment, and safety for rural works [6]. The management plan must include preventive measures for the workers' health (medical examinations) and other actions catering to specific needs, SESTR—Specialized Service on Safety and Health for Rural Work and CIPATR—Internal Commission for Rural Work Accident Prevention.

According to the risks in the workplace, the risk management program should also contemplate the Hearing Conservation Program (HCP), the Respiratory Protection Program (RPP), the Dermatoses Occupational Program (DOP), and the Ergonomic Action Program (EAP) [14].

As internal and specific standard, each company must have in written form the operating procedure (OP) or operating instructions (OI), based on the manuals for machines and pesticide application equipment (NR 31), and the service order (SO), as set out in NR 1 [5] for each OP.

Companies should also have other internal rules to regulate the health and safety of workers, such as hygiene, cleaning, and maintenance of machine and equipment. To meet the requirements of NR 31, the preventive safety procedures also include training workers on prevention of accidents with pesticides, ergonomic measures, safety of machinery, and equipment. The workers should also be granted access roads to workplaces, transportation of workers and cargo, living areas for meals in the field and toilets, and collective and personal protection measures [6].

3.1.3.1. Pesticide packaging

The Decree Law no. 4074 [10] states that pesticide containers shall be designed and constructed to prevent leakage, evaporation, loss, or alteration of its content, and to facilitate the cleaning, sorting, reuse, recycling, and proper disposal. The packages should be resistant to the contents and not able to form harmful or dangerous compounds. Packages must be resistant everywhere and adequately meet the conservation requirements.

Packages must have sealing wax or another external device to ensure visually the package has not been violated. When stacking of rigid packaging is allowed, the maximum number of units that can be stacked should be stated.

The rigid packaging containing formulations miscible or dispersible in water must be submitted to triple washing operation, or equivalent technology, by the user according to the instructions on their labels, leaflets, or brochure supplement.

Users should return the empty containers of water miscible pesticides and their lids, triple washed, to the shop of purchase at the latest 1 year from the date of purchase. Users should make available to the supervisory authorities the empty containers return vouchers, provided by the shops, receiving stations or gathering centers for at least 1 year after the packaging has been returned.

Packaging containing products unfit for use or unused should be disposed of following the guidelines informed in the package leaflet. It is the responsibility of the company that registered, produced, and commercialized the product to collect and dispose of the products.

3.1.3.2. Pesticide labels and package leaflets

The pesticide registration legislation, Decree Law no. 4074 [10], requires that warnings regarding the danger of pesticides should be placed on the label and package leaflet. The pesticide labels should have on the bottom a distinctly colored band separated from the rest of the label, with a height equivalent to 15% of the label/package height. The colors of the bands correspond to different toxicological classes established by the Ministry of Health, in Ordinance no. 03 [8], for pesticides: red, extremely toxic products (Class I); yellow, highly toxic (Class II); blue, moderately toxic (Class III); and green, slightly toxic (Class IV).

A white circle with a diameter equal to the band height containing the skull and crossbones in black on white background should be included on the front panel of the label, with the words "caution poison." Specific pictograms, internationally accepted, should be placed along the colored band from the center to the edge occupying 50% of the band height (Figure 3).

The label central column shall contain the manufacturing and expiration dates, indications whether the content is explosive, flammable, oxidizing, corrosive, irritant, or subject to applied sales. The following warnings should also be on the label: "The use of personal protective equipment is required. Protect yourself" and "The return of the empty package is required," along with the toxicological and potential environmental hazard classification.

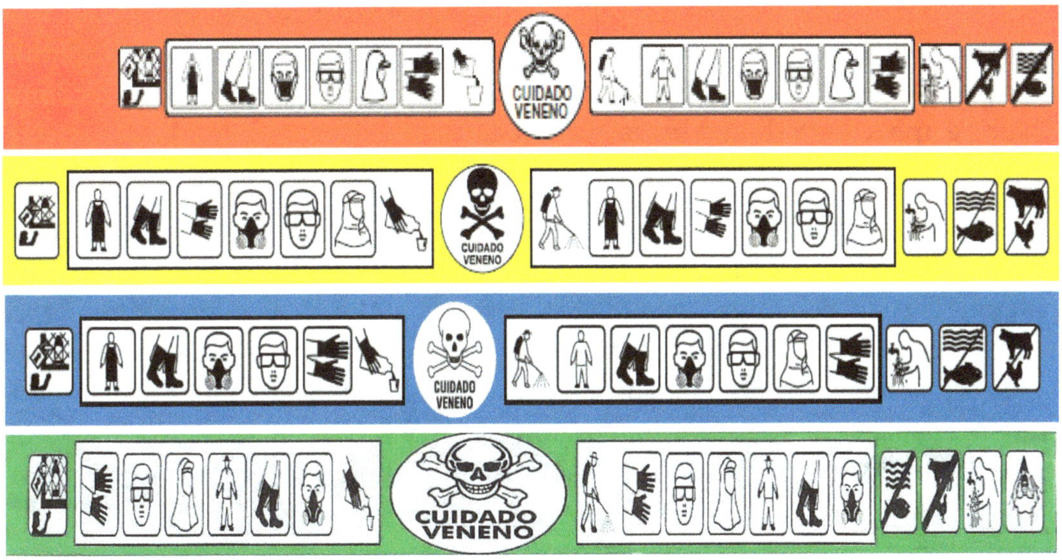

Figure 3. Warning band required at the bottom of the label, colored according to the toxicological class and pictograms about environmental and worker safety.

The labor legislation NR 31 [6] prohibits the handling of any pesticide not registered and not authorized by the relevant government agencies, complementing the preventive safety measures established in the legislation for pesticide registration. It prohibits the handling by persons under 18 and over 60 years old and pregnant women. It prohibits the handling of any pesticides in the workplace at odds with the indications and the instructions on the label and package leaflet.

It prohibits working on newly treated areas before the end of the reentry interval set on the label, except with the use of recommended protective equipment. It also prohibits any person to enter and stay, during aerial spraying, in the area to be treated.

3.1.3.3. Mandatory precaution measures in the package leaflet of pesticides

Decree Law no. 4074 [10] requires that the precaution measures against the poisoning risk of workers should be on the labels and in the package leaflet. Sample data related to the protection of human health are stated on the label and in the package leaflet of the herbicide Front™ follows [15].

The herbicide Front™ is registered by the company Du Pont of Brazil SA, in the Ministry of Agriculture, Livestock and Supply—MAPA, under number 10110, containing the following herbicides: diuron (603 g/kg), hexazinone (170 g/kg) and sulfometurom methyl (14.5 g/kg), and other inert ingredients (212.5 g/kg). To prevent spraying drift and reducing the occurrence of worker exposure, the herbicide package leaflet recommends the following:

Winds: Windspeed higher than 10 km/h or situations when the absence of winds causes a thermal inversion increases the potential for drift. The wind conditions and many factors, such as droplet diameter and type of equipment determine the potential spray drift. Do not apply if there are gusts of wind. Do not perform aerial application when there is no wind.

Reentry interval for people in the treated crops: People are not allowed to enter the area where the product was applied before it is completely dried (at least 24 hours after application). If it is necessary to enter during this period, the personal protective equipment (PPE) recommended for use during application should be used as well.

Instructions for product storage, conservation, and accident prevention: Keep the product always closed in its original packaging. The site should store exclusively toxic products, away from food, drink, feedstock, or other materials. The construction must be masonry or noncombustible material. The location must be ventilated, covered, and have waterproof floors. Warning signs such as "CAUTION: POISON" should be placed in the area. The place should be locked to prevent access of unauthorized persons, especially children. There must always be adequate packaging available to wrap broken packaging or to collect leaked product. In case of warehouses, the instructions of ISO 9843, ABNT—Brazilian Technical Standards Association should be followed. Observe the provisions of state and local legislation.

Data related to the protection of human health: Read the instructions carefully before use. Dangerous product. Use personal protective equipment as indicated.

General precautions: Product exclusively for agricultural use. Do not eat, drink, or smoke while handling and applying the product. Do not handle or apply the product without the recommended PPE. Recommended PPE must be worn in the following order: overalls, boots, apron, respirator, goggles, hood, and gloves. Do not use damaged PPE. Do not use equipment with leaks or defects. Do not unclog spray tips, nozzles, and valves with your mouth. Do not carry the product together with food, medicine, feed, animals and people.

Precautions when preparing the product for application: Product extremely irritating to the eyes. In the event of accidental contact with the product, follow the guidelines outlined in first aid procedures and quickly seek emergency medical service. Open the package carefully to avoid dispersion of dust. Use PPE: water-repellent cotton overalls with long sleeves going over the gloves and pants legs over the boots, rubber boots, waterproof apron, respirator with mechanical filter class P2, safety glasses with side shields, hood, and nitrile gloves. Handle the product in open and ventilated area.

Precautions during application: Avoid as much as possible contact with the treated area. Do not apply the product in the presence of strong winds and the hottest hours of the day. Do not apply product against the wind, when using a backpack herbicide applicator. When using a tractor (or plane), apply product against the wind. Apply the product only at recommended doses and observe the safety interval (time interval between the last application and harvest). Use personal protective equipment (PPE): water-repellent cotton overalls with long sleeves going over the gloves and trouser legs over the boots, rubber boots, respirator with mechanical filter class P2, safety glasses with side shields, hood, and nitrile gloves.

Precautions after application: Flag the treated area with the words "Entry prohibited. Treated area." Keep the warnings until the end of the reentry period. If you need to enter the area treated during this period, use the PPE recommended during application. Keep the remaining product properly closed in the original packaging and locked away from children and animals. Before removing PPE, wash the gloves while still dressed to avoid contamination. Recommended PPE must be removed in the following order: hood, goggles, aprons, boots, overalls, gloves, and respirator. Take a bath immediately after applying the product. Change and wash protective clothing separately from regular family laundry. When washing the clothes, use gloves and waterproof apron. Maintain and wash protective equipment after each product application. Follow correctly the manufacturer's specifications regarding filter usage time. Do not reuse the empty package. Use the PPE during package disposal: water-repellent cotton overalls with long sleeves, nitrile gloves, and rubber boots.

First aid: Go to an emergency medical center and take the packaging, label, package leaflet and agronomic prescription for the product. *Ingestion*: If the product has been swallowed, do not induce vomiting. If vomiting occurs naturally, lay the person sideways. Do not give anything to drink or eat. *Eyes*: In case of contact, wash with plenty of running water longer than 15 minutes. Prevent the wash water from entering the other eye. *Skin*: In case of contact, remove contaminated clothing and wash the skin with running water and mild soap. *Inhalation*: If the product has been inhaled, take the person to an open and ventilated place.

3.1.3.4. Training of workers

Even with technical training, the worker can make mistakes that result from carelessness, inattention, overconfidence, lack of technical expertise, and mechanical and emotional factors [3]. The employee must be trained, in detail, about the correct storage, transportation, and use of pesticides as described on the label and in the package leaflet.

The employee must also be trained on proper equipment maintenance of both backpack and mechanized applicators. Workers must be able to apply the pesticide with the least possible contact. On the other hand, the employer must select the least toxic products and create conditions to mechanize and automate operations to minimize contact between worker and pesticide.

The training on pesticide handling and application in field conditions is essential to reduce risks and prevent poisoning. Labor legislation NR 31 [6] states that the machinery and implements must be used according to the manufacturer's technical specification, within the operational limits and restrictions indicated. Therefore, equipment must be operated by qualified and adequately trained workers.

The NR 31 [6] also requires that rural employers, or equivalent, must provide training on how to prevent accidents with pesticides to all workers directly exposed to them. The NR 31 requires that training must be provided to workers with direct exposure, and the program should consist of a minimum twenty hours distributed in a maximum of eight hours during normal working hours. This training should provide minimum knowledge about direct and indirect exposure to pesticides; signs and symptoms of intoxication and first aid procedures; labeling and safety signs; hygienic procedures during and after work; use of clothing and personal protective equipment; and cleaning and maintenance of clothing and personal protective equipment.

The NR 31 also provides that the rural employer must inform all employees about the use of pesticides in the establishment, such as the treated area: description of the general characteristics of the location area, type of application, including equipment to be used; trade name of the product used; toxicological classification; date and time of application; reentry interval; withdrawal period/grace period; protection measures required for workers in direct and indirect exposure; and measures to be taken in case of poisoning [6].

3.1.3.5. Emergency medical procedures

Labor legislation NR 31 [6] states that the rural employer must preserve the occupational health of workers, prevent, and control the injuries resulting from work accidents. The actions should be planned and implemented based on the identification of risks and paid by rural employers.

The rural or similar employer must ensure medical examinations and meet the deadlines and the schedule required. The required medical examinations are as follows: admission, held during the hiring process, before the worker takes on his responsibilities; periodic medical examination, held annually; medical examination upon return to work, held on the first day when the employee returns to work after being absent for longer than 30 days due to any illness or accident; medical examination upon changing function, provided that the worker is going to be exposed to a specific risk different than the previous; and dismissal medical examination, performed at the end of the employment contract [6].

Medical tests include clinical evaluation and complementary exams when necessary and depending on the risks. After each medical examination, the Occupational Health Certificate (OHC) must be issued in duplicate, containing the following data: full name of the worker, worker ID and function; exposure to occupational risks; indication of medical procedures that the worker underwent and when they were performed; and whether the worker is fit or unfit for the specific function to be performed. The OHC should have the doctor's registration number issued by the Medicine Regional Council and be dated and signed by the doctor who performed the examination. The first part of the OHC should be filed and be available for inspection while a copy is compulsorily given to the employee, upon receipt of signing the first via [6].

Other health actions at work must be planned and executed according to the needs and peculiarities. All rural establishments must be equipped with the necessary first aid material, according to the characteristics of the activity to be performed.

The employer should ensure the removal of the injured in an emergency, without cost to the employee. The employer must also allow workers access to health agencies for the purpose of prevention and prophylaxis of endemic diseases and the application of tetanus vaccine.

3.1.4. Hygiene, cleaning, maintenance, and safety of the environment

Occupational hygiene measures consist of actions and procedures to prevent, or minimize, environment and worker contamination with pesticides. These actions should be applied at all working stages.

The hygiene and cleaning measures are applied to machinery, pesticide application equipment, handling of pesticides, materials, and clothing. The occupational hygiene is also applied to workers, who must turn them into habits to reduce exposures and prevent contamination of the materials, equipment, and tools with pesticides.

Workers should be instructed to clean immediately after contamination occurs and to keep all components sanitized and clean. There are actions that should be performed before and after working with pesticides. For example, gloves should be decontaminated immediately after getting contaminated with pesticides during work.

Preventive health and environment safety after use of pesticides is also present in the Brazilian legislation for pesticide registration and labor. In the pesticide registration legislation, Decree Law no. 4074 [10] states that as a preventive safety measure, the agronomic prescription must have the diagnosis of plant health problem, the recommendation to read carefully the label, and the package leaflet of the recommended pesticides. The packaging and labeling of pesticides cannot be confused with toiletries, pharmaceuticals, food, diet, beverage, cosmetics, and perfumes. The package leaflet must be present in single packs and contain all the information on the label and instructions for use, poisoning signs, symptoms, and treatment.

The labor legislation NR 31 [6] states that all workers should be informed regarding the use of pesticides about the treated area, description of the general characteristics of the area and the location; type of application, including the equipment used; trade name of pesticide; toxicological classification; date and time of application; reentry interval; protective measures required for workers in direct and indirect exposure; and the measures to be taken in case of intoxication.

The preservation, maintenance, cleaning, and use of the equipment may only be performed by previously trained and protected persons. Equipment should be cleaned without contaminating wells, rivers, streams, and any other water collections NR 31 [6].

3.2. Protective measures

If the working conditions remained unsafe (MOS < 1) after the pesticide registration and labor legislation requirements were met and the preventive measures were put in place, the protective measures should be implemented intensively enough to make the working environment safe (MOS ≥ 1).

Protective measures aim to isolate or neutralize the risks. They are grouped into collective that control the risk at the source (generation) and on the path (propagation or trajectory) and individual, which controls the risk directly on the exposure routes in the worker's body (receiver).

Unsafe working conditions are compromised by defects, failures, technical irregularities, and lack of safety devices, therefore exposing to danger the physical integrity and/or health of the workers, facilities, and equipment. For example, lack of adequate protection when operating machinery and equipment [3].

For unsafe working conditions (MOS < 1), the need for exposure control (NEC) can be calculated using the formula proposed by Machado-Neto [23]:

$$NEC = \left(1 - MOS < 1\right) \times 100 \left(\%\right).$$

NR 31 requires that the employer must adopt collective protection measures to control the risks at the source, followed by personal protective measures at no cost to the worker, to complement when risk factors persist temporarily [6].

3.2.1. Collective protection

Collective protection measures can act on toxicity and/or exposure, considering the two main risk factors of poisoning with pesticides.

3.2.1.1. Controlling herbicide toxicity

The pesticide toxicity is controlled by replacing the pesticide with a less toxic one, with higher NOEL value (Table 2). The higher the NOEL value, the greater the safe dose and greater MOS value.

Pesticide formulation	Common name	g i.a. /L	NOEL, mg/kg/day	Registration holder
Gesapax 500 SC	Ametryn	500.0	2.0	Syngenta Proteção De Cultivos Ltda.
Aurora 400 EC	Cafentrazona-ethyl	400.0	3.0	FMC Química Do Brasil Ltda
Gamit Star EC	Clomazone	800.0	14.0	FMC Química Do Brasil Ltda
Roundup Original SL	Glyphosate	480.0	30.0	Monsanto Do Brasil Ltda
Dual Gold EC	Metolachlor	960.0	7.5	Syngenta Proteção De Cultivos Ltda.
Boral 500 SC	Sulfentrazone	500.0	12.0	FMC Química Do Brasil Ltda
Butiron SC	Tebutiurom	500.0	7.0	Milenia Agrociências S.A.
Combine 500 SC	Tebutiurom	500.0	7.0	Dow Agrosciences Industrial Ltda
DMA 806 BR SL	2.4D	806.0	1.0	Dow Agrosciences Industrial Ltda.
Callisto SC	Mesotrione	480.0	1.8	Syngenta Proteção De Cultivos Ltda.

Table 2. Commercial formulations of herbicides, active ingredients, and their concentrations in the formulations, NOEL values TGA [31], and registration holders in Brazil.

3.2.1.2. *Controlling worker exposure to herbicides*

The collective protective measures that control exposure are applied to the components of the working environment. The first may be the automation of potentially contaminating operations performed by the worker; however, very rarely this action can be applied. For example, closed systems for preparing and supplying the mixture of pesticide with the carrier.

The main measure of collective protection, when working with pesticides in field conditions, is to isolate the risk areas or the worker doing the job. The isolation of the risk area can be achieved by using a bar protection adapted to the sprayer bar pulled by the tractor used for applying nonselective herbicide in eucalyptus culture (Figure 4). The spray bar was reduced to 2.5 m in length and covered with sturdy plastic blades at the front, sides, and rear (Figure 4). The bar has been adapted to apply nonselective pesticide over a 2.0-m-wide area on the weeds between the rows in areas planted with 1.0-m-tall young eucalyptus plants [24].

The total exposure of the tractor driver without individual protection, but with protected spray bar, was 838.88 mg/day of glyphosate and MOS of 8.62 [24]. Therefore, the protection of the spray bar made the tractor driver work safe, with acceptable poisoning risk and tolerable exposure levels.

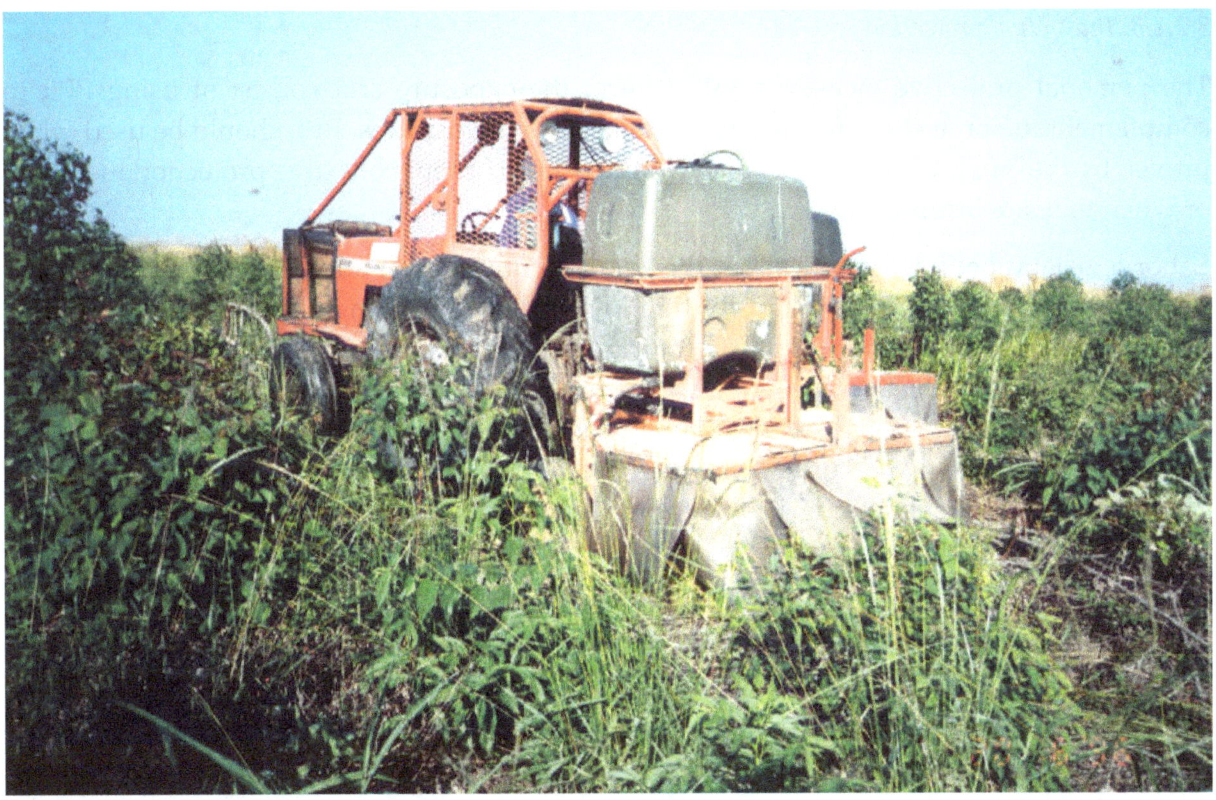

Figure 4. Sprayer bar protected with plastic blades attached to the bar used to apply nonselective herbicide between plant rows in eucalyptus plantation areas [24].

Although affected by several factors, occupational exposure to pesticides is directly related to the concentration of active ingredient in the sprayed mixture and the effective exposure time during the work day [1]. Therefore, another way of changing an unsafe working condition to safe is to limit the working hours to the number of hours during which it is safe to perform the activity (TST). This parameter can be calculated using the following formula proposed by Machado-Neto [23]:

$$\text{SWT} = \text{MOS} \times \text{eet},$$

where SWT indicates safe working time (h); MOS, margin of safety; and eet, effective exposure time (h).

The calculated SWT values lead to two situations:

1. If MOS $\geq$ 1, the SWT is greater than the considered exposure time and reaffirms the safety of working conditions under study. For safe conditions, the SWT expresses their safety levels.
2. If MOS $<$ 1, the SWT is less than the exposure time of the workday. Therefore, the calculation enables to restrict daily exposure to the SWT, using it as a collective safety measure.

3.2.1.3. Individual protection

The personal protective measures only control the exposure and consist of using PPE to complement the protection of collective and preventive measures. PPE should be used when proven by the employer that is technically unfeasible to adopt collective protection measures or when they are insufficient [6].

Labor legislation NR 31 provides that the rural employer must adopt at least the following personal protective measures: supply the PPE and work clothing appropriate to the risks undertaken without causing thermal discomfort to the worker. Provide PPE and work clothing in perfect working order and properly cleaned, replacing them as necessary. It should be made clear that their decontamination at the end of each workday is the responsibility of the rural employer. Instruct on the correct use of protective devices. Provide a suitable place for safekeeping of personal clothing. Provide water, soap, and towels for personal hygiene. Ensure that any protection device or contaminated clothing be taken out of the workplace. Ensure that no device or protective clothing is reused before due decontamination. Forbid the use of personal clothing when applying pesticides [6].

The same legislation further states that it is mandatory to supply PPE to the workers for free in the following circumstances: when the collective protection measures are technically proven unfeasible or when they do not offer complete protection against the risks resulting from work and while the collective protection measures are being implemented and to meet emergency situations. PPE should be appropriate to the risks and kept in perfect condition and operation. The employer must require and train the employee to use PPE [6].

PPE control exposures on the workers' body surface via dermal and respiratory routes. Respiratory exposure is controlled with respirators equipped with filters for particles or particles and vapors, with activated carbon. Dermal exposure is controlled with PPE made of porous and nonporous materials, or impervious. Waterproof materials are plastic coated, laminated, and rubberized; for hand protection, waterproof gloves; feet protection, waterproof rubber boots; leg protection, aprons; and plastic goggles with side shield. The porous materials are various types of fabric impregnated with carbon-fluorine compounds, which repel the water droplets of the spray mist. These porous materials are used to make the hood, long-sleeved shirts, and pants.

There is no need to use any PPE when working conditions are classified as safe (MOS ≥ 1); however, PPE could always be recommended as accident preventive measure. The noncontrolled dermal exposure was reduced by 99%, from 838.88 to 8.62 mg/day of glyphosate in the case of the tractor driver applying glyphosate in eucalyptus plantations with the protective plastic cover over the sprayer bar (Figure 4) and wearing PPE consisting of a set of water-repellent parts (hood, long-sleeved shirt and pants), gloves, and waterproof boots. MOS increased from 8.62 to 103.24 [24]. The use of PPE made the working condition of the tractor driver even more secure.

Author details

Joaquim G. Machado-Neto

Address all correspondence to: joaquim@fcav.unesp.br

São Paulo State University, Jaboticabal, Brazil

References

[1] Bonsall, J L. Measurement of occupational exposure to pesticide. In: Turnbull, G I. Occupational hazards of pesticide use. London: Taylor e Francis; 1985. pp. 13–33.

[2] Borsano, P R; Barbosa, R P Soares, S P S. Equipamentos de segurança. São Paulo, 1st ed. Editora Érica Ltda; 2014. 120 p.

[3] Borsano, P R.; Rivers, R; Fusco, M. Proteção e prevenção de perdas no ambiente organizacional. São Paulo, 1st ed. Editora Érica Ltda; 2014. 120 p.

[4] Brazil. Decree no. 349—Convenção no. 012—Indenização por acidentes de trabalho (agricultura). Brasília, 1991. Available from: http://portal.mte.gov.br/legislacao/convencao-n-12.htm. [Accessed: 2015-04-30].

[5] Brazil. NR 1—Disposições gerais. Brasília, 2009. Available from: http://portal.mte.gov.br/data/files/FF8080812BE914E6012BEF0F7810232C/nr_01_at.pdf. [Accessed: 2015-05-20].

[6] Brazil. NR 31—Segurança e saúde no trabalho na agricultura, pecuária silvicultura, exploração florestal e aquicultura. Brasília, 2013. Available from: http:// portal.mte.gov.br/data/files/8A7C812D33EF459C0134561C307E1E94/NR31%20(atualizada%202011).pdf. [Accessed: 2015-05-20].

[7] Brazil. NR 9—Programa de prevenção de riscos ambientais. Brasília, 2014. Available from: http://portal.mte.gov.br/data/files/FF80808148EC2E5E014961B76D3533A2/ NR-09%20 (atualizada%202014)%20II.pdf. [Accessed: 2015-05-20]

[8] Brazil. Ordinance no. 03/MS/SNVS, de 01/16/1992. Brasília, 1992. Available from: http://www.aenda.org.br/fito/PortAnvisa3-92.pdf. [Accessed: 2015-05-20].

[9] Brazil. Ordinance no. 3.214—Convenção no. 184—Convenção relativa à segurança e saúde na agricultura. Brasília, 1978. Available from: http://portal.mte.gov.br/legislacao/convencao-n-184.htm [Accessed: 2015-04-30].

[10] Brazil. Decree Law no. 4074. Brasília, 2002. Available from: http://www.planalto.gov.br/ccivil_03/decreto/2002/d4074.htm. [Accessed: 2015-05-20].

[11] Bronaugh, R L. In vitro methods for the percutaneous absorption of pesticides. In: Honeycutt, R C; Zweig, G; Ragsdale, N N, editors. Dermal exposure related to pesticide use—discussion of risk assessment. Washington: ACS. 1985, p. 33 – 41..

[12] Brouwer, D H; Brouwer, R; De Vreede, J A F; De Mik, G; Van Hemmen, J J. Respiratory exposure to field-strength dusts in greenhouses during application and after reentry. Zeist: TNO Health Research—Annual report 1990; 1990. p. 183–184.

[13] Byers, M E; Kamble, S T; Witkowski, J F; Echtenkams, G. Exposure of a mixer-loader to insecticides applied to corn via a center-pivot irrigation system. Bulletin of Environmental Contamination and Toxicology. 1992; 49: 58–65.

[14] Campos, A. Cipa—Comissão Interna de Prevenção de Acidentes: uma nova abordagem. 20th ed. São Paulo,. Editora Senac; 1999. 375p.

[15] Du Pont do Brasil S.A. 2015. Front™—package leaflet. Available from: http:// www.dupont.com.br/content/dam/assets/products-and-services/cropprotection/ assets/ ptBR/Front_Bula.pdf. [Accessed: 2015-05-20]

[16] Durhan, W F; Wolfe, H R. Measurement of the exposure of workers to pesticides. Bulletin of the World Health Organizatioon. 1962; 26: 75–91.

[17] Eldoradobrasil. 2015. Available from: http://www.painelflorestal.com.br/noticias/ mercado/ eldorado-brasil-busca-profissionais-em-agua-clara-e-tres-lagoas?utm_campaign=newsletter_gabarito _13052015_floresta&utm_medium=email&utm_source=RD±Station. [Accessed: 2015-05-12].

[18] Franklin, C A, Muir, N I, Greenhagh, R. The assessment of potential health hazards to orchardists spraying pesticides. In: Plimmer, J R. editor. Pesticide residues and exposure. Washington: ACS; 1982. p. 157–168.

[19] Guy, R H., Hadgraft, J, Maibach, H I. Transdermal absorption kinetics: a physicochemical approach. In: Honeycutt, R C, Zweig, G, Ragsdale, N N, editors. Dermal exposure related to pesticide use—discussion of risk assessment. Washington: ACS; 1985. p. 19 – 31.

[20] Jensen, J K. The assumptions used for exposure assessments. In: Siewierski M. editor. Determination and assessment of pesticide exposure. New York: Elsevier; 1984. pp 147–152.

[21] Larini, L, Cecchini R. A intoxicação como fenômeno biológico. In: Larini L. Toxicologia. São Paulo: Editora Manole Ltda; 1987. p. 1–40.

[22] Machado-Neto J G, Matuo T. Avaliação de um amostrador para o estudo da exposição dérmica potencial de aplicadores de defensivos agrícolas. Ciência Agronômica. Jaboticabal: FCAV-UNESP; 1989. 4/2: 21–22.

[23] Machado-Neto J G. Estimativas do tempo de trabalho seguro e da necessidade de controle da exposição ocupacional dos aplicadores de agrotóxicos [thesis]. Jaboticabal: São Paulo State University; 1997.

[24] Machado-Neto J G, Bassini A J, Aguiar L C. Safety of working conditions of glyphosate applicators on eucalyptus forests using knapsack and tractor powered sprayers. Bulletin of Environmental Contamination and Toxicology.2000; 64: 309–15.

[25] Mathias C G T, Hinz R S, Guy R H, Maibach H T. Percutaneous absorption: interpretation of in vitro data and risk assessment. In: Honeycutt R C, Zweig G, Ragsdale N N, editors. Dermal exposure related to pesticide use—discussion of risk assessment. Washington: ACS; 1985. p. 13 – 17.

[26] Oliveira M L. Segurança no trabalho de aplicação de agrotóxicos com turboatomizador e pulverizador de pistolas em citros [thesis]. Jaboticabal: Universidade Estadual Paulista; 2000.

[27] Saliba T M. Manual de higiene ocupacional e PPRA. 4th ed. São Paulo: LTr; 2013. 368 p.

[28] Saliba T M, Corrêa M A C, Amaral L S. Higiene do trabalho e programa de prevenção de riscos ambientais. São Paulo: LTr, 2002. 262p.

[29] Scaldelai A V, Oliveira C A D, Milaneli E, Oliveira J B C, Bolognesi P R. Manual prático de saúde e segurança do trabalho. 2th ed. São Caetano do Sul: Yendis Editora Ltda; 2012. 433p.

[30] Severn D J. Use of exposure data for risk assessment. In: SIEWIERSKI M. editor. Determination and assessment of pesticide exposure. New York: Elsevier; 1984. p. 13–19.

[31] TGA—Therapeutic Goods Administration. ADI List: Accept daily intakes for agricultural and veterinary chemicals. Australian Government, Department of Health and

Ageing. Canberra, 2008. Available from: http://www.ag.gov.au/cca. [Accessed: 2012-05-20]

[32] Turnbull G L. Current trends and future needs. In: Turnbull, G L. Occupational hazards of pesticide use. London: Taylor and Francis; 1985. p. 99–116.

[33] USEPA—United State Environmental Protection Agency. Glossary of terms relates to health, exposure, and risk assessment. Washington: EPA/450/3-88/016; 1989. 34p.

[34] Van Hemmen J J. Agricultural pesticide exposure data bases for risk assessment. Bulletin of Environmental Contamination and Toxicology. 1992; 126: 1–85.

[35] Wolfe H R, Armstrong J F, Staiff D C, Comer S W. Exposure of spraymen to pesticide, Archives Environmental Health. 1972; 25: 29–31.

[36] WHO—World Health Organization. Field surveys of exposure to pesticide standard protocol. Document VBC/82.1. 1982. Available from: http://www.who.int/iris/handle/10665/112732. [Accessed: 2015-05-20]

3

Occupational Exposure to Coal, Genotoxicity, and Cancer Risk

Grethel León-Mejía, Milton Quintana Sosa,
Paula Rohr, Katia Kvitko,
João Antonio Pêgas Henriques and Juliana da Silva

Abstract

Coal is a heterogeneous mixture containing large quantities of organic and inorganic matter, including carbon, hydrogen, oxygen, sulfur, nitrogen, and organometallic forms. The presence of mineral matter in coal may result in a number of environmental and human health problems related to its mining, preparation, and combustion. During coal mining activities, large quantities of coal dust, ashes, polycyclic aromatic hydrocarbons (PAHs), and heavy metals are released into the environment, forming a complex mixture. This mixture becomes one of the most important occupational risks for the health and safety of workers due to its synergistic, additive, and enhancing effects. Once inside the organism, this cocktail-like mixture can interact with cellular mechanisms related to the production of reactive oxygen species (ROS) and can cause damage in important macromolecules such as DNA, lipids, and proteins. In this review, human populations exposed to coal and coal burning were analyzed. Data from different studies were evaluated in relation to the effect of complex mixture exposure on DNA damage and mechanisms, and the background factors, such as gender, age, or smoking habit. The high temperatures that occur in combustion processes affect the characteristics of the resulting particles. The coal fly ash is released by combustion and its composition varies depending on the coal type and the method of collection used such as electrostatic precipitators. Compounds such as PAHs once activated by the organisms have been shown to have mutagenic and carcinogenic activity due to its ability to form adducts with purines. Moreover, metals that commonly are evaporated during the cooling process increase its toxicity. The particles when inhaled can pass from the alveoli into the bloodstream and affect extrapulmonary organs. Several studies have described the inflammatory cascade that triggers exposure to coal and coal fly ash particles; they have a complex composi-tion capable of generating a persistent inflammatory process, resulting in diseases widely described as emphysema, bronchitis, pneumoconiosis, asthma, and cancer. Several human biomonitoring studies have been conducted evaluating the inflammatory process and the release of cytokines, polymorphisms involved in detoxification mechanisms, different biomarkers associated with occupational exposure, DNA damage, and the influence of oxidative stress in disease development. The relationship between chronic exposure to coal and coal ash particles and cancer is still widely debated. This review gave us a broad assessment about the associated mechanisms between cancer and exposure to coal and different findings around the world.

Keywords: coal, biomonitoring, DNA damage, ROS, PAHs, diseases

1. Introduction

In the last decades, the human population genetics integrity has been compromised by the great industrial activity, which exposes people to a variety of chemicals and genotoxic agents. As a result, it is important to determine what is considered as an "acceptable" level of genetic damage in a concrete population, carry out assay genotoxicity as a routine and also monitor those who, by their occupation or lifestyle, are more exposed or with a bigger risk of having alterations on their genetics stability [1].

One method to quantify the exposure to those substances, as well as its possible impact on the organism, is the use of biological monitoring procedures, or biomonitoring, through biomarkers. Biomonitoring studies try to establish a connection between the environmental factors and the diseases. They detect first alterations in nonmalignant phases, so as to prevent health problems by recognizing the environmental cause of them.

The biological markers, or biomarkers, are the measurable changes (biochemical, physiological, or morphological) that associate to a toxic exposure or any early biochemical alteration, whose study on the biological fluids, tissues, or exhaled air that allow to assess the health risk exposure intensity. The identification of genotoxicity markers believed to cause genome damage is useful, since it can define a prepathogenesis state, such as cancer. It is of vital importance for different diseases prevention, which is the final goal of biomonitoring. In order to achieve it, there must be two stages: 1) detecting human exposure to environment carcinogenic agents; 2) determining genotoxic effects *in vivo* [2].

The combined use of genetic biomarkers and classic epidemiology tools (clinic history and questionnaires) has enabled the identification of early effects to the occupational exposure to distinct pollutant around the world [2–4]. Many biomarkers are used to assess genotoxic effects on human populations exposed to complex mixtures of chemicals. Although there are different possibilities, micronuclei (MN) frequency, chromosomal aberrations (CAs), and comet assay are the most commonly chosen biomarkers. MN originates from chromosome fragments or whole chromosomes that are not included in the main daughter nuclei during nuclear division [5, 6]. MN induction reflects clastogenic and aneugenic damage and is a predictive biomarker of cancer risk [7]. Comet assay detects DNA lesions in individual cells obtained under a variety of experimental conditions; the technique can also be used to evaluate DNA repair [8, 9].

The large inter-individual variability in the capacity to activate or inactivate potential genotoxic and carcinogenic compounds is probably influenced by polymorphisms of the genes encoding the metabolizing enzymes. Genes and proteins involved in metabolization/detoxification of xenobiotics, as well as those involved in DNA repair, are usually used as potential markers of susceptibility for the development of several diseases in which the etiology is related to exposure to environmental hazards. Polymorphisms in such genes have been linked with an increased risk of cancer in several case-control studies [10].

Biomonitoring studies in populations exposed to complex mixtures of chemicals considering individual susceptibility are quite complicated due to inadequate toxicity data, and the unpredictable nature of interaction effects that may be synergistic, additive, or enhancers.

2. Occupational exposure to coal

The coal reserves in a worldwide level is up to 847.5 billion of tons, enough amount to serve the current production for 119 years. This prediction is different from the ones related to oil and gas, which have available supplies for less time [11]. According to data from the International Energy Agency (IEA), coal is the most used resource for energy generation in the world, responsible for 41% of the total production. Nowadays, the main application of mineral coal is to generate energy through thermal power plants. These reserves are considered to have a 109-year lifespan and their coalfields are located in 75 countries. The main world coal producers are China, the United States, India, Australia, Indonesia, Russia, South Africa, Germany, Poland, and Kazakhstan, which are responsible for 91% of the world's production [12]. If those projections are right, the consequences of coal mining and combustion will have large effects in the environment. Thus, the exposed populations monitoring is fundamental with the aim of contributing to the state of knowledge about the health risk and motivate the establishment of control, hygiene, and prevention strategies.

It is well known that coal mining activities are one of the biggest resources of contamination due to the large quantity of substances liberated in the environment. The content of the coal dust and ashes produced by burning are not always homogeneous and this depends on the source and rank of the coal [13, 14]. Coal dust is constituted from carbon, hydrogen, oxygen, nitrogen, quartz (crystalline silica), and inorganic minerals, such as beryllium, cadmium, cobalt, chromium, iron, boron, copper, nickel, antimony, zinc, aluminum, titanium, magnesium, manganese, mercury, and lead [15]. As observed, coal is a mixture of a variety of chemicals, including hydrocarbons, which may raise polycyclic aromatic hydrocarbons (PAHs). All technological processes associated with open fire or temperatures between 400 and 600°C, that may lead to PAHs, should be considered potentially hazardous [16, 17].

In relation to coal mining residues exposure, studies in which biomarkers of effect, susceptibility, and exposure are used as epidemiological tools remain rare and a big part of them come from studies on underground coal mining [18, 19]. The effects generated by open coal mining are little explored, though. In open coal mining, the residues pass directly to the atmosphere, where complex mixtures are formed, and the coal exposure to environmental factors such as sunlight facilitates the processes of spontaneous combustion and, therefore, the release of PAHs [20].

Studies about the coal exposure and its harmful effects have been conducted around the world [21–23]. The main way for exposure of the coal mining workers to the potentially dangerous residues is through the inhaling of coal dust particles from mining and manipulation. It is a known fact that the coal mining continuous exposure can cause a variety of diseases, such as coal workers pneumoconiosis (CWP), silicosis, cancer, and chronic obstructive pulmonary disease (COPD), as emphysema and chronic bronchitis [24].

Many studies have established that some of those diseases could have been originated from the genotoxic damage generated by the inhalation of those mineral particles, able to interact with macrophages, epithelial cells, and other cells generating the production of large amount of reactive oxygen species (ROS) [24–26]. The continuous inhalation of coal dust and fly ashes particles is an important cell and non-cell source of ROS in the lung. This may be associated to the damage of target cells of that tissue and other cell lines, after spreading through the bloodstream [27].

Coal-induced DNA damage is related to macrophage activation and the recruitment of polymorphonuclear cells. This cell activation induces the release of inflammatory mediators, such as cytokines, ROS and reactive nitrogen species (RNS). The proinflammatory properties of ROS and RNS include endothelial cell damage, lipid peroxidation and oxidation, the release of chemostatic factors, the recruitment of neutrophils, and DNA damage [26, 28]. Interaction of ROS with DNA can result in DNA structural and transcriptional errors [29, 30]. Damage caused by ROS is recognized by DNA glycosylases, apurinic/apyrimidinic endonucleases of the base excision repair (BER) mechanism, and in some cases, by the nucleotide excision repair (NER) machinery, leading to DNA strand-breaks [31, 32].

Although chronic exposure may continue to damage the DNA, it has been suggested that inorganic elements can induce DNA single-strand breaks, possibly via the generation of ROS and that this type of damage is soon repaired. Metals are also known to modulate gene expression of enzymes [33]. In addition, PAHs can induce DNA lesions as single-strand breaks via DNA repair mechanisms, related with increased adduct formation and electrophilic metabolites [34–36]. Electrophilic metabolites covalently interact with the DNA [37, 38], and adducts are formed with purines, especially guanine, after metabolic activation by enzymatic complex P450 [39]. The International Agency for Research on Cancer (IARC) classified quartz, main constituent of coal, into IARC Group 1 (carcinogen), due to sufficient evidence for carcinogenicity in experimental animals and in humans [40, 41]. The other factor that could lead to different results in coal dust exposure, with positive and negative results, might be explained by the possible differences in composition, in which the proportion of the metals, PAHs, and silica (quartz) content may have an influence on the genotoxicity. Despite those findings, coal dust remains classified as non-carcinogen for human (Group 3) in IARC [40, 41]. The importance of coal as an energy source makes its characterization and estimation of risks of extreme importance to the safety of those individuals and the environment.

Several factors may explain conflicting results among different studies with human exposed to coal, e.g. cigarettes smoked, age, gender, nutritional status, and individual polymorphisms [6, 42]. Susceptibility is critical to an understanding of coal diseases, including cancer, and many xenobiotic agents act to alter susceptibility. Unknown individual susceptibility, inadequate toxicity data, and the unpredictable nature of interaction effects make the implementation of a human biomonitoring assessment for complex mixtures of chemicals extremely complicated.

3. Oxidative stress and genotoxic damage related with coal exposure

One important aspect to consider about the coal exposure is the amount of products generated during the coal combustion. The burning of coal, in order to generate electricity, produces flue gasses and particulate materials like coal fly ashes and residues as scoria and bottom ash. The finer particles (coal fly ash) are obtained by mechanical or electrostatic precipitation of the dust in suspension in the gases produced by combustion, while the coarser particles fall to the bottom by gravity and are removed at the bottom of the boiler [43, 44].

The combustion temperature is an important factor that determines the physical properties of the particles. In the combustion of conventional high temperature (>1400°C), the main aluminosilicate melts and condenses to form spherical particles. The coal fly ash particles produced are mostly irregularly shaped and contain a complex mixture consisting of unburned carbon; oxides; quartz; elements such as aluminum, silicon, calcium, iron, nickel, arsenic, chromium, copper, lead, cadmium, zinc [45, 46], and PAHs [47].

The coal fly ash has a relatively low toxicity as compared with coal or quartz [45]. Studies have determined the role of coal fly ash particle size and the release of iron, which leads to generation of radicals and oxidative stress. In this context, it was demonstrated the ability of coal fly ash release of bioavailable iron, which triggers processes and redox oxidant production [48]. In addition, it was shown that interleukin 8 (IL-8) levels in human lung epithelial cells are increased in response to coal fly ash and vary with the bioavailability of iron, as a function of source of coal and particle size [49]. The smaller size fraction had more stimulatory activity, which may be related to the fact that iron is more concentrated in this fraction. Particle size is a critical factor because a larger surface area allows more significant transport of metal and other adsorbed components, increasing the pulmonary toxicity of particulate matter (PM) [50].

The particles are classified according to their aerodynamic diameter (in micrometer) in coarse (PM 10), fine (PM 2.5), ultrafine (PM 0.1) [51]. The smaller particles are more harmful with respect to health effects because of their very high alveolar deposition fraction, large surface area, chemical composition, ability to induce inflammation, and potential to translocate to the circulation to extrapulmonary organs [52–54]. These particles could trigger persistent lung inflammation compared to the coarse particles in addition to the exposure to genotoxic compounds, which are contained in the particles [26, 55].

Depending on the toxicity, the chemical properties, and the concentration in air, coal and coal fly ash particles can constitute a risk to exposed workers. When these particles are inhaled and deposited in the lungs, they can lead to health risks due to the leaching of genotoxic compounds and altered immunological mechanisms affecting the lung parenchyma causing diseases [56]. These nanometric particles are very small, which allows them to penetrate the biological organs and affect its normal function. More specifically, as the particle load in the lung increases the alveolar macrophages and epithelial cells are activated, leading to the release of inflammatory mediators, ROS, enzymes (elastases, proteases, collagenases), cytokines [tumor necrosis factor alpha (TNF-α), interleukins], and growth factors (TGF-β) that control and stimulates the fibrosis, genotoxic events, and cell death [45, 57, 58].

Persistent inflammatory processes have been accepted as a crucial factor in the pathogenesis. In Zhai et al. [59], was investigated whether systemic TNF-α, soluble TNF-α receptors (p55, p75), IL-6, and soluble IL-6 receptor could be markers of biological activities of Chinese CWP. Interestingly, those results suggest that serum levels of TNF receptors and IL-6 are associated with the fibrotic process of CWP and serum cytokine levels may be correlated with the severity of CWP. In the pathogenesis of these respiratory diseases related with coal exposure, oxidative damage plays a key role. Either acting in association or independently, the chemical and physical characteristics can lead to the generation of ROS and oxidative stress [60, 61].

These particles are chemically heterogeneous and can be a source of oxidants by themselves ("acellular" mechanisms), due to their composition, such as oxides, metals, and PAHs [26]. Soluble metals (transition) associated to the particle can increase the generation of ROS by Haber-Weiss reactions. PAHs may be metabolically activated and induce ROS and oxidative stress, also forming bulky adducts or strand breaks on DNA [50, 62, 63].

Another way of generating oxidants is via cellular. Once in the lungs, alveolar macrophages are activated and generate large amounts of ROS, and chemoattractant factors of other inflammatory cells such as monocytes and neutrophils are released, which amplify this response generating more oxidants [64]. The particle size is a critical factor, because very large particles are difficult to phagocytose, leading to the process of incomplete or "frustrated" phagocytosis aggravating the response [65, 66].

Considering three different scenarios with respect to exposure to particles, the generation of oxidative stress, inflammation, and oxidative DNA damage, several authors questioned whether the lung inflammation may be related to secondary genotoxic effects. They also questioned if phenomena of oxidative stress, inflammation and DNA damage are independent or interrelated, whether oxidative stress stimulates inflammatory processes, or inflammation mediated by particles cause oxidative stress, or even if it is possible that particles may cause both phenomena of oxidative stress and inflammation but for different mechanisms of action [26, 61].

In normal physiological conditions, there is a balance between ROS generation and antioxidant defenses. However, the continuous inhalation of particles may interfere in this equilibrium leading to oxidative stress process in the lung. Consequently, a high loading of particles alters the oxidant-antioxidant balance, leading to oxidative damage and the beginning of pathological processes [67]. The most important effects of ROS in the lung include damage to cell membranes by lipid peroxidation process, protein oxidation, and DNA damage in target cells [27].

As seen in **Figure 1**, oxidative DNA damage can have many consequences, from cell death and tissue destruction to cell proliferation. Furthermore, ROS can also act as regulators in signaling pathways intracellularly and transcription factors of a variety of genes including those of proinflammatory cytokines, adhesion molecules, and proto-oncogenes [68].

In vitro effects induced by coal exposure have been described in different cells such as murine alveolar type II epithelial cells (C10) [69] and in 7TD1 cells [70]. ROS generation and oxidative damage by coal fly ash particles have been described in different cell lines, in human peripheral blood mononuclear cells [71], in rat alveolar macrophages (NR8383) [72], in BEAS-2B human lung epithelial cells [73], and in rat lung epithelial (RLE) cells [74].

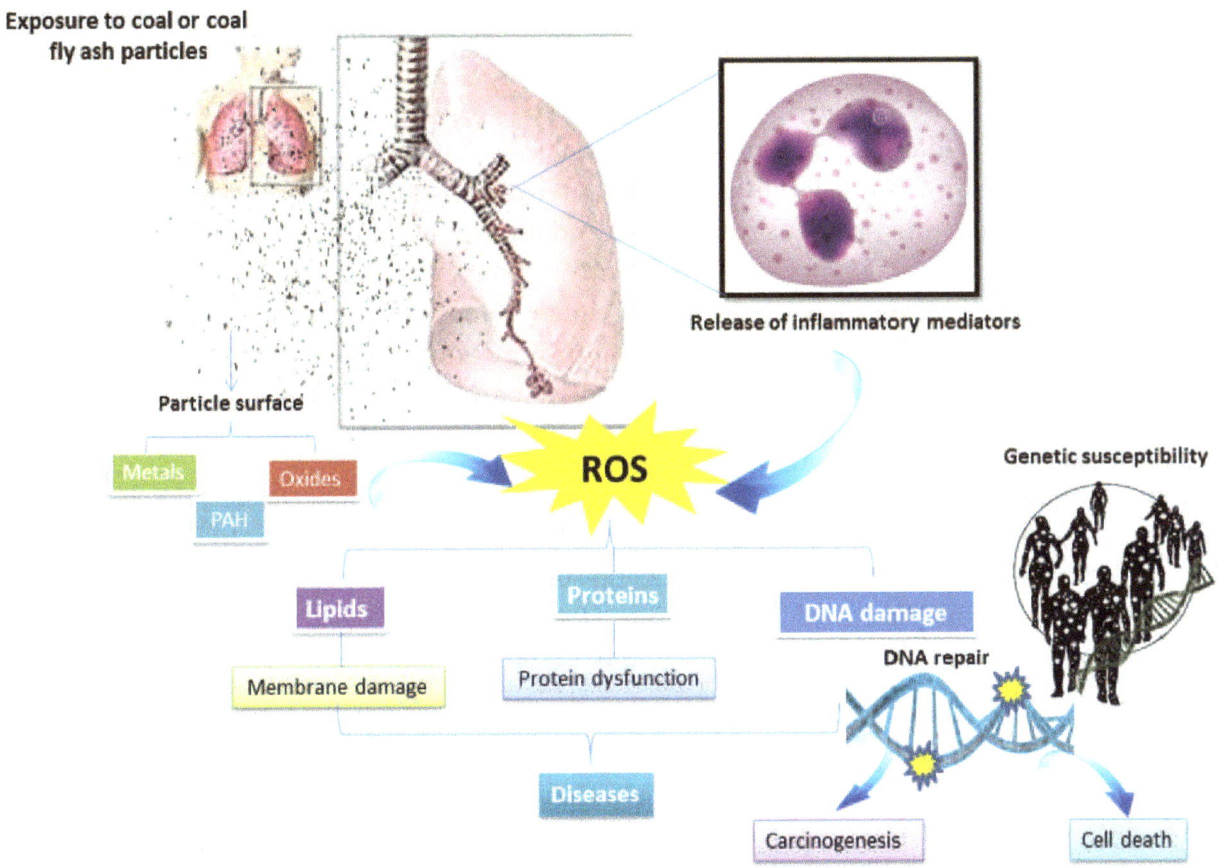

Figure 1. Main pathways associated with the generation of oxidative damage and the development of diseases induced by coal and coal fly ash particles.

ROS induce point mutations and CAs in cells. Many inhaled toxic substances contained in the particles contribute to oxidative modification that has as target of attack specific components of the cytoplasm and the nucleus. Such changes include DNA breakage, DNA oxidative modification, base modifications, alterations in the DNA sequence, poly-ADP ribosylation, activation of kinases, activation of proto-oncogenes, and inactivation of tumor suppressor genes. Persistent generation of ROS generated by mineral particles indestructible or engulfed incompletely leads to damage to organelles keys [59, 61, 75]. The oxidation of C8 deoxyguanosine (dG), resulting in 7-dihydro-8-oxo-2′-deoxyguanosine (8-oxodG), is the most common oxidative lesion generated by ROS. The proportion of 8-oxodG/dG has been considered as a biomarker of oxidative stress and has been studied in relation to exposure to mineral particles *in vitro* and *in vivo* [76].

Human biomonitoring studies about the effects of exposure to coal and residues using different biomarkers have been conducted around the world. In this context, our group has obtained interesting findings in workers exposed to coal mining in Colombia and Brazil. In Rohr et al. [77], was found that Brazilian workers with occupational exposure to coal had significantly increased genetic damage in peripheral blood lymphocytes compared with unexposed individuals. Exposed workers presented lower average levels of thiobarbituric acid reactive substances (TBARS) and catalase activity (CAT). In addition, DNA damage evaluated by human buccal micronucleus cytome (BMCyt) assay was observed in mine workers, which could be a consequence of oxidative damage resulting from exposure to coal residue mixtures [78].

In Colombia, DNA damage in lymphocytes of coal open-cast mining workers using the cytokinesis-blocked micronucleus test and the comet assay were observed [79]. Also, in buccal mucosa samples, the micronucleus frequencies and nuclear buds were significantly higher in the exposed group than in non-exposed control group. Interestingly, blood samples of Colombian mining workers analyzed showed higher values of silicon and aluminum characteristic elements of coal particles, compared with the control group [80]. All these studies converge to a point: the compounds contained in the particles may be related to ROS generation, DNA damage, and formation of pro-mutagenic adducts.

These are important findings if we consider that oxidative DNA damage can lead to long-term risk of cancer and other diseases caused by air pollution by these particles. In **Table 1**, can be observed an overview of key studies on the genotoxicity in human population exposed to coal and coal combustion products. These studies demonstrated DNA damage using different methods, related with inorganic elements and oxidative stress.

References	Country	Exposure(s)	Biomarker	Outcome(s)
[81]	Slovenia	_	Sister-chromatid exchanges (SCE), unstable chromosome and chromatid aberrations and micronuclei in blood lymphocytes	Significantly higher levels of chromosomal aberrations, SCE and micronuclei in exposed group compared with the control group.
[82]	Brazil	Underground workers directly exposed, surface	Oxidative stress biomarkers (TBARS, GSH/GSSG, α-tocopherol, GST, GR, GPx, SOD, CAT).	The results showed that subjects directly and indirectly exposed to coal dust face an oxidative stress condition. They also indicate that people living in the

References	Country	Exposure(s)	Biomarker	Outcome(s)
		workers indirectly exposed, residents living near the mines.		vicinity of the mine plant are in health risk regarding coal mining-related diseases.
[22]	Turkey	Coal combustion products	Chromosomal aberrations (CAs), polyploidy, sister-chromatid exchanges (SCEs), and micronuclei (MN) in blood cells.	Significantly higher levels of CA, polyploidy, SCE, and MN in peripheral blood lymphocytes of workers compared with controls.
[83]	Turkey	Underground coal mining	SCE, CA, and micronuclei frequencies in peripheral lymphocytes.	Increase in sister chromatid exchanges, chromosomal aberrations, and micronucleus frequencies found in underground coal miners as compared to control group.
[21]	China	Indoor smoky coal emissions that contain high levels of polycyclic aromatic hydrocarbons (PAHs)	GSTM1 and GSTT1 genotypes. Expression of p53 protein in sputum samples.	The GSTM1 null genotype may enhance susceptibility to lung cancer due to these indoor coal combustion emissions. Smoky coal use was strongly associated with overexpression of p53 in tumor cells among highly exposed women.
[79]	Colombia	Open cast mining	(MN) frequency and DNA damage (comet assay) in lymphocytes.	The biomarkers evaluated showed statistically significant higher values in the exposed group compared to the non-exposed control group.
[80]	Colombia	Open cast mining	Micronucleus (MN) frequencies, nuclear buds, karyorrhectic and karyolytic cells in buccal mucosa samples and content of inorganic elements in blood samples by PIXE.	MN frequencies and nuclear buds in buccal mucosa samples were significantly higher in the exposed group than in the non-exposed control group. In addition, karyorrhectic and karyolytic cells were also significantly higher in the exposed group (cell death). Blood samples showed higher values of silicon (Si) and aluminum (Al) in the exposed group.
[84]	Russian	Underground coal	Chromosomal and chromatid type	A higher frequency of chromosomal aberrations in the exposed group

References	Country	Exposure(s)	Biomarker	Outcome(s)
		mining	aberrations in blood lymphocytes	compared with the control group.
[77]	Brazil	Open coal mining	MN and nucleoplasmic bridge frequencies in peripheral lymphocytes, damage index and damage frequency (comet assay).	Increased MN and nucleoplasmic bridge frequencies in peripheral lymphocytes, increased damage index and damage frequency (comet assay). Lower average levels of TBARS and catalase activity (CAT), while the mean superoxide dismutase activity (SOD) levels were higher in the exposed group.
[78]	Brazil	Open coal mining	Buccal micronucleus cytome (BMCyt) DNA damage, cell death, and basal cell frequency in buccal cells.	The exposed group presented a significantly higher frequency of basal cells, micronuclei in basal and differentiated cells, and binucleated cells compared to the non-exposed group. No correlation between DNA damage and metal concentration in the blood of mine workers.
[19]	Peru	Underground coal mining	Chromosomal aberrations in peripheral lymphocytes	Miners occupationally exposed to underground mining activity have an increased frequency of chromosomal aberrations compared with the controls.
[85]	–	Coal fly ash particles	SCE frequencies in peripheral blood lymphocytes.	No increased SCE frequencies were found in PBLs of workers potentially exposed to coal fly ash when compared to the control group. No differences were observed between the exposed and control groups for frequencies of gene mutations at the HPRT locus in PBLs, for micronucleus frequencies using the cytokinesis block method, or for urinary mutagen excretion measured with *Salmonella typhimurium* tester strains TA98 and TA97.
[86]	Germany	Underground coal mining	Structural chromosomal aberrations in peripheral lymphocytes	Coal miners had significantly higher frequencies of chromosomal aberrations compared with controls.
[87]	Turkey	Underground coal	Sister chromatid exchange (SCE) and	SCE and MN frequencies in CWP patients were found significantly higher than

References	Country	Exposure(s)	Biomarker	Outcome(s)
		mining	micronucleus (MN) frequency in lymphocytes of Turkish CWP patients.	in coal workers and unexposed groups.

Table 1. Overview of key studies on the genotoxicity in human population exposed to coal and coal combustion products.

4. Conclusions

The coal mining activities generate different types of compounds that are released into the environment. Once into the atmosphere, these compounds form a complex mixture that consists of metals, oxides, and PAHs. These compounds can interact with "acellular" and cellular mechanisms related with ROS production. The metals found in the coal fly ash and coal particles by different ways lead to the ROS formation. Important macromolecules as DNA, proteins, and lipids can suffer oxidative modifications. The PAHs contained in the particles also influence the particles toxicity. A second indirect way for excessive ROS formation is related to cellular mechanisms, which is consequence of oxidative burst of macrophages and neutrophils during phagocytosis of particles and inflammation produced.

If we think in exposed populations, we cannot ignore the social and environmental impact associated with coal mining. The continuous inhalation, the high load of particles in phagocytic cells, the oxidant-antioxidant imbalance which are linked to the origin of pathological processes; this whole scenario is worrisome to biologic level for these populations. In addition, in recent years, coal mining had a remarkable increase in demand; international mining companies have increased their investments in exploration around the world. For this reason, human biomonitoring studies in exposed populations become really necessary to contribute to knowledge state about the risk for those people in order to motivate the design of control, hygiene, and prevention strategies, besides epidemiological surveillance.

Author details

Grethel León-Mejía [1,2], Milton Quintana Sosa [2], Paula Rohr [3], Katia Kvitko[4], João Antonio Pêgas Henriques [1,5*] and Juliana da Silva [6*]

*Address all correspondence to: pegas.henriques@gmail.com and juliana.silva@ulbra.br

1 Laboratory of Molecular Radiobiology, Center of Biotechnology, Postgraduate Program in Cell and Molecular Biology (PPGBCM), Federal University of Rio Grande do Sul (UFRGS), Porto Alegre, Rio Grande do Sul, Brazil

2 Simon Bolivar University, Faculty of Basic Sciences, Unit of Research, Development and Innovation in Genetics and Molecular Biology, Barranquilla, Colombia

3 Laboratory of Celular and Molecular Biology, Academic Unit of Health Sciences, Universidade do Extremo Sul Catarinense (UNESC) – Criciúma SC), Brazil

4 Postgraduate Program in Genetics and Molecular Biology (PPGBM), Federal University of Rio Grande do Sul (UFRGS) Porto Alegre, Rio Grande do Sul, Brazil

5 Laboratory of Molecular Radiobiology, Center of Biotechnology, Federal University of Rio Grande do Sul (UFRGS) Porto Alegre, Rio Grande do Sul, Brazil

6 Laboratory of Genetic Toxicology, Postgraduate Program in Molecular and Cell Biology Applied to Health (PPGBioSaúde), Lutheran University of Brazil (ULBRA), Canoas, Rio Grande do Sul, Brazil

References

[1] Zalacain, M; Sierrasesumaga, L; Patino, A. (2005). The cytogenetic assay as a measure of genetic instability induced by genotoxic agents. An Sist Sanit Navar. 28(2);227–36.

[2] Pastor, S; Lucero, L; Gutierrez, S; Durban, R; Gomez, C; Parron, T; et al. (2002). A follow-up study on micronucleus frequency in Spanish agricultural workers exposed to pesticides. Mutagenesis. 17(1);79–82.

[3] Martino-Roth, M.G; Viegas, J; Roth, D.M. (2003). Occupational genotoxicity risk evaluation through the comet assay and the micronucleus test. Genet Mol Res. 2(4); 410–7.

[4] Cassini, C; Calloni, C; Bortolini, G; Garcia, SC; Dornelles, MA; Henriques, JÁ; Erdtmann B; Salvador M. (2011). Occupational risk assessment of oxidative stress and genotoxicity in workers exposed to paints during a working week. Int J Occup Med Environ Health. 24(3);308–19.

[5] Fenech, M; Morley, A. (1985). Solutions to the kinetic problem in the micronucleus assay. Cytobios. 43;233–46.

[6] Mateuca, R; Lombaert, N; Aka, P.V; Decordier, I; Kirsch-Volders, M. (2006). Chromosomal changes: induction, detection methods and applicability in human biomonitoring. Biochimie. 88(11);1515–31.

[7] Bonassi, S; Znaor, A; Ceppi, M; Lando, C; Chang, W.P; Holland, N; et al. (2007). An increased micronucleus frequency in peripheral blood lymphocytes predicts the risk of cancer in humans. Carcinogenesis. 28(3);625–31.

[8] Tice, R.R; Agurell, E; Anderson, D; Burlinson, B; Hartmann, A; Kobayashi, H; et al. (2000). Single cell gel/comet assay: guidelines for in vitro and in vivo genetic toxicology testing. Environ Mol Mutagen. 35(3);206–21.

[9] Collins, A.R. (2014). Measuring oxidative damage to DNA and its repair with the comet assay. Biochim Biophys Acta 1840;794–800. doi: 10.1016/j.bbagen.2013.04.022.

[10] International Agency for Research on Cancer (IARC), Monographs on the Evaluation of Carcinogenic Risk to Humans, Reevaluation of Some Organic Chemicals, Hydrazine and Hydrogen Peroxide Agency for Research on Cancer, Toluene, World Health Organization. (1999). Lyon 71;829–864. Online: http://monographs.iarc.fr/ENG/Monographs/vol71/mono71.pdf

[11] Cerrejón-responsible mining. Uses of coal. (2013). Online, in Spanish: http://www.cerrejon.com/site/mas-sobre-el-carbon/usos-del-carbon.aspx

[12] International Energy Agency (IEA). (2016). Online: http://www.iea.org/

[13] Aneel- National Electric Energy Agency. Atlas Electric Power in Brazil. Chapter 9 – Mineral Coal. (2009). Online, in Portuguese: www.aneel.gov.br/arquivos/pdf/atlas_par3_cap9.pdf

[14] Caballero, A.L; Médico, O.A. (2013). Characterization and possible use of coal ash resulting from coal combustion in thermocentral of bed fluidized. Río Turbio (Argentina). National University of Austral Patagonia. Online, in Spanish: http://www.redisa.uji.es/artSim2013/CaracterizacionDeResiduosSolidos/Caracterizacion%20Cenizas%20Combustion%20Carbon.pdf

[15] Kalkreuth, W; Holz, M; Kern, M; Machado, G; Mexias, A; Silva, M.B; Willett, J; Finkelman, R; Burger, H. (2006). Petrology and chemistry of permian coals from the Paraná basin: Santa Terezinha, Leão-Butiá and Candiota Coal fields, Rio Grande do Sul, Brazil. Intern. J. Coal Geol. 68;79–116.

[16] Kvitko, K; Bandinelli, E; Henriques, J; Heuser, V; Rohr, P; Da Silva, F; Schneider, N; Fernandes, S; Ancines, C; Da Silva, J. (2012). Susceptibility to DNA damage in workers occupationally exposed to pesticides, to tannery chemicals and to coal dust during mining. Genet. Mol. Biol. 35;1060–68.

[17] Jarvis, I.W; Dreij, K; Mattsson, Å; Jernström, B; Stenius, U. (2014). Interactions between polycyclic aromatic hydrocarbons in complex mixtures and implications for cancer risk assessment. Toxicology. 3(321);27–39.

[18] Agostini, J; Otto P; Wajntal A. (1996). Chromosome damage in underground coal miners: detection by conventional cytogenetic techniques and by submitting lymphocytes of unexposed individuals to plasma from at-risk groups. Braz J Genet. 19;641–6.

[19] Santa Maria, S.R; Arana, M; ,Ramirez O. (2007). Chromosomal aberrations in peripheral lymphocytes from male native miners working in the Peruvian Andes. Genet Mol Biol. 30;1135–8.

[20] León, G; Perez, L.E; Linares, J.C; Hartmann, A; ,Quintana M. (2007). Genotoxic effects in wild rodents (*Rattus rattus* and *Mus musculus*) in an open coal mining area. Mutat Res. 630;42–9.

[21] Lan, Q; ,He X. (2004). Molecular epidemiological studies on the relationship between indoor coal burning and lung cancer in Xuan Wei, China. Toxicology. 198;301–5.

[22] Celik, M; Donbak, L; Unal, F; Yüzbasioglu, D; Aksoy, H; Yilmaz, S. (2007). Cytogenetic damage in workers from a coal-fired power plant. Mutat Res. 627(2);158–63.

[23] Karami, S; Boffetta, P; Brennan, P; Stewart, P.A; Zaridze, D; Matveev, V; Janout, V; Kollarova, H; Bencko, V; Navratilova, M; Szeszenia-Dabrowska, N; Mates, D; Gromiec, J.P; Sobotka, R; Chow, W.H; Rothman, N; Moore, L.E. (2011). Renal cancer risk and occupational exposure to polycyclic aromatic hydrocarbons and plastics. J Occup Environ Med. 53(2);218–223; 1076–2752.

[24] Petsonk, E.L; Rose, C; ,Cohen R. (2013). Coal mine dust lung disease. New lessons from old exposure. Am J Respir Crit Care Med. 187(11);1178–85.

[25] Vallyathan, V; Shi, X; Castranova, V. (1998). Reactive oxygen species: their relation to pneumoconiosis and carcinogenesis. Environ Health Perspect. 106(Suppl. 5);1151–5.

[26] Knaapen, A.M; Borm, P.J; Albrecht, C; ,Schins R.P. (2004). Inhaled particles and lung cancer. Part A: Mechanisms. Int J Cancer 109;799–809.

[27] Schins, R.P; ,Borm P.J. (1999). Mechanisms and mediators in coal dust induced toxicity: a review. Ann Occup Hyg. 43(1);7–33.

[28] Ba, X; Aguilera-Aguirre, L; Rashid, QT; Bacsi, A; Radak, Z; Sur, S; Hosoki, K; Hegde, ML; Boldogh I. (2014). The role of 8-oxoguanine DNA glycosylase-1 in inflammation. Int J Mol Sci. 15(9);16975–97.

[29] Schottenfield, D; Bebe-Dimmer, J. (2006). Chronic inflammation: a common and important factor in the pathogenesis of neoplasia. CA: Cancer J. Clin. 56;69–83.

[30] Svilar, D; Goellner, EM; Almeida, KH; Sobol, RW. (2011). Base excision repair and lesion-dependent subpathways for repair of oxidative DNA damage. Antioxid Redox Signal. 14(12);2491–507.

[31] Sander, M; ,Wilson S. (2005). Base Excision Repair, AP Endonucleases and DNA Glycosylases, John Wiley & Sons Ltd, Chichester.

[32] Storr, S.J; Woolston, C.M; Zhang, Y; ,Martin S.G. (2013). Redox environment, free radical, and oxidative DNA damage. Antioxid Redox Signal. 18(18);2399–408.

[33] Jomova, K; ,Valko M. (2011). Advances in metal-induced oxidative stress and human disease. Toxicology. 283;65–87.

[34] Brescia, G; Celotti, L; Clonfero, E; Neumann, G.H; Forni, A; Foa, V; Pisoni, M; Ferri, G.M; Assennato, G. (1999). The influence of cytochrome P450 1A1 and glutathioneS-

transferase M1 genotypes on biomarker levels in coke-oven workers. Arch. Toxicol. 73;431–9.

[35] Rojas, M; Cascorbi, I; Alexandrov, K; Kriek, E; Auburtin, G; Mayer, L; Kopp-Schneider, A; Roots, I; Bartsch, H. (2000). Modulation of benzo[a]pyrene diolepoxide-DNA adduct levels in human white blood cells by CYP1A1, GSTM1 and GSTT1 polymorphism. Carcinogenesis 21;35–41.

[36] Pavanello, S; Pulliero, A; Lai, A; Gaiardo, A; Mastrangelo, G; Clonfero, E. (2005). Anti-B[a]PDE-DNA formation in lymphomonocytes of humans environmentally exposed to polycyclic aromatic hydrocarbons, G. Ital. Med. Lav. Ergon. 27;312–4.

[37] Pereira-Neto, A.D; Moreira, J.C; Dias A.E.X.O; Arbilla G; Ferreira L.F.V; Oliveira A.S; Barek J. (2000). Assessment of human contamination by polycyclic aromatic hydrocarbons (PAHs) and nitrated derivatives (NPAHs): a methodological review. Quim. Nova 23;9. In Portuguese.

[38] Singh, R; Sram, R.J; ,Binkova B; Kalina, I; Popov, T.A; ,Georgieva T; ,Garte S; Taioli, E; ,Farmer P.B. (2007). The relationship between biomarkers of oxidative DNA damage, polycyclic aromatic hydrocarbon DNA adducts, antioxidant status and genetic susceptibility following exposure to environmental air pollution in humans. Mutat. Res. 620;83–92.

[39] Baird, W.M; Hooven, L.A; ,Mahadevan B. (2005). Carcinogenic polycyclic aromatic hydrocarbon-DNA adducts and mechanism of action. Environ. Mol. Mutagen. 45;106–14.

[40] International Agency for Research on Cancer (IARC). (2012). Arsenic, metals, fibres, and dusts: a review of human carcinogens. Lyon. 100C;526. Online: http://monographs.iarc.fr/ENG/Monographs/vol100C/mono100C.pdf

[41] International Agency for Research on Cancer (IARC). (1997). Silica, some silicates, coal dust and para-aramid fibrils, IARC Monographs on the Evaluation of the Carcinogenic Risks of Chemicals to Humans. Lyon. 68;528. Online: http://monographs.iarc.fr/ENG/Monographs/vol68/mono68.pdf

[42] Bonassi, S; Coskun, E; Ceppi, M; Lando, C; Bolognesi, C; Burgaz, S; et al. (2011). The HUman MicroNucleus project on eXfoLiated buccal cells (HUMN(XL)): the role of life-style, host factors, occupational exposures, health status, and assay protocol. Mutat Res. 728(3);88–97.

[43] Silva, L; Ward, C.R; ,Hower J; ,Izquierdo M; ,Waanders F; ,Oliveira M; ,Li Z; Hatch, R; ,Querol X. (2010). Mineralogy and leaching characteristics of coal ash from a major Brazilian power plant. Coal Combust Gasificat Prod. 2;51–65.

[44] Martinez, J. (2012). Coal fly ash and bottom ash or scoria. Technical file, Spain. On line, in Spanish: http://www.cedexmateriales.es/catalogo-de-residuos/24/cenizas-volantes-de-carbon-y-cenizas-de-hogar-o-escorias/

[45] Borm, P.J. (1997). Toxicity and occupational health hazards of coal fly ash (CFA). A review of data and comparison to coal mine dust. Ann Occup Hyg. 41;659–76.

[46] Swaine, D.J; ,Goodarzi F. (1997). Environmental Aspects of Trace Elements in Coal. Kluwer, Dordrecht.

[47] Ruwei, W; Jiamei, Z; Jingjing, L; Liu, G. (2013). Levels and patterns of polycyclic aromatic hydrocarbons in coal-fired power plant bottom ash and fly ash from Huainan, China. Arch Environ Contam Toxicol. 65(2);193–202.

[48] Ball, B.R; Smith, K.R; Veranth, J.M; ,Aust A.E. (2000). Bioavailability of iron from coal fly ash: mechanisms of mobilization and of biological effects. Inhal Toxicol. 12(Suppl. 4);209–25.

[49] Smith, K.R; Veranth, J.M; Hu, A.A; Lighty, J.S; ,Aust A.E. (2000). Interleukin-8 levels in human lung epithelial cells are increased in response to coal fly ash and vary with the bioavailability of iron, as a function of particle size and source of coal. Chem Res Toxicol. 13(2);118–25.

[50] Mazzoli-Rocha, F; Fernandes, S; Einicker-Lamas, M; Zin, W.A. (2010). Roles of oxidative stress in signaling and inflammation induced by particulate matter. Cell Biol Toxicol. 26(5);481–98.

[51] Donaldson, K; ,Stone V. (2003). Current hypotheses on the mechanisms of toxicity of ultrafine particles. Ann Ist Super Sanità;. 39;405–10.

[52] Oberdörster, G; Sharp, Z; Atudorei, V; Elder, A; Gelein, R; Kreyling, W; Cox, C. (2004). Translocation of inhaled ultrafine particles to the brain. Inhal Toxicol. 16(6–7);437–45.

[53] Schins, R.P; Lightbody, J.H; Borm, P.J; ,Shi T; Donaldson, K; ,Stone V. (2004). Inflammatory effects of coarse and fine particulate matter in relation to chemical and biological constituents. Toxicol. Appl. Pharmacol. 195;1–11.

[54] Mani, U; Prasad, A.K; ,Suresh Kumar V; Lal, K; Kanojia, R.K; Chaudhari, B.P; Murthy R.C. (2007). Effect of fly ash inhalation on biochemical and histomorphological changes in rat liver. Ecotoxicol Environ Saf. 68(1);126–33.

[55] Donaldson, K; Tran, L; Jimenez, L.A; Duffin, R; Newby, D.E; Mills, N. (2005). Combustion-derived nanoparticles: a review of their toxicology following inhalation exposure. Part Fibre Toxicol. 2;10.

[56] Carbone, F; Pagliara, R; Barone, A.C; Beretta, F; D'Anna, A. (2009). Characterization of nano-ashes generated during pulverized coal combustion. Report Ricerca Sistema Elettrico. Online: http://www.enea.it/it/Ricerca_sviluppo/documenti/ricerca-di-sistema-elettrico/centrali-carbone-rendimenti/rse109.pdf.

[57] Gilmour, M.I; O'Connor, S; Dick, C; Miller, C.A; ,Linak W.P. (2004). Differential pulmonary inflammation and in vitro cytotoxicity of size-fractionated fly ash particles from pulverized coal combustion. J Air Waste Manag Assoc. 54;286–95.

[58] Sambandam, B; Devasena, T; Islam, V.I; Prakhya, B.M. (2015). Characterization of coal fly ash nanoparticles and their induced in vitro cellular toxicity and oxidative DNA damage in different cell lines. Indian J Exp Biol. 53(9);585–93.

[59] Zhai, R; Liu, G; Ge, X; Bao, W; Wu, C; Yang, C; Liang, D. (2002). Serum levels of tumor necrosis factor-alpha (TNF-alpha), interleukin 6 (IL-6), and their soluble receptors in coal workers' pneumoconiosis. Respir Med. 96(10);829–34.

[60] Bonner, J.C. (2007). Lung fibrotic responses to particle exposure. Toxicol Pathol. 35(1); 148–53.

[61] Møller, P; Danielsen, P.H; Karottki, D.G; ,Jantzen K; ,Roursgaard M; Klingberg, H; Jensen, D.M; Christophersen, D.V; Hemmingsen, J.G; Cao, Y; ,Loft S. (2014). Oxidative stress and inflammation generated DNA damage by exposure to air pollution particles. Mutat Res Rev Mutat Res. 762;133–66.

[62] Risom, L; Møller, P; Loft, S. (2005). Oxidative stress-induced DNA damage by particulate air pollution. Mutat. Res. 592;119–37.

[63] Valavanidis, A; Vlachogianni, T; Fiotakis, K; Loridas, S. (2013). Pulmonary oxidative stress, inflammation and cancer: respirable particulate matter, fibrous dusts and ozone as major causes of lung carcinogenesis through reactive oxygen species mechanisms. Int J Environ Res Public Health. 10;3886–907.

[64] Fubini, B; ,Hubbard A. (2003). Reactive oxygen species (ROS) and reactive nitrogen species (RNS) generation by silica in inflammation and fibrosis. Free Radic Biol Med. 34;1507–16.

[65] Champion, J.A; ,Mitragotri S. (2006). Role of target geometry in phagocytosis. Proc Natl Acad Sci U S A. 103(13);4930–4.

[66] Schinwald, A; ,Donaldson K. (2012). Use of back-scatter electron signals to visualise cell/nanowires interactions in vitro and in vivo; frustrated phagocytosis of long fibres in macrophages and compartmentalisation in mesothelial cells in vivo. Particl Fibre Toxicol. 9;34.

[67] Porter, D.W; Leonard, S.S; Castranova V. (2006). Particles and Cellular Oxidative and Nitrosative Stress. Chapter 6. National Institute for Occupational Safety and Health. pp. 119–138

[68] Porter, D.W; Leonard, S.S; Castranova V. (2006). Particles and Cellular Oxidative and Nitrosative Stress. Chapter 6. National Institute for Occupational Safety and Health. Particle toxicology. Chapter 6. pp 119–138.

[69] Albrecht, C; Borm, P.J.A; Adolf, B; Timblin, C.R; ,Mossman B.T. (2002). In vitro and in vivo activation of extracellular signal-regulated kinases by coal dusts and quartz silica. Toxicol Appl Pharmacol. 184;37–45.

[70] Gosset, P; Lassalle, P; Vanhée, D; Wallaert, B; Aerts, C; Voisin, C; Tonnel, A.B. (1991). Production of tumor necrosis factor-alpha and interleukin-6 by human alveolar macrophages exposed in vitro to coal mine dust. Am J Respir Cell Mol Biol. 5;431–6.

[71] Dwivedi, S; Saquib, Q; Al-Khedhairy, A.A; Ali, A.Y; Musarrat, J. (2012). Characterization of coal fly ash nanoparticles and induced oxidative DNA damage in human peripheral blood mononuclear cells. Sci Total Environ. 15;331–8.

[72] Diabaté, S; Mülhopt, S; Paur, H.R; Wottrich, R; Krug, H.F. (2002). In vitro effects of incinerator fly ash on pulmonary macrophages and epithelial cells. Int J Hyg Environ Health. 204;323–6.

[73] Diabaté, S; Bergfeldt, B; Plaumann, D; Ubel, C; Weiss, C. (2011). Anti-oxidative and inflammatory responses induced by fly ash particles and carbon black in lung epithelial cells. Anal Bioanal Chem. 401(10);3197–212.

[74] van Maanen, J.M; Borm, P.J; ,Knaapen A; van Herwijnen, M; Schilderman, P.A; Smith, K.R; Aust, A.E; Tomatis, M; Fubini, B. (1999). In vitro effects of coal fly ashes: hydroxyl radical generation, iron release, and DNA damage and toxicity in rat lung epithelial cells. Inhal Toxicol. 11;1123–41.

[75] Liou, G.Y; ,Storz P. (2010). Reactive oxygen species in cancer. Free Radic Res. 44(5);479–96.

[76] Haghdoost S, Czene S, Näslund I, Skog S, Harms-Ringdahl M. (2005). Extracellular 8-oxo-dG as a sensitive parameter for oxidative stress in vivo and in vitro. Free Radic Res. 39(2);153–62.

[77] Rohr, P; Kvitko, K; da Silva, F.R; Menezes, A.P; Porto, C; Sarmento, M; Decker, N; Reyes, J.M; Allgayer, Mda C; Furtado, T.C; Salvador, M; Branco, C; da Silva, J. (2013a). Genetic and oxidative damage of peripheral blood lymphocytes in workers with occupational exposure to coal. Mutat Res. 758(1–2); 23–8.

[78] Rohr, P; da Silva, J; da Silva, F.R; Sarmento, M; Porto, C; Debastiani, R; Dos Santos, C.E; Dias, J.F; Kvitko, K. (2013b). Evaluation of genetic damage in open-cast coal mine workers using the buccal micronucleus cytome assay. Environ Mol Mutagen. 54(1);65–71.

[79] León-Mejía, G; Espitia-Pérez, L; Hoyos-Giraldo, L.S; Da Silva, J; Hartmann, A; Henriques, J.A; Quintana, M. (2011). Assessment of DNA damage in coal open-cast mining workers using the cytokinesis-blocked micronucleus test and the comet assay. Sci Total Environ. 409(4);686–91.

[80] León-Mejía, G; Quintana, M; Debastiani, R; Dias, J; Espitia-Pérez, L; Hartmann, A; Henriques, J.A; Da Silva, J. (2014). Genetic damage in coal miners evaluated by buccal micronucleus cytome assay. Ecotoxicol Environ Saf. 107;133–9.

[81] Al-Sabti, K; Lloyd, D.C; Edwards, A; ,Stegnar P. (1992). A survey of lymphocyte chromosomal damage in Slovenian workers exposed to occupational clastogens. Mutat. Res. 280;215–23.

[82] Avila Júnior,S; Possamai, FP; Budni, P; Backes, P; Parisotto, EB; Rizelio, VM; Torres, MA; Colepicolo, P; Wilhelm Filho, D. (2009). Occupational airborne contamination in south Brazil: 1. Oxidative stress detected in the blood of coal miners. Ecotoxicology 18(8);1150-7.

[83] Donbak, L; Rencuzogullari, E; Yavuz, A; Topaktas, M. (2005). The genotoxic risk of underground coal miners from Turkey. Mutat Res. 588(2);82–7.

[84] Minina, V.I; Kulemin, I.E; Tolotchko, T.A; Meĭer, A.V; Savtchenko, I.A; Volobaev, V.P; Gafarov, N.I; ,Semenikhina M.V. (2015). Genotoxic effects of occupational environment in Kuzbass miners. Med. Tr. Prom. Ekol. 5; 4–8.

[85] Stierum, R; Hageman, G; Welle, I; Albering, H; Schreurs, J; Kleinjans, J. (1993). Evaluation of exposure reducing measures on parameters of genetic risk in a population occupationally exposed to coal fly ash. Mutat Res. 319;245–55.

[86] Wolf, G; Arndt, D; Kotschy-Lang, N; Obe, G. (2004). Chromosomal aberrations in uranium and coal miners. Int J Radiat Biol. 80(2);147–53.

[87] Ulker, O; Ustundag, A; Duydu, Y; Yucesoy, B; Karakaya, A. (2008). Cytogenetic monitoring of coal workers and patients with coal workers' pneumoconiosis in Turkey. Environ Mol Mutagen. 49;232–7.

4

Rehabilitation of Patients with Prostate Cancer

Meral Huri, Burcu Semin Akel and Sedef Şahin

Abstract

Cancer rehabilitation involves helping an individual with cancer to regain maximum psychological, physical, cognitive, social, and vocational functioning with the limits up to disease and its treatments in an interdisciplinary team concept. Prostate cancer is one of the most frequent male malignancies in the world. Prostate cancer treatment options have the risk of some side effects including loss of muscle strength, fatigue, pain, urinary incontinence, erectile dysfunction, cognitive problems, decrease in bone density, weight loss, gynecomastia, and hot flushes with stress-related psychosocial problems. Relative to other cancers, the prognosis of men with prostate cancer is much better and the potential treatment-related side effects have important implications which can affect the health-related quality of life (QOL) of this population. Recent studies support the efficiency of multimodal treatment to recognize, prevent, and increase functional recovery with an interdisciplinary rehabilitation team which includes physical and occupational therapists. This chapter describes briefly cancer rehabilitation and rehabilitation approaches at every stage of patients with prostate cancer for minimiz-ing the morbidity rate associated with prostate cancer treatment to increase occupa-tional participation and improve QOL.

Keywords: prostate cancer, rehabilitation, physiotherapy, occupational therapy

1. Introduction

Cancer rehabilitation involves helping an individual with cancer to regain maximum psychological, physical, cognitive, social, and vocational functioning with the limits up to disease and its treatments in an interdisciplinary team concept [1]. Prostate cancer is one of the most frequent male malignancies in the world [2]. The development of serum prostate-specific antigen (PSA) and advanced cancer treatment modalities increased 10-year survival rates from ~60% to >70%. Prostate cancer can occur as a local disease or an advanced metastatic disease. Surgical removal of the prostate gland, hormonal therapy, radiation therapy, cryoablation, and expectant monitoring are some of the treatment options for patients with prostate cancer [3].

These treatment options are associated with the risk of some side effects including fatigue, pain, urinary incontinence, erectile dysfunction, cognitive problems, decrease in bone density, weight loss, gynecomastia, and hot flushes with stress-related psychosocial problems [4]. Relative to other cancers, the prognosis of men with prostate cancer is much better, and the potential treatment-related side effects have important implications which can affect the health-related quality of life (QOL) of the patients; besides, these treatment-related side effects are significant in this population [5].

Increased rates of survival and support required for functional, physical, and psychological status led to a considerable interest in rehabilitation needs and the approaches used to increase the QOL of the patients with prostate cancer [5]. Recent studies support the efficiency of multimodal treatment to recognize, prevent, and increase functional recovery with an interdisciplinary rehabilitation team which includes physical and occupational therapists. These professionals provide inpatient care, outpatient follow-up and education, and services in home care, palliative, and hospice care settings [6].

Physical therapists play a vital role in the rehabilitation of patients with prostate cancer by teaching and implementing weight-bearing and gentle exercise, resistive exercises, and vibration exercises which transmit energy to the body with special techniques that strengthen the posture, balance, and body fitness, maintain or improve bone density, and prevent falls [6, 7]. In addition, pelvic floor training helps alleviate symptoms of urinary incontinence and maintain normal pelvic floor muscle functions [8]. Physical therapy also focuses on restoring the cardiovascular system which helps improve blood flow; this has been shown to improve symptoms associated with cancer-related fatigue and erectile dysfunction. Physical therapists assess the patients and develop individualized intervention programs including exercise programs to increase the endurance, muscle strength, mobility, and balance of patients with prostate cancer [6–8].

Occupational therapists play a vital role in increasing the occupational participation of the patients with prostate cancer [5]. Occupational therapists use training in activities of daily living, assistive technology approaches, education of energy conservation techniques, management of treatment-related problems such as pain, fatigue, and nausea. Moreover, occupational therapists give occupational balance training for regaining value of engagement in meaningful activities with a holistic view of creative and therapeutic use of activity [5, 9]. Occupational therapists focus on adaptations and offer education assistance for sexual activity for patients where certain sexual positions are limited or impossible due to pain, fatigue, or positioning issues. This complication in prostate cancer treatments is one of the most important limitations of activities of daily living that men face [9]. Occupational therapists offer ways to help patients with prostate cancer to confirm, express, accept, and use problem-solving techniques to present the changes due to prostate cancer and its treatment. Effective stress management must include relaxation and social support in a supportive environment. Such interventions decrease treatment-related symptoms, reduce the physiological accompaniments of stress, and improve mood. Patients who participate in such rehabilitation interventions are shown to have improved mental health by feeling more controlled and experiencing reduced interpersonal conflicts and distress related to cancer-related intrusive thinking [5]. In addition, cognitive therapy and changing life style with cognitive behavioral therapy are the mostly used occupational therapy interventions for patients with prostate cancer [5]. Futhermore, remaining in or returning to work is increasingly important for patients with and survivors of prostate cancer. Occupational therapists support men to remain in or return to work by providing fast-track care, counseling, and monitoring the men in work environment [10].

This chapter describes briefly cancer rehabilitation and rehabilitation approaches for prostate cancer patients at every stage of the disease for minimizing the morbidity rates associated with prostate cancer treatment to increase occupational participation and improve QOL. The chapter also focuses on physical and occupational therapy approaches for patients with prostate cancer with psychosocial and vocational rehabilitation after prostate cancer treatment.

2. Cancer rehabilitation

Conventionally, function is the most important indicator of activity and is strongly associated with physical performance and interrelated areas such as range of motion, muscular strength, and endurance [11]. The more contemporary function is a perspective that encompasses individual's physical conditions, emotional and psychological states, and the environmental and social circumstances of the individual [12]. The World Health Organization's International Classification of Functioning, Disability and Health (ICF) describes a framework that focuses this multidimensional or biopsychosocial approach for a deeper understanding of function [11, 12]. Within the ICF framework, function is defined as the interactions between an individual, their health conditions, and the social and personal situations in which they thrive [13]. The complex interactions between these variables determine function and disability. In the context of prostate cancer, morbidity associated with the disease and its treatments can lead to functional problems or impairments in physiological, psychological, or behavioral attributes (body functions and structures), potentially leading to limitations in the ability to execute desired tasks (activity) and participation in social demands (participation) [14]. A variety of approaches and a framework for cancer rehabilitation are based on the ICF to diagnosis and treatment of function for prostate cancer survivors [15].

The overall aim in rehabilitation of all cancer types is to overcome all symptoms causing functional difficulties and increase QOL [16]. De Lisa mentioned the importance of maintaining QOL at a high level; therefore, rehabilitation should not only focus on improving function and prognosis [17]. In general, cancer rehabilitation goals are classified as restorative, supportive, palliative, and preventive according to progression and the nature of cancer. *Restorative care* aims at maximal recovery of residual function of the patients. *Supportive* efforts seek to increase ability in daily life and mobility using effective methods such as decrease in functional difficulties and compensate for permanent deficits. In this stage, rehabilitation also aims to prevent disuse for secondary problems such as contractures and loss of muscle strength. *Palliative treatment* aims to reduce or eliminate symptoms such as pain and dyspnea. In the terminal stage of the patient, physical, psychological, and social high QOL as well as wishes of the patient are important, and positioning, heat modalities, low-frequency therapy, breathing– relaxation exercises, or assistive devices can be used. The primary goal of *preventive rehabilitation* is to prevent impairments. Rehabilitation in this stage must include preoperative education, maintenance of strength, and range of motion after treatment. This rehabilitation process starts right after diagnosis [18]. This framework can guide a therapist in all types of cancer.

Body functions and body structures
Somatic
Direct operation sequences (wound healing, lymphocele, urinary retention, urinary)
Radiation effects (cystitis, proctitis, lymphedema)
Treatment-related hormone deficiency symptoms
Urinary incontinence
Post-therapeutic pain syndromes
Sequelae cytostatic chemotherapy (polyneuropathy), myelosuppression
Sexual dysfunction (erectile dysfunction)
Psychosocial
Problems of coping
Depression
Relapse fears
Sleep disorders
Partnership problems
Fatigue syndrome
Post-traumatic stress disorder
Activities
Reduction in exercise capacity
Restriction in the field of transportation (incontinence, bone pain, edema)
Social withdrawal
Participation
Problems in integrating into the social environment
Problems with the reintegration
Limitation of mobility and participation in cultural life (incontinence)

Table 1. Impairment of functional health in prostate cancer.

General rehabilitation goals	Evaluation instruments
Physical performance	WHO Activity Index, Karnofsky Performance Score, Harvard Step Test, Ergometry, Muscle Strength Measurement (Vigorimeter, Digimax Muscle Testing), Quality of Life Questionnaires (EORTC-QLQ-C30), Functional Assessment of Cancer Therapy (G: General, F: Fatigue, P: Prostate-FACT)
Function-related treatment goals	Direct Assessment of Functional Abilities (DAFA) Direct Assessment of Functional Status (DAFS)
Reducing post-surgical problems (scars discomfort, seroma)	Clinical observation
Reducing symptoms after radiotherapy (cystitis, proctitis)	Micturition, Chair Diary
Reducing hormone deficiency symptoms (vasomotor reactions, osteoporosis)	Visual Analog Scale (VAS) *Osteodensitometry must be checked
Reducing symptoms after cytostatic chemotherapy (polyneuropathy)	Common Toxicity Criteria of the National Cancer Institute (NCI-CTC), Sensitivity Measurement, Vibration Sense
Reduction of fatigue	Multidimensional fatigue Inventory (MFI), Functional Assessment of Cancer Therapy, Fatigue (FACT-F), Visual Analog Scale (VAS), EORTC-QLQ-C30, Fatigue Module
Reducing pain	Visual Analog Scale (VAS), Pain Diary
Reduction of lymphedema	Clinical observation, Rating scale
Bladder in post therapeutic Urge symptoms	Voiding diary *Must be checked with the urologist
Improvement in urinary incontinence	Miktions protocol, PAD test, Biofeedback, *Residual urine and results of uroflowmetry must be checked with the urologist.
Dealing with sexual dysfunction, improvement of erectile dysfunction	Diary, International Index of Erectile Function (IIEF)
Improvement of functional disorders of the musculoskeletal system	Range of motion
Improving self-sufficiency	Detailed activity analysis, Functional Independence Measure (FIM), Barthel Index (BI), Instrumental Activities of Daily Living Scale (IADL), Role Checklist (RL)
Reduction of long-term care	Functional Independence Measure (FIM), Barthel Index (BI)
Learning proper movement, sporting and leisure activities	OQ (Occupational Questionnaire), Interest Checklist and Activity Checklist (ICAC)
Improvement of cognitive performance	d2-test (attention stress test), Benton test (visual memory-BT), Multiple Choice Vocabulary Intelligence Test (MWT-B),

General rehabilitation goals	Evaluation instruments
	Loewenstein Occupational Therapy Cognitive Assessment (LOTCA)
Promoting disease management, improving self-awareness and self-acceptance, emotional stabilization	EORTC, SF-36, Functional Assessment of Cancer Therapy (G: General, F: Fatigue, P: Prostate-FACT),
Coping with stress and anxiety depressive states and relaxation	"Stress thermometer", Hospital Anxiety and Depression Scale (HADS-D), Beck Depression Inventory (BDI), Beck Anxiety Inventory (BAI), Visual Analog Scale (VAS)
Reduction of Progression	Fear of Progression Questionnaire
Assistance in transition and when dealing with stroke-related disabilities (incontinence, erectile dysfunction)	QLQ-C30, prostate module
Breakdown of family and partnership problems	Interview, Couples Climate Scales
Reduction of insomnia	SF, Diary
Construction of meaning and objective perspectives	Interview
Treatment goals in the social sphere and Preparation of reintegration, possibly initiating professional promotions	CIO Community Integration Questionnaire, ISSI (Interview Schedule For Social Interaction)
Obtaining self-sufficiency, financial management and participation in social life and counseling and assistance for reintegration, placement of self-help groups	Reintegration to Normal Living Index, Instrumental Activities of Daily Living Scale (IADL)
Learning to continence training and transfer in activities of daily living	Miktions protocol, Diary, Barthel Index (BI), Instrumental Activities of Daily Living Scale (IADL)
Reduction of risk behavior (smoking alcohol abuse, overwork)	Life Habits Assessment (LIFE-H), Questionnaires
Positive influence of eating habits within the meaning of health promotion	Diet Protocol, Body Mass Index (BMI), Bioelectrical Impedance Analysis (BIA)
Vocational rehabilitation	Worker Role Interview, Valpar Component Work Samples (VCWS), COPM

Table 2. Rehabilitation goals and the evaluation instruments mostly used for patients with prostate cancer.

In patients with prostate cancer, fatigue, urinary incontinence, sexual dysfunction, impaired physical performance, psychological distress, weight gain, and changes in male body image are stated as the long-term sequelae of disease. Therefore, while considering general rehabilitation framework, special attention has to be given and specific methods must be used while making a treatment plan for patients with prostate cancer.

The evaluation for rehabilitation program of patients with prostate cancer for determining the individual rehabilitation needs can be identified after completion of the primary treatment of prostate cancer to verify the success of rehabilitation intervention [19]. During the follow-up treatment in patients who are taken directly from the acute care settings, the results of the current status of malignancy and PSA levels must be recorded in addition to the results of special rehabilitation evaluation tests, instruments, or interviews on the day of admission to check the rehabilitation capacity of patients with prostate cancer. Patients must be evaluated by functional and goal-oriented evaluation instruments in the somatic, psychosocial, and vocational rehabilitation and participation in daily living activities and public life with contextual factor areas; thus, the therapist can obtain a top-down view of these patients [20]. **Table 1** shows the impairment areas of functional health in prostate cancer which must be analyzed by rehabilitation therapists.

Evaluation tests for assessing body structure and functions, activity, and participation conducted at the beginning and end of rehabilitation to assess the level of achieving success in terms of the rehabilitation goals. **Table 2** shows the rehabilitation goals and the evaluation instruments which are mostly used by the therapists for patients with prostate cancer.

Cancer rehabilitation must include different therapies from different specialists to improve muscle strength and cardiopulmonary endurance, preserve energy for daily living activities, decrease stress, and especially decrease the effects of prostate cancer and its treatments. Physical therapy and occupational therapy specialists may be involved in the care of prostate cancer patients from the beginning of treatment to the end of a patient's life. They provide evidence-based interventions during inpatient care, outpatient follow-up, education, and services in home care and hospice care settings.

3. Physical therapy

Herein, it is important to remember that rehabilitation programs are driven for men with prostate cancer. Therefore, physical therapists should also be aware of the factors threatening men's health. These factors are stated as obesity, overweight, and bad habits (smoking and drug or alcohol abuse). Epidemics in many diseases are directly related to smoking, poor diet, excess alcohol consumption, and sedentary lifestyles [21]. For a man with prostate cancer and life-threatening habits, the rehabilitation program must also include preparation of a healthy life plan for him as well as his partner. Smoking and other substance abuse should be avoided and such patients can be referred to psychotherapy or cognitive behavioral therapy to redesign their lifestyle. A coordinated plan of rehabilitation team aiming at a healthy diet and lifestyle can lead to good recovery after cancer diagnosis. The main role of physical therapy is to inhibit sedentary behavior and maintain adequate exercise for patients with prostate cancer.

3.1. Muscle strength and loss of bone mineral density

Prostate cancer and its treatments can cause inactivity and disuse syndrome which must be avoided, while fitness and active lifestyles should be encouraged [16]. It is important to preserve and restore function through exercise as exercise has several, evident positive effects on patients with cancer. Graded exercise has been suggested as a treatment strategy for cancer-related fatigue that has the strongest evidence [22]. Aerobic exercise has been found to have effects on not only fatigue but also psychological well-being, QOL, physical performance, and weight control [16, 22, 23]. Improvements in the sense of personal worth, self-esteem, self-image, and confidence have also been stated as good results of exercise. Therefore, exercise improves the positive mood of people and decreases negative moods such as depression and anxiety [16, 22–24]. Some studies also stated the reduced risk of disease recurrence [22–24].

It is stated that aerobic exercise is helpful if it is given in low to moderate intensity (50–70 heart rate%), starting from 15 minutes to 30 minutes duration 3–5 times a week in a progressive way. The current exercise guidelines indicate that cancer survivors should achieve 150-min aerobic exercise per week and resistance (strength) training twice weekly [24, 25]. Most importantly, exercise needs to become a habit. Patients can be encouraged to start exercise with a short duration (15 min a day, several times a week) and then shape the pattern. Electronic monitoring bracelets can be helpful while following this pattern [21]. The patient can also control himself via this bracelet.

Berglund offered a physical training program for men with prostate cancer for an hour lasting for 7 weeks. This training started with light physical training, breathing exercises, and relaxation, and then included exercises of the pelvic floor [26]. The participants stated the benefit of this exercise program. The physical therapist should prepare a patient-specific aerobic exercise plan. Strengthening and endurance exercises should be performed in addition to aerobic training to improve participation in the activities of daily living [16]. Pelvic floor exercises must be added to physical therapy program for prostate cancer patients. These exercises will be mentioned during the management of urinary incontinence.

3.2. Incontinence

Urinary incontinence is common in patients with prostate cancer who underwent surgery or radiation therapy. Stress incontinence characterized with loss of urine with a cough, sneeze, or laugh is the most common type of urine leakage after prostate surgery, while the need to frequently urinate with episodes of leakage is the most common type seen after radiation therapy [27]. The treatments are as follows:

a. *Pelvic floor exercises*: Pelvic floor muscle training was found to be evident in speeding the recovery of continence [27, 28]. Recovery of normal urinary control after surgery normally takes 1 or 2 years. Pelvic-floor reeducation should be used for treating incontinence effectively [16]. First, it is important to train men to control their ability to hold in their urine. For this purpose, men are instructed on the identification and function of the pelvic floor muscles. Training men prior to prostate surgery can help men use their muscles more actively following surgery [27]. Kegel exercises are taught to men to strengthen the pelvic floor muscles. These exercises consist of repeated, high-intensity contractions of the muscles. Similar to providing training, introducing the exercises before surgery is also very beneficial. If possible, the patient is advised to start exercises before the medical treatment. Pelvic floor exercises can be combined with biofeedback programs. In a study, the authors showed positive results on incontinence after a single session of biofeedback-assisted behavioral training. The use of biofeedback may improve a man's ability to isolate the pelvic floor muscle and differentiate between muscle contraction and relaxation [29, 30].

b. *Supportive care, behavioral therapy*: This treatment includes behavior modification to prevent urine leakage. Men are advised to drink fewer fluids, avoid caffeine, alcohol, or spicy foods, and limit drink before bedtime. Patients must be encouraged to urinate regularly and not wait until the last moment possible. Conservative behavioral treatments by changing patients' behavior or environment or by teaching new skills can make improvements in symptoms [31].

c. *Neuromuscular electrical stimulation*: Stimulation can be used to retrain and strengthen weak urinary muscles and improve bladder control. A probe is inserted into the anus and a current is passed through the probe at a level below the pain threshold, causing a contraction. The patient is instructed to squeeze the muscles when the current is on. After the contraction, the current is switched off [28, 30].

3.3. Fatigue management

Most cancer patients experience fatigue and loss of energy. This severe and activity-limiting symptom is also common among patients with prostate cancer. Fatigue is mostly related with cancer treatment [16, 31]; however, it may also be present after or before treatment due to cancer [32, 33]. From our experience, in the presence of fatigue, patients, their relatives, and even some professionals suggest to rest and slow down activities. During the day time, many patients sleep a lot and cannot sleep well at night. Prolonged rest and inactivity induces muscular catabolism and the time of being fatigue increases [16]. Therefore, cancer patients suffering from primary fatigue should not be advised to increase the amount of daily rest. As we have mentioned earlier, exercise has a positive effect on fatigue. Therefore, patients should not be advised to rest more but carry out aerobic exercise [34]. It is supported that an 8-week cardiovascular exercise program in patients with localized prostate cancer undergoing radiotherapy improved the overall QOL and helped prevent fatigue [31].

Occupational therapists follow other strategies in terms of physical, psychological, cognitive, and social dimensions of fatigue. Graded activity and diversional should be planned in the manner of giving exercise [33]. Other interventions to reduce the degree of fatigue are stress management, nutritional management, and energy conservation techniques [16]. During energy conservation, patients should be taught to spread out activities through the use of timetables, organize activities to the energy level required, ensure breaks during activities, and use adaptive devices [33]. Providing good rest/sleep patterns, teaching structured sleep is also an important role of a therapist [16]. The patient should be recommended to maintain a schedule of sleeping and waking times, avoid sleeping constantly during day time, open curtains in the morning, and avoid doing things that can affect night sleep [33]. Therapists should remember that fatigue is an important symptom of cancer and help their patients to manage this symptom.

3.4. Lymphedema management

Lymphedema can be observed in patients with prostate cancer as a result of radiation damage or following the removal of lymph nodes during surgery. It is characterized with the collection of fluids in the lower extremities, and compression therapy helps the fluid to move and reduce swelling which can help the patient move easily and comfortably [34, 35].

Both occupational and physical therapists may decide the kind of compression therapy and the effective manual techniques for patients with prostate cancer. Elevation, exercise, and using custom-fitted compression wear can help increase the lymph flow in the early stages of lymphedema. Compression wears are worn continuously throughout the day and removed at night. They are reapplied as soon as the patient awakens in the early morning. Additionally; to drain the lymph from the extremity pneumatic pump compression which provides sequential, active compression can be used in the home [34, 35]. For severe edema, compression bandaging after manual lymphatic drainage using light massage (complete decongestive therapy) can be effective. Manual massage can help collateral lymph vessels to milk the lymphedema. To determine the effectiveness of the treatment, the size of the extremity always must be monitored by the therapist [36–38].

3.5. Peripheral neuropathy

Peripheral neuropathy is one of the side effects of chemotherapy. It is characterized with tingling, burning, or shooting pain sensation of hands and feet depending on nerve damage. Patients with prostate cancer may also experience loss of sensation which can cause problems on somatosensory perception, finger movements and grasping problems, balance problems, tripping, and/or decreased reflexes. Physical and occupational therapy can help the patients with prostate cancer to improve coordination, balance and gait, fine motor skills, and dexterity. The primary aim of treating peripheral neuropathy is to decrease the risk of falling and injuries [39].

3.6. Scar tissue management

Radiation therapy can cause scar tissue which may increase pain and decrease the flexibility of the skin. Physical therapists can use manual therapy and tissue techniques for stretching and tissue and nerve mobilization to decrease pain and increase the tissue mobility of the patients with prostate cancer [39].

3.7. Early ambulation

If patients underwent surgery, early postoperative ambulation and improving physical functions is the main goal of physical therapy [22]. During chemotherapy, physical strength tends to diminish; hence, rehabilitation aims to encourage ambulation consistent with the patient's condition even during chemotherapy and prevent disuse syndrome and maintain physical and muscle strength by performing early ambulation [24, 26].

4. Occupational therapy

Occupational therapy (OT) offers a client-centered approach to patients with prostate cancer. OT clinical reasoning assessments and interventions focus on functioning and participation by rehabilitating the abilities of the patients with prostate cancer. Therapists guide goal-directed activities that give meaning to the patient's life [40]. According to the ICF, the affected performance areas of prostate cancer on which OT focuses are shown in **Table 3**.

ICF			
Body structure/body function	**Impairment**	**Activity**	**Participation**
Prostate	Sensory	Basic ADL* Instrumental ADL*	Loss of sense of self as a sexual being
	Cognitive		Loss of ability to participate in activities (self-care, sport, and leisure)
	Psychological		Loss of occupational roles: work/ family
	Motor		Inability to be independently involved in daily occupations

*ADL = Activities of Daily Living.

Table 3. Affected performance areas and occupational therapy focus in patients with prostate cancer.

As shown in **Table 3**, OT mainly focuses on activity and participation limitations in the rehabilitation phase. Patients with prostate cancer generally require activity education, sensory training breathing and relaxation education, stress management education, sensory stimuli and praxis skills, cognitive therapy, erectile dysfunction and sexual rehabilitation, cognitive therapy, vocational rehabilitation, patient education and counseling, and also rehabilitation during palliative care and supportive care to engage in activities independently.

4.1. Daily living activities education

Reasons of limitation of activity are both dysmotility and muscle weakness. Activity limitation interventions are important for improving the activity performance of patients with cancer. The occupational therapist describes and measures activity performance necessitated to be carried out by patients with prostate cancer. After the activity for individual needs is identified, intervention strategies may be determined. The practitioner must determine the appropriate intervention approach for each patient. These strategies are divided into four parts: restoration, compensation, environmental modification, and education of patient [41].

4.1.1. Restoration

Patients have many different activities related to their roles. It is important to determine the most important activities for their life. The focus of the restorative approach is to develop patient skills and abilities or restore the activity performance of the patient with prostate cancer. A restorative approach is planned specifically to the situation of the patient. In this stage, grading of the activity level can be done. Grading can be done according to the following parameters:

- *Physical assistance*: If the patient with prostate cancer is in need of help, practitioner or caregiver can provide assistance. In this way, patients' skill to complete task may be increased. The presence of some symptoms such as fatigue or pain can cause the patient with prostate cancer to take physical support. This support does not mean that caregiver do all of the tasks instead of the patient.
- *Supervision and cuing*: This involves a number and types of cues. For example, if the patient forgets some tasks of activity due to cognitive impairment, patient can be supported by verbal, tactile, and written material cues to help the patient with cancer finalize the activity.
- *Activity demands*: The activity can be changed due to complexity of performance skills. Generally, for patients with prostate cancer, it will be better to select an activity with low-motor and high-cognitive demands by the reason of symptoms. In activity education, the motor and cognitive demands of the activity can be increased step by step.
- *Sequencing of activity*: Activity is divided in order of priority and sequence. The number of steps in tasks and the total number of steps can be purposed to increase. Thus, patient with prostate cancer can complete the activity easily without fatigue or pain.
- *Type of activity*: During activity education, activities can be graded from familiar to unfamiliar or from former to new. This method can help the patient with prostate cancer feel more comfortable during activity education.
- *Environment*: Activity environment can affect participation in the activities. For instance, patients with prostate cancer may have urinary incontinence. Therefore, patients may need to use toilet frequently. This situation can affect men in a negative way. To avoid negative symptoms such as stress or unhappiness, patients may limit themselves to only familiar environments to find a toilet. In intervention programs, the activity can be graded from a familiar to unfamiliar environment.

4.1.2. Compensation

The compensation approach focuses on using the patients' skills to achieve the highest possible stage of functioning in the activities. Therapists may teach the patients with prostate cancer new methods for modifying task performance to compensate for deficient areas of occupation, performance, and individual factors. If the patients still require help for participation in new activities, the occupational therapist should also give some advice regarding the use of adapted techniques or equipment. Patients with prostate cancer may need to use some assisted technology devices such as activity facilitator or computer-aided software to perform the activities. These instruments can help decrease symptoms (i.e., fatigue and pain) of cancer and increase participation in the activities of patients.

4.1.3. Environmental modification

Environmental modifications consist of compensation, modification, and adaptation strategy. The compensation approach directly influences patient functioning. However, environmental modification approach influences patients' functioning indirectly. Patients with prostate cancer will need help for home or work environment. Occupational therapists should give advice to redesign the home or work environment of the patient with prostate cancer where the patients can participate in activity easier than before. Modifications can include low-cost and easily accessible strategies to improve participation in domestic and community activities. Patients can also have problems in a social environment. They might not want to participate in social activities owing to general reluctance to do any activities. Besides, they may be exposed to stigma and pity from other people. For these reasons, occupational therapists must consider both physical and social aspects. Daily living activity education needs to be holistic and must integrate the activity, environment, and the patient with prostate cancer. Using occupation-based activity, education improves participation and supports wellness and QOL of patients with prostate cancer.

4.2. Sensory training

Treatment modalities such as surgery (e.g., radical prostatectomy), androgen deprivation therapy, radiation therapy, and chemotherapy affect the sensory–neural ways in body. After treatment, some deficiencies can occur in sensory skills. In particular, body composition may be affected if patients receive ADT. The generally observed side effects such as fatigue and pain might negatively affect patient body. Literature evidence demonstrates that sensory training is an important part of intervention program in patients with prostate cancer [42]. The purpose of sensory training is to develop body image by increasing body awareness. The body awareness includes these trainings and sensory stimuli, breathing, and relaxation techniques.

4.3. Breathing and relaxation education

Cancer and its treatment can be stressful for patients with prostate cancer and their partners and caregivers. Relaxation techniques and other body/mind practices can help calm the patient's mind, reduce stress, and sharpen the ability to focus to maintain inner peace. Some patients with prostate cancer use these techniques to help themselves relax while they wait for the results of treatments or tests. Breathing techniques include slow inhalation and exhalation to reduce tension in the shoulders, trunk, and abdomen. The process begins with focusing on normal breathing in a quiet and comfortable place when the patients feel stressful. Patients should perform deep inhalation and slow exhalation. During this phase, the abdominal muscles should be relaxed during inhalation; the abdominal muscles should be contracted during exhalation [41]. Relaxation techniques involve teaching the patient with prostate cancer to cope with stress which results in deficiency of body composition. During relaxation education, the patient with prostate cancer is instructed to contract and relax his major skeletal muscles systematically and then asked to repeat phases silently and finally asked to use purposeful images to achieve the goals [41]. OT practitioners have a core role in providing therapeutic activities that enable the patients with sensory problems to develop body imagination in occupational performance.

4.4. Stress management

Occupational therapists help patients with prostate cancer to acknowledge, express, accept, and use problem-solving techniques to address the changes that result from prostate cancer and its treatments. Effective stress management can include relaxation training, education, a supportive environment, social support, and participation in daily living activities. It is supported that these interventions can help decrease the treatment-related symptoms, the physiological accompaniments of stress, and improve mood of the patient with prostate cancer. Patients who participate in such rehabilitation programs are shown to control and experience reduced interpersonal conflicts and distress related to cancer-related intrusive thinking and have improved mental health [5].

4.5. Sensory stimuli

The patients involve in many activities which include various sensory stimuli. The basic activities involve tactile and proprioceptive inputs. Occupational therapists impart sensory training to patients with prostate cancer and also suggest somatosensoriel perception activities that involve tactile and proprioceptive inputs especially after chemotherapy or hormonal therapy. Patients use these senses during routines of activity in daily life. In addition, mirror activities and visual perception skills must be added to intervention programs to promote sensorial perception, harmony with the environment, and the body imagination of patients with prostate cancer [43–45].

4.6. Cognitive therapy

Cognitive therapy approach was generally used in patients with mental health problems. However, patients with prostate cancer may have some deficiencies in cognitive skills owing to cancer and its treatments [16]. OT intervention should focus on cognitive skills and activity function, and it includes orientation, memory, attention, motor planning, and executive functions of the patient with prostate cancer [44, 45].

Orientation is the ability to understand the self and the relationship between self and past–present environment time. After receiving the cancer treatments, patients might have orientation problems about place or time. In the intervention, verbal and external cues are used as reminders and therapy advances by changing numbers and types of cues [46]. *Memory* is described in terms of sensory memory, working or immediate memory, and long-term memory. If there are any problems on these types of memory, patients' tasks may be affected. Occupational therapists evaluate and improve memory abilities. They may also advice to use verbal, visual, and external cues for activity independently [46]. *Attention* is a multidimension that includes five components: sustained attention (concentration), selective attention, divided attention, alternating attention, and shifting of attention. Patients may have problems pertaining to not only each component of attention but also several components of attention [46]. The occupational therapist provides examples of basic and complex tasks for each component of attention. *Motor planning or praxis* is the ability of individuals to point at how to get their body to do what they want it to do. Motor planning involves the cognitive skills of intending to move, selecting a goal, planning the movement, and anticipating the end result. Impaired motor planning is disabling in cancer patients so that they may not be able to initiate or follow through on tasks [46]. The occupational therapist may give information about the functional properties of an activity. Besides, they might inform about conceptual errors related to creating the idea of the movement, involving object usage information, and sequencing of activity. When evaluating or treating patients with prostate cancer for motor planning abilities, it is important to identify the patients' activities. A series of cues (visual, verbal, or tactile) may be used if the patient experiences difficulty in performing an activity demand in the OT [46]. *Executive functions* consist of organization, problem-solving, and coping skills. It may significantly influence performance of activities of daily living. Occupational therapist using a dynamic interactional approach to the intervention of executive functions and organizational, problem- solving, and coping skills would focus on self-awareness and ability to perform new, unexpected or routine tasks [46]. In conclusion, cognitive impairments can be seen, caused either by cancer or its treatments in patients with prostate cancer. Hence, cognitive skills of prostate cancer patients should not be ignored.

4.7. Erectile dysfunction and sexual rehabilitation

Rehabilitation approach to erectile dysfunction is focused on pelvic floor muscle training and the muscle strength at the base of the penis. After the initial examination and determining an intervention plan, the physical therapist may guide the patient to perform specific pelvic floor muscle exercises and indirectly related muscles such as abdominal and gluteal muscles. These exercises help increase oxygen supply to the tissues. Vacuum therapy can also be used to generate negative pressure that increases the blood flow to the penis [47].

Sexual rehabilitation is one of the most important components of rehabilitation of patients with prostate cancer and significantly related to quality of life. Men with prostate cancer are more stressed about sexual dysfunction if they are younger. Both younger and older men are in need of physical, social, emotional, and psychological treatment assistance for this issue [28].

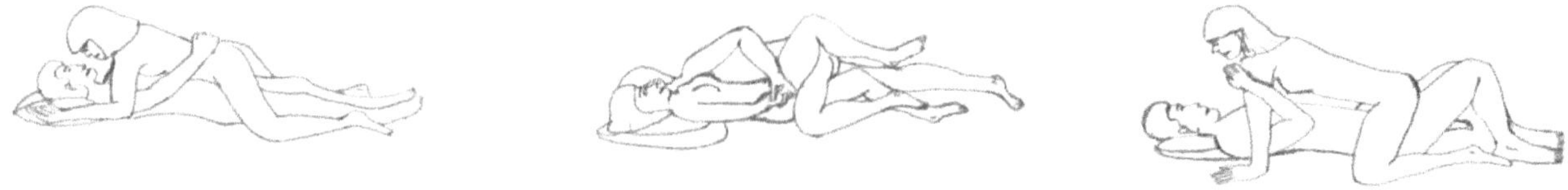

Figure 1. Safe and less fatigue sex positions for patients with prostate cancer.

Sexuality is an intimate issue and occupational therapy practitioners can examine both societal attitudes toward patients with prostate cancer and their own beliefs, values, and attitudes about sexuality. Patients can be emotionally vulnerable and recessive. The occupational therapists may provide information about the sexual rehabilitation. Rehabilitation should consists of an interdisciplinary team including nurses, physiotherapists, occupational therapists, social workers, sexologists, dieticians, massage therapists and psychologists. Die Perink et al. had conducted a rehabilitation program, with a 4-day course developed based on the experience with rehabilitation of more than 7000 cancer survivors, included physical activity, pelvic floor exercises, couples massage and relaxation, diet, and education of sexuality. They advise to practice sexual rehabilitation about sexual dysfunction [28]. Occupational therapists may give physically advice not only patients, but also partners regarding favorable sex positions (**Figure 1**). These positions can be more comfortable and safe for men. Thus, the occurrence of symptoms such as fatigue and pain will be reduced with occupational therapy intervention. Patients with prostate cancer will thus have normal sexual function. The patients and their partners should be informed about social support. It has many dimensions, including emotional, material assistance, and information. The occupational therapist should give lifestyle advice to patients for applying to their daily life. Thus, the patients and their partners will be improved.

4.8. Vocational Rehabilitation

Long survival with good quality of life make the patient with prostate cancer to think about returning to work after prostate cancer treatment and also 6 months after the radical prostatectomy surgery, men can return to their work. This may be a big positive step for men, and men might look forward to re-establishing his usual routine and it is understandable if they feel anxious or worried. But from a view of occupational therapy, having a return-to-work plan can help the patient to make the transition easier. Most of the mentally and physically healthy prostate cancer survivors do not require a job change, while others need some adjustments such as reduced working hours, modified duties, trying to do similar jobs, making self to do lists with time use with fatigue management, or the use of assistive technology. An occupational therapist can help the man determine if he is ready to go back to work, identify accommodations that will help him do his job, and help him get training or seek new employment if needed. In addition, improving self-management skills of prostate cancer survival helps him identify his needs and borders which can help him prepare for independent daily life and social reinteraction [48].

4.9. Patient education and counseling

Patient, partner, family, and caregiver education are an important part of occupational therapy because nearly all of the approaches (restoration, compensation, environmental modification, etc.) involve learning new strategies and combining these strategies into persons' lifestyles. Education contains information about prostate cancer; symptoms create and raise awareness about management skills. At the same time, an occupational therapist can use various materials such as demonstration, written format, pictures, and videotapes to help the patient and family participate in their activities. In addition to general education, it is supported that the main education resource of the patient with prostate cancer is internet but this way may not be helpful for psychosocial healing of the patient with prostate cancer or the survivor. Hence, in recent studies, new education programs were designed such as "Between men," which offers group online therapy sessions and education. The aims of these programs were to give the patients all the available information about prostate cancer, treatment, side effects, and how to deal with the side effects. Program planned once a week for 7 weeks and it included patients' experiences and reactions, patients' communication difficulties especially sexual and emotional effects, prostate cancer disease and treatments, incontinence, sexuality, importance, and problem solving. Online education programs must be improved and generalized for patients and survivors with prostate cancer [5, 49].

5. Rehabilitation in palliative care and hospice care

In palliative and hospice care, both physical and occupational therapists support men with prostate cancer by minimizing the secondary symptoms related to cancer and its treatments. The role of the occupational therapist and physical therapist in palliative and hospice care is quite similar and important.

At the end of life, physical therapy offers functional training, therapeutic exercise, and soft tissue mobilization. The goals of physical therapy are to improve overall strength, range of motion, and endurance of the patient with prostate cancer. Physical therapists may use heat, cold, and TENS (transcutaneous electrical nerve stimulation) for pain relief and design exercises that improve endurance and positioning regimens that help the patient maintain functional range of motion [50, 51].

In this stage, occupational therapists identify the roles and activities which are meaningful to the patient with prostate cancer and try to present the barriers that limit their performance. Occupational therapists support the patient both for physical and psychosocial/behavioral health requirements and pay close attention to what is most important for the patient. They look at the available activity and environmental resources to increase patient participation. The main goal of occupational therapy is to improve the quality of life according to patients' values and maximize residual functional abilities [50].

6. Conclusion

Patients with prostate cancer can face problems about body structure and functions, activity, and participation which may limit their participation to life. Patients with prostate cancer require skilled rehabilitation and supportive care from the initial process of diagnosis through clinical reasoning and treatment to posttreatment periods. Qualified interdisciplinary rehabilitation interventions may help men regain their performance and independency and maintain the highest quality of life.

Author details

Meral Huri*, Burcu Semin Akel and Sedef Şahin

*Address all correspondence to: meralhuri@yahoo.com

Hacettepe University, Faculty of Health Sciences, Department of Occupational Therapy, Ankara, Turkey

References

[1] Cheville AL. Cancer rehabilitation. Semin Oncol. 2005; 32 (2): 219–224. DOI:10.1053/j.seminoncol.2004.11.009

[2] Jemal A, Bray F, Center MM, Ferlay J, Ward E, Forman D. Global cancer statistics. CA Cancer J Clin. 2011; 61: 69–90. DOI: 10.3322/caac.20107.

[3] Bray F, Lortet-Tieulent J, Ferlay J, Forman D, Auvinen A. Prostate cancer incidence and mortality trends in 37 European countries: an overview. Eur J Cancer. 2010; 46 (17): 3040–3052. DOI:10.1016/j.ejca.2010.09.013

[4] Heidenreich A, Bastian PJ, Bellmunt J, Bolla M, Joniau S, Kwast TV. EAU guidelines on prostate cancer. Part 1: screening, diagnosis, and treatment of clinically localised disease. Eur Urol. 2011; 59: 61–71. DOI: 10.1016/j.eururo.2013.09.046

[5] Huri M, Huri E, Kayihan H, Altuntas O. Effects of occupational therapy on quality of life of patients with metastatic prostate cancer: a randomized controlled study. Saudi Med J. 2015; 36 (38): 954–61. DOI: 10.15537/smj.2015.8.11461

[6] Keogh J W, Patel A, MacLeod RD, Masters J. Perceived barriers and facilitators to physical activity in men with prostate cancer: possible influence of androgen deprivation therapy. Eur J Cancer Care. 2014; 23 (2): 263–273. DOI: 10.1111/ecc.12141.

[7] Friedenreich C, Kopciuk K, Wang Q, McGregor S, Angyalfi S, Courneya K. Pre-and post-diagnosis physical activity and survival after prostate cancer. J Sci Med Sport. 2012; 15: 334–335.

[8] Baumann FT, Zopf EM, Bloch W. Clinical exercise interventions in prostate cancer patients—A systematic review of randomized controlled trials. Supp Care Cancer. 2012; 20 (2): 221–233. DOI 10.1007/s00520-011-1271-0

[9] Silver JK, Gilchrist LS. Cancer rehabilitation with a focus on evidence-based outpatient physical and occupational therapy interventions. Am J Phys Med Rehabil. 2011; 90 (5): 5–15.

[10] Knoll N, Wiedemann AU, Schultze M, Schrader M, Heckhausen J. Prostate cancer patients gradually advance goals for rehabilitation after radical prostatectomy:

applying a lines-of-defense model to rehabilitation. Psychol Aging. 2014; 29 (4): 787. DOI: 10.1037/a0038311.

[11] Chasen M, Jacobsen PB. Rehabilitation in cancer. In: Olver IN, editor. The MASCC Textbook of Cancer Supportive Care and Survivorship. New York: Springer; 2011. P. 389–396.

[12] Dalton SO, Johansen C. New paradigms in planning cancer rehabilitation and survivorship. Acta Oncol. 2013; 52 (2): 191–194. DOI:10.3109/0284186X.2012.748216

[13] Egan MY, McEwen S, Sikora L, Chasen M, Fitch M, Eldred S. Rehabilitation following cancer treatment. Disabil Rehabil. 2013; 35(26): 2245–2258. DOI: 10.3109/09638288.2013.774441

[14] Weis J, Giesler JM. Rehabilitation for cancer patients. In: Goerling U, editor. Psycho-Oncology. Berlin Heidelberg: Springer; 2014; 87–101.

[15] Holm LV, Hansen DG, Kragstrup J, Johansen C, dePont Christensen R, Vedsted P. Influence of comorbidity on cancer patients' rehabilitation needs, participation in rehabilitation activities and unmet needs: a population-based cohort study. Supp Care Cancer. 2014; 22(8): 2095–2105.

[16] Fialka-Moser V, Crevenna R, Korpan M, Quittan M. Cancer rehabilitation particularly with aspects on physical impairments. J Rehabil Med. 2003; 35: 153–162. DOI 10.1080/16501970310000511

[17] DeLisa JA. A history of cancer rehabilitation. Cancer. 2001; 92(4): 970–974. DOI: 10.1002/1097-0142

[18] Dietz JJ. Adaptive rehabilitation in cancer. Postgrad Med. 1980; 68: 145–153.

[19] Ture M, Barth J, Angst F, Aeschlimann A, Schnyder U, Zerkiebel N. Use of inpatient rehabilitation for cancer patients in Switzerland: who undergoes cancer rehabilitation? Swiss Med Wkly. 2014; 145: 14214. DOI:10.4414/smw.2015.14214

[20] Lehmann C, Beierlein V, Hagen-Aukamp C, Kerschgens C, Rhee M, Frühauf S. Psychosocial predictors of utilization of medical rehabilitation services among prostate cancer patients. Die Rehabil. 2012; 51 (3): 160–170. DOI: 10.4414/smw.2015.14214

[21] Pelman RS, Elterman DS. Lifestyle and disease, male health and risks. Rev Med Clin Condes. 2014; 25(1): 25–29. DOI:10.1016/S0716-8640(14)70006-9

[22] Shin KY, Guo Y, Konzen B, Fu J, Yadav R, Bruera E. Inpatient cancer rehabilitation: the experience of a national comprehensive cancer center. Am J Phys Med Rehabil. 2011; 90 (5): 63–S68. DOI: 10.1097/PHM.0b013e31820be1a4

[23] Bourke L, Homer KE, Thaha MA, Steed L, Rosario DJ, Robb KA. Interventions to improve exercise behaviour in sedentary people living with and beyond cancer: a systematic review. Br J Cancer. 2014; 110: 831–841. DOI: 10.1038/bjc.2013

[24] Bourke L, Sohanpal R, Nanton V, Crank H, Rosario DJ, Saxton JM. A qualitative study evaluating experiences of a lifestyle intervention in men with prostate cancer undergoing androgen suppression therapy. Trials. 2012; 13: 208. DOI: 10.1186/1745-6215-13-208

[25] Hunter EG, Baltisberger J. Functional outcomes by age for inpatient cancer rehabilitation: a retrospective chart review. J Appl Gerontol. 2013; 32(4): 443–456. DOI: 10.1177/0733464811432632

[26] Berglund G, Petersson LM, Eriksson KRN, Häggman M. "Between men": patient perceptions and priorities in a rehabilitation program for men with prostate cancer. Patient Educ Counsel. 2003; 49 (3):285–292. DOI:10.1016/S0738-3991(02)00186-6

[27] Newman DK, Guzzo T, Lee D, Jayadevappa R. An evidence-based strategy for the conservative management of the male patient with incontinence. Curr Opin Urol. 2014; 24: 553–559. DOI:10.1097/MOU.0000000000000115

[28] Dieperink KB, Mark K, Mikkelsen TB. Marital rehabilitation after prostate cancer – a matter of intimacy. Int J Urol Nurs. 2016; 10 (1): 21–29. DOI: 10.1111/ijun.12091

[29] Mina DS, Au D, Alibhai SMH, Jamnicky L, Faghani N, Hilton WJ. A pilot randomized trial of conventional versus advanced pelvic floor exercises to treat urinary incontinence after radical prostatectomy: a study protocol. BMC Urol. 2015; 15: 94. DOI 10.1186/s12894-015-0088-4

[30] Wang W, Huang QM, Liu FP, Mao Q. Effectiveness of preoperative pelvic floor muscle training for urinary incontinence after radical prostatectomy: a meta-analysis. BMC Urol. 2014; 14: 99. DOI: 10.1186/1471-2490-14-99

[31] Donna B, Greenberg MD, Jennifer L, Gray BA, Catherine M, Mannix RN. Treatment-related fatigue and serum interleukin-1 levels in patients during external beam irradiation for prostate cancer. J Pain Sympt Manage. 1993; 8 (4): 196–200. DOI: 10.1016/0885-3924(93)90127-H

[32] Monga U, Garber SL, Thornby J, Vallbona C, Kerrigan AJ, Monga TN. Exercise prevents fatigue and improves quality of life in prostate cancer patients undergoing radiotherapy. Arch Phys Med Rehabil. 2007; 88(11): 1416–22. DOI: 10.1016/j.apmr.2007.08.110

[33] Cooper J. Occupational therapy in oncology and palliative care. In: Lowrie D. Occupational Therapy and Cancer Related Fatigue. John Wiley Sons, 2006.

[34] Courneya KS, Keats MR, Turner AR. Physical exercise and quality of life in cancer patients following high dose chemotherapy and autologous bone marrow transplantation. Psychooncology. 2000; 9: 127–136. DOI:10.1002/(SICI)1099-1611

[35] Wollin DA, Makarov D. Extended pelvic lymph node dissection for prostate cancer: do more nodes mean better survival? Oncology. 2014; 8 (7): 601–601.

[36] Rasmusson E, Kjellén E, Blom R, Björk-Eriksson T, Nilsson P, Gunnlaugsson A. EP-1081: low rate of lymphedema after pelvic lymphadenectomy followed by pelvic

irradiation of node positive prostate cancer. Radiother Oncol. 2013; 106 (2): 410. DOI: 10.1016/S0167-8140(15)33387-9

[37] Shaitelman SF, Cromwell KD, Rasmussen JC, Stout NL, Armer JM, Lasinski BB. Recent progress in the treatment and prevention of cancer-related lymphedema. Cancer J Clin. 2015; 65 (1): 55–81. DOI: 10.3322/caac.21253

[38] Preston, NJ, Seers, K, Mortimer, PS. Physical therapies for reducing and controlling lymphoedema of the limbs. Cochrane Database Syst Rev, 2004; 4.

[39] Choi, M, Craft, B, Geraci, SA. Surveillance and monitoring of adult cancer survivors. Am J Med. 2011; 124 (7): 598-601.

[40] Burhardt A. Oncology. In: Pendleton HM, Schultz-Krohn W, editors. Pedretti's Occupational Therapy Practice Skills for Physical Dysfunction. 6th ed. USA: Elsevier; 2006; 1157–1168.

[41] Pergolotti M, Deal AM, Williams GR, Bryant AL, Reeve BB, Muss HB. A randomized controlled trial of outpatient CAncer REhabilitation for older adults: the CARE Program. Contemporary Clinical Trials. 2015; 44: 89–94. DOI:10.1016/j.cct.2015.07.021

[42] Keogh JWL, MacLeod RD. Body composition, physical fitness, functional performance, quality of life, and fatigue benefits of exercise for prostate cancer patients: a systematic review. J Pain Sympt Manage. 2012; 43 (1): 96–110. DOI: 10.1016/j.jpainsymman.2011.03.006

[43] Rhodes VA, McDaniel RW, Hanson B, Markway E, Johnson M. Sensory perception of patients on selected antineoplastic chemotherapy protocols. Cancer Nurs. 1994; 17 (1): 45–51.

[44] Dolhi C, Leibold ML, Schreiber J. Interventions to improve personal skills and abilities, sensorimotor techniques. In: Crepeau EB, Cohn ES, Schell BAB, editors. Willard and Spackman's Occupational Therapy. 1st ed. Baltimore: Lippincott Williams and Wilkins; 2003. 595–606.

[45] Waylett-Rendall J. Interventions to improve personal skills and abilities, sensory reeducation. In: Crepeau EB, Cohn ES, Schell BAB, editors. Willard and Spackman's Occupational Therapy. 1st ed. Baltimore: Lippincott Williams & Wilkins; 2003.579–580.

[46] Giles GM. Learning perspectives, cognitive therapy. In: Crepeau EB, Cohn ES, Schell BAB, editors. Willard & Spackman's Occupational Therapy. 1st ed. Baltimore: Lippincott Williams and Wilkins; 2003.259–260.

[47] Bernardo-Filho M, Barbosa ML, da Cunha Sá-Caputo D, de Oliveira Guedes E, Pacheco Carvalho de Lima R. The relevance of the procedures related to physiotherapy in interventions in patients with prostate cancer: short review with practice approach. Int J Biomed Sci. 2014; 10 (2): 73–84.

[48] Tamminga SJ, De Boer AGEM, Verbeek JHAM, Frings-Dresen MHW. Return-to-work interventions integrated into cancer care: a systematic review. Occup Environ Med. 2010; 67 (9): 639–648. DOI:10.1136/oem.2009.050070

[49] Klemm P, Bunnell D, Cullen M, Soneji R, Gibbons P, Holecek A. Online cancer support groups: a review of the research literature. Comp Inform Nurs. 2003; 21 (3): 136–142. DOI: 10.1097/00024665-200305000-00010

[50] Prochnau C, Liu L, Boman, J. (2003). Personal–professional connections in palliative care occupational therapy. Am J Occup Ther. 2003; 57 (2): 196–204.

[51] Kealey P, McIntyre, I. An evaluation of the domiciliary occupational therapy service in palliative cancer care in a community trust: a patient and carers perspective. Eur J Cancer Care. 2005; 14(3): 232–243.

5

How does Botulinum Toxin Injection and Physiotherapy Complement Each Other in Cerebral Palsy?

Ayşe Numanoğlu Akbaş

Abstract

Cerebral Palsy (CP) is a clinical condition that describes impairments of motor and sensory systems due to a lesion in immature brain. CP-related disorders effect movements, balance and posture of the child. Spasticity is most frequent motor disorder seen in CP and effects 70–80% of the children with CP. Spasticity can lead to abnormalities in all motor system levels involving muscles, joints, bones and tendons. If spasticity exists for long period of time, immobilization of muscles in short position and changes in the connective tissue around joints lead to shortening of the muscles and connective tissue. Various methods are used for spasticity management in children with CP. Botulinum neurotoxin (BoNT) injections, oral medications, selective dorsal rhizotomy and intrathecal baclofen applications are the foremost among them. BoNT injections are most prevalently used one among these applications. BoNT, which is a neurotoxin obtained from *Clostridium botulinum* bacteria, is frequently used in children with CP to decrease muscle tone for a certain period in the selected muscles, prevent contractures, postpone surgery and decrease frequency of surgeries. During this time frame that muscle tone decreased, it is very important to increase activity and participation levels of children. For achieving better motor outcomes and functional independence, BoNT injections should be combined with physiotherapy (PT) and occupational therapy (OT).

Keywords: botulinum toxin, cerebral palsy, physiotherapy, spasticity, occupational therapy

1. Introduction

BoNT/A injections are one of the most frequently used methods to reduce muscle tone in individuals with CP. Given with clinical precision, BoNT/A has reversible chemo-denervation effects, such that focal applications in selected muscles ensure selective muscle relaxation to intended muscles. BoNT/A was used in CP for the first time in 1993 by Koman et al. [1]. It has been used in gradually increasing rates since the day it was first used and in wider age ranges. The purpose of this section is to explain how BoNT injections and physiotherapy (PT) approaches complement each other. In this section, general information about CP, changes that occur in muscles due to spasticity, outcome measurements related with BoNT/A applications, combined usage of BoNT/A applications with PT and occupational therapy (OT) approaches, target muscles for injection, appropriate age range and side effects of injections will be discussed.

2. Cerebral palsy definition and classification

Cerebral palsy (CP) defines a group of permanent disorders of movement and posture development that causes activity limitation; these disorders are related with nonprogressive influence, lesion or anomalies that occur in developing brain. Disorders of communication and behavior, sensation, perceptional, cognitional problems and epilepsy generally accompany motor disorders of CP [2, 3]. These disorders affect body movements, balance and posture negatively [4–6].

Surveillance of Cerebral Palsy in Europe (SCPE) [2] classifies CP as spastic, dyskinetic and ataxic type based on the predominant neurologic findings. Majority (70–80%) of children with CP have spastic clinic characteristics. Increased muscle tone of the effected extremities, increased deep tendon reflexes, muscular weakness, tremor, abnormal posture and movement patterns, increased coactivation of antagonistic muscles, abnormal control of voluntary movement and associated movements and stereotypical movements are seen in spastic type [7–9].

Classification of children with CP according to anatomic pattern and special neuromotor effect is crucial for the treatment of motor disorders [10]. The most important major classification in children with CP is the classification made according to the anatomic pattern of effect. Hemiparesis, where only half of the body is affected; diparesis, where lower extremities are affected basically and upper extremities are affected slightly; and quadriparesis, where all extremities are affected, are the most widespread definitions [10]. In recent years, the idea suggested by SCPE for the spastic type has started to be accepted for CP classification; as "unilateral spastic CP" where a single side of the body is affected or "bilateral spastic CP" where both sides are affected [2].

3. Spasticity

Spasticity, widely seen in CP, is the increase of physiologic muscle tone. Spasticity can occur in different forms depending on the formation time, location, size and diffuseness of the lesion in the developing central nervous system [11].

Fibrous contractures inside muscle or connective tissue around joints originating from spastic extremity posture, which are forming over time, compromise the increased response of the muscle against passive stretch and are one of the reasons of increased muscle tone. Muscle contractures and spasticity generally complicate patient care and reduce extremity functions and motor capacity [11–13].

CP is caused by nonprogressive lesion in the brain but accompanying spasticity, reduced muscle strength, muscle length changes, abnormalities in joint movements, functional capacity deficiencies and many situations like this are not static and can change over time with growth. Musculoskeletal system pathologies may start to cause greater problems as child grows. For normal muscle growth, elongation of the muscle under physiological overload is necessary. A hypertonic muscle, unable to relax, will eventually fail to grow and develop with the normal elongation of the bone in a child. Increase in height and weight of the child can contribute to musculoskeletal system problems. Spasticity can cause contractures and torsional deformities due to the growth in bones and muscles not being in proportion. Moreover, instability and early osteoarthritic changes can be observed in joints. As the individuals with CP grow, abnormal biomechanical situations affecting joints and static postures can cause pain formation. As the child grows old, chronic pain, social isolation, functional limitations and dependency can affect mental status negatively [7, 14].

4. Tone inhibition in children with CP

BoNT/A injections relax muscles by blocking acetylcholine release, with pharmacologic effect occurring in 48–72 h, but which wanes 3–4 months later [7]. However, this period when tone decreases gives an opportunity for therapeutic approaches [7, 15]. BoNT/A injections in children with CP are generally combined with PT and OT, while trying to achieve better rehabilitation outcomes. This complementary application has been accepted generally because it can be applied to the spastic muscles directly and the amount of the toxin can be adjusted per muscle, and it has rapid effect and has only a few side effects [16, 17]. But tone reduction alone is not enough for gaining functional outcomes. Applications such as stretching and strengthening the muscles, weight bearing on extremities and practicing daily life activities are essential. Children need to continue an intensive physiotherapy program before and after the BoNT/A application for achieving functional improvements [18].

Many studies investigate to maximize this effect of BoNT/A injections. In this perspective, combined usage of PT and BoNT/A has been discussed. This temporary effect of BoNT/A can be increased by activity-based physiotherapy and rehabilitation programs [15]. The decrease of tone by selective chemodenervation of overactive muscles presents an opportunity to extend muscle length, prevent contracture formation, strengthen antagonistic muscles, introduce new movement strategies to children and improve motor and functional skills [19, 20].

It was reported that PT and OT approaches that are used in children with CP in combination with BoNT/A injections are conventional PT, conventional OT, constrained induced movement therapy (CIMT), hand-arm bimanual intensive training (HABIT), casting, active/passive stretching exercises, strengthening exercises, neurodevelopmental approach (Bobath), robotic rehabilitation and mobility and walking training [15, 21–25].

Although the benefits of BoNT/A injections with PT and OT combinations are mentioned in many studies, optimal intensity and dosage of the therapies to be applied is not known [16]. According to expert opinion and consensus reports, PT following BoNT/A injections must consist of functional motor training, serial casting, stretching and strengthening exercises [26–28]. According to the literature, PT and OT programs can be followed-up as individualized therapy, group therapy, distance learning or a home program by family education [29–31].

5. Classification in CP

Classification systems have been developed to determine the severity of functional limitations in CP. The most important and widely used one of these systems is the Gross Motor Function Classification System (GMFCS) developed by Palisano et al. (1997). This system comprises five levels: level I expresses the best level of gross motor function and level V expresses the most influence in motor function. According to this system, the children in level I can walk independently, and the children in level V cannot sit independently without a support and cannot protect their head and body postures against gravity [32].

It is reported that BoNT/A application is used generally in ambulant hemiplegic and diplegic children with mild or moderate motor influence. The reason for an increase usage in this population depends on the acquisition of greater functional gains of these children [33]. In mildly affected children, tone of the spastic, active and nonfibrotic muscles can be decreased until 12–16 weeks [27, 34, 35]. In children with severe motor disorders, on the other hand, this gain is more limited. In children who are at GMFCS level 4–5, even very simple tasks used in daily life could generate problems and affect quality of life negatively [36, 37]. Although BoNT/A injections are used in these children to facilitate active movement, to ease their care and to decrease pain, there are not adequate evidences reporting the effect of these applications [33].

Researchers report that small children with CP at GMFCS level I–II show better development in gross motor function, on the other hand, older children in GMFCS level III–IV show less development in gross motor function or no development at all. The possibility of development of contractures in older children with worse gross motor function level diminishes benefiting possibility from BoNT/A injection. Especially in GMFCS level IV–V children, dysphagia, respiration problems, brain stem pathology and cranial nerve influence accompany more and therefore it is reported that BoNT/A dose for these children must be adjusted very carefully [27, 34].

6. Physiotherapy and occupational therapy approaches frequently used in CP

The purpose of therapy in CP is to improve functionality, support skill development and locomotion, sustain health in terms of social interaction and independency and to prevent possible deformities. Best results are achieved by early intense intervention. For an effective treatment program, team approach including physiotherapy, occupational therapy, behavioral therapy, pharmacological and surgical treatment, adaptive equipment and therapy and treatment of related health problems is necessary. The purpose of all treatment methods is to improve independency of the child [7, 10].

PT and OT applications start at birth and continue through life span to minimize sensory and motor disorders, to support normal motor development of the children, to improve activity and participation, to facilitate activities of daily life and to reduce load of family and caretakers. However, increased muscle tone, whose negative effects were mentioned in detail above, complicates physiotherapy and OT applications and is shown as one of the reasons of unresponsiveness to PT in children with CP [19]. Therefore, PT and OT approaches must be combined with applications helping tone control such as BoNT/A injections. Most frequently used physiotherapy approaches in children with CP are neurodevelopmental treatment (Bobath); based on normal sense-motor development of children, Vojta; using reflex stimulus points, Avres; suggesting that sensory-motor integration and organization is the basic of psychomotor development and conductive education (Peto), where intensive training programs are applied in the management by a leader and Goal Directed Therapy determining individual targets [18]. Numerous different therapy methods including electrotherapy applications, muscle strengthening and stretching exercises, orthotics, adaptive equipment and serial casting can also be used along with these approaches.

7. Evidences on physiotherapy approaches in combination with BoNT/A injections

BoNT/A injection in CP is considered as a selective tool to reduce spasticity. Appropriate selection of the patient, treatment dosage and muscles is crucial for effective injections [19]. In the scope of the International Classification and Functioning (ICF), BoNT/A injections affect body structures and functions; however, when it is combined with physiotherapy, it causes changes in the activity level as well [16]. The effectiveness of physiotherapy programs changes based on the application period and intensity [15]. Moreover, experience and knowledge level of physiotherapist, context of home program and conformity of the families to home program is crucial for the effectiveness of the treatment. There is no consensus on the type of exercises, or rehabilitation methods should be used to maximize the effects of tone reduction following BoNT/A applications. It is reported that orthotic management, serial casting and intensive physiotherapy are the most significant factors to benefit the most from the injection effect [19, 38].

It is reported that age of the patient, therapy applications and casting are crucial factors improving success following BoNT/A injections [39]. Inclusion of especially strengthening exercises and targeted motor training within the physiotherapy program is suggested [27].

The effects of PT + BoNT/A injections are reported as the reduction in spasticity, increase in dynamic and passive range of motion, improvement in selective motor control, improvement in strength, improvement in function and task performance and reduction in pain [27].

There are numerous studies in the literature investigating the usage of PT and BoNT/A applications together. In a study, the effectiveness of BoNT/A injections in long term with and without physiotherapy was determined. One of the groups received regular PT (two times a week) while other group received intensive PT. It was reported that gross motor function showed more improvement in the intensive PT group at the end of 1 year. Although tone increased after a period, gross motor function scores were preserved. It has been emphasized that BoNT/A injections decreased muscle tone in children with CP and when combined with PT the benefits of this application improved (Jianjun, Shurong et al. 2013).

In a study comparing the influence the two different PT methods, an intense physiotherapy program consisting of NDT (focusing on motor development and function) was applied to a group while conventional intense physiotherapy program (focusing on muscle length and strength) was applied in the other group. It was reported that the children benefited from both interventions; however, the success in NDT group was higher in terms of reaching the determined targets [19].

Chaturvedi et al. compared two groups of children with CP; one group received PT and other group received PT + BoNT/A injection. After 6 months of rehabilitation, they reported that gross motor function improved in both groups and also there was increase in the sensory and motor fiber diameter measured by diffusion tensor tractography; in other words, brain plasticity improved. They discussed that BoNT/A injections made as an addition to PT did not affect the result in 6 months [15].

Improvement of hip abduction angle, popliteal angle and passive dorsal flexion was reported in individuals who received intense physiotherapy including use of ankle foot orthosis (AFO) after BoNT/A application [40]. In a research conducted on 29 children with CP and spastic equinus deformity, it was reported that tone reduction and dorsal flexion improvement was good in cases which were applied BoNT + PT and serial casting and their effects were preserved in the long terms in comparison to the cases which were applied only BoNT + PT. However, in this study, PT program only includes stretching for ankle. Lack of an extensive physiotherapy program may have affected the results. In this study, the authors reported the pressure ulcers in three patients as negative effects of casting and failure to do exercise when casting was made was reported to be a disadvantage. They suggested to apply weight-bearing and isometric exercises during the casting period [41].

In a study measuring muscle activation patterns with surface electromyography (sEMG) after BoNT/A application combined with intensive PT, it was reported that this combination had positive effects on walking kinematics but had no effect on muscle activation patterns [42].

In 47 children with spastic CP who were applied PT (stretching of flexor muscles, strengthening extensor muscles, functional mobility training) for 12 weeks following multilevel BoNT/A injections for lower extremity muscles, it was reported that gross motor function measured by Gross Motor Function Measurement (GMFM) improved, and this improvement was preserved up to 1 year; however, there was no change in energy consumption [38].

PT applied in 71 children with CP consists of stretching of flexor muscles, balance training and walking training (five times a week in the first 3 weeks and three times a week during the following 8 weeks); along with multilevel BoNT/A injections at the lower extremities, it was reported that the muscle tone decreased in the follow-up in the first 3 months; however, this was not preserved in the follow-up in the 6 months and the improvement in gross motor function that was measured by GMFM was sustained in both 3 and 6 months [43].

According to a review conducted in 2009, it was reported that BoNT/A is an effective application for decreasing spasticity and functional improvements can be achieved with time limitation. However, the follow-up periods were up to 6–24 weeks in many studies and this made it difficult to determine long-term effects and the effects of the repeating injections [44]. In contradicting with the former review we mentioned, in a systematic review conducted in 2011, BoNT/A injections made separately or in combination with casting were not suggested; it has been discussed that there is not adequate evidence on the combinations of BoNT/A injections with PT and usual care [45].

In researches where BoNT/A injections are applied along with PT, failure to explain adequately the content and period of the applied physiotherapy approaches, which modalities were used and who performed the PT applications makes it difficult to select the most correct therapy approach to be combined with BoNT/A injections. Methodological differences can explain the different results obtained in these studies. However, as proven in the above given studies, it is observed that the integration of the two applications resulted with especially improvement in gross motor function in children with spastic CP.

8. Evidences on occupational therapy approaches in combination with BoNT/A injections

The greatest problem faced when working with children with unilateral spastic CP is the rehabilitation of paretic upper extremities. These children manage to stand up and walk more easily and spontaneously in general. Numerous different reasons such as spasticity, shortness and weakness of upper extremity muscles, limited joint movement, rotational deformities in the forearm and wrist bones, decreased unilateral skills, inadequate motor control and sensory problems affect functional development of the affected extremity in children with unilateral CP [46].

CIMT aiming to facilitate intense usage of the affected extremity and limiting the healthy extremity usage; HABIT facilitating combined usage of both extremities, and Goal Directed Therapy, determining individual targets have been reported during the recent years as evidence-based applications improving upper extremity activities following BoNT/A injections [47–49].

The purpose of the post injection therapy is to ensure motivation and new experiences and form an environment where the children can use their affected arm [50]. There are studies reporting that usage of the affected upper extremity in children with unilateral CP does not improve when BoNT /A injections are made separately without combining with the therapy [51].

In a study comparing the two groups who were applied modified CIMT and OT approach supporting bimanual activity following BoNT/A injections in children with unilateral CP, improvement was achieved in upper extremity performance, functional skills, occupational performance and goal attainment, and the groups were not superior to one another. Therefore, it is suggested that clinicians divert to specific goals and select the family friendly and comfortable application [52].

In a randomized controlled study, a group which was applied OT following BoNT/A injection and another group which was only applied OT was compared, and it was reported that more successful result in terms of bimanual performance was obtained in the group which was applied OT in combination with BoNT/A. The authors reported that there was improvement in terms of activated range of motion and goal performance in both the groups. However, they reported that in the ICF framework, the improvement in each domain was observed only in the group applied OT after BoNT/A injection [53].

According to a Cochrane systematic review published in 2010, it was emphasized that BoNT/A injection combined with OT in children with CP and having unilateral influence was more effective in reducing the disorder and improving activity level in comparison to only OT [51].

9. Appropriate muscle selection in CP

Existing pathologies of the children are considered for the selection of the muscles to be injected, and generally BoNT/A injection need to be made for more than one muscle at the same time in general to obtain change in walking and other functional activities [34, 54]. BoNT/A injections are applied most frequently for equinus and equinovarus deformities, knee and hip flexion spasticity, adductor spasticity and spasticity of the upper extremity (e.g. finger flexion, wrist flexion, ulnar deviation, elbow flexion and shoulder adduction injection). In ambulant children with CP, generally walking pathologies are considered for the selection of the muscles to be injected. In children those who have spastic equinus, injections are made mostly to gastrocnemius and soleus muscles; in those who have jump gait to gastrocnemius, soleus and hamstring muscles; in those who have scissoring and jump gait to gastrocnemius, soleus, hamstrings and adductor muscles; in those who have scissoring to hamstrings and adductor muscles; in those who have spastic knee flexion to hamstrings and in those who have only scissoring to adductor muscles [15, 22, 35, 55].

The reason for more frequent usage of BoNT/A injections in lower extremities is explained as containing fewer fine skills, improving movement and gaining better functionality to the children during their daily life activities [33]. Complexity of neural motor control during upper extremity functions limits the usage of BoNT/A injections in upper extremities [56].

10. Evaluation in CP

Various assessment methods are used in CP to evaluate combined effects of PT, OT and BoNT/A applications. Tone assessments are the major ones among these. There are various clinic scales, biomechanical evaluation tools and neurophysiologic evaluation methods to

ICF domain	Assessment tool
Body structures and function	Active and Passive ROM Ashworth/Modified Ashworth Scale Dynamic Sonoelastography Electromyography Goal Attainment Scale (GAS) Gross Motor Function Measurement (GMFM) Manuel Muscle Testing The Quality of Upper Extremity Skills Test (QUEST) Physician's Rating Scale (PRS) Selective Motor Control Assessment Tardieu/Modified Tardieu Scale Three-Dimensional Gait Analyses Visual Analogue Scale (VAS) WeeFIM_ (Functional Independence Measure)
Activity/participation	Gross Motor Function Measurement (GMFM) *Assisting Hand* Assessment (AHA) ABILHAND-Kids Questionnaire Bimanual Fine Motor Function (BFMF) Child Health Questionnaire (CHQ) Edinburgh Visual Gait Score (EVGS) Energy Expenditure Measures Goal Attainment Scale (GAS) Manual Ability Classification System (MACS) Observational Gait Scale Physician's Rating Scale (PRS) Six-Minute Walk Test The Quality of Upper Extremity Skills Test (QUEST) The *Canadian Occupational Performance Measure* (COPM) Three-Dimensional Gait Analyses Visual Analogue Scale (VAS) WeeFIM_ (Functional Independence Measure)
External/personal factors	*Goal Attainment Scaling* (GAS)

Table 1. Outcome measurements used in children with CP to assess effects of BoNT/A injections.

evaluate spasticity; however, there is no consensus about how spasticity can be evaluated the best. The most frequently used clinical scales are Ashworth/Modified Ashworth and Tardieu/Modified Tardieu scales [57, 58]. However, reliability of these scales is questioned. In a study, it was reported that for assessing medial hamstrings spasticity, MTS and MAS were less sensitive in comparison to the sEMG in the determination of changes following BoNT/A injection [59].

In addition, there are scales such as Spasticity Grading, Modified Composite Spasticity Index, Duncan Ely Test, New York University Tone Scale and the Hypertonia Assessment Tool (HAT) [60–62]. As biomechanical evaluation tools, myotonometer, sensors, Wartenberg Pendulum Test, dynamometer, goniometric measurement and robot supported evaluation tools are used [61, 63–67]. Electromyography, tonic stretch test and soleus muscle Hoffmann reflex (H-reflex) are neurophysiologic evaluation methods that could be used in spasticity evaluation [61, 68, 69].

In addition to spasticity, changes in muscle length, normal motor development and functions are also evaluated. According to the literature, the most frequently used measurement tools in this respect are Gross Motor Function Measure evaluating gross motor function, Three-Dimensional Gait Analyses, Six-Minute Walk Test and Physician's Rating Scale (PRS) evaluating walking parameters, electromyography evaluating muscle activations, dynamic sonoelastography evaluating intrinsic characteristics of muscles, *Assisting Hand* Assessment (AHA), The *Canadian Occupational Performance Measure* and The Quality of Upper Extremity Skills Test evaluating upper extremity functions, *Goal Attainment Scaling* evaluating the level of reaching the determined targets and The Pediatric Evaluation of Disability Inventory measuring functional independency. Also active and passive range of motion, selective motor control and manual muscle strength measurement are in use for this population. The distribution of the measurement tools that are used most frequently in publications based on ICF dimensions is shown in **Table 1** [17, 19, 24, 25, 34, 38, 49, 52, 53, 55, 70–75].

11. Changes occurring in the intrinsic structure of muscle with BoNT/A injection

It was reported that increased stretch reflex response of spasticity had both neural and nonneural components. Motor unit and reflex activity formed against muscle length growth is indicated as the neural foundation, and mental status, stress, fatigue, decreased sarcomere number and decreased flexibility, muscle stiffness and high collagen content in spastic muscle are indicated as the nonneural components [76, 77].

Positive effects targeted with BoNT/A injections on neural characteristics of muscles and therapy targeted on passive and active characteristics; therefore, combinations of these applications are suggested [33].

In a child with spastic diparetic CP, it was reported that muscle stiffness diminished, gross motor function improved and tone measured with MAS decreased after BoNT/A injection to gastrocnemius muscle combined with physiotherapy including electro stimulation, stretching and strengthening exercises applied twice a day for 4 weeks [70]. In another study conducted on children with spastic diparetic CP with the same design, it was reported that intrinsic stiffness of muscles decreased at the end of 4 weeks [77]. Some authors discussed that spastic muscle relaxation facilitates extremity growth and decreases fixed contracture development [57, 77, 78].

In animal experiments, it was shown that muscle and tendon growth and function was close to normal following BoNT/A injection; however, it caused reduction in bone mineral density [79]. It was reported that in some animals, BoNT/A injections made to nonspastic muscles prevented normal growth of muscle and caused progressive and persistent atrophy of muscle. In another study, it was reported that atrophy caused by BoNT/A injection was not reversed by exercise training [80, 81]. There are studies reporting that injections can cause decrease in muscle strength in children with CP; nevertheless, it was reported that there was 4–5% decrease in muscle volume by injections made to gastrocnemius muscle in 15 children with CP, and this was not as dramatic as in animal experiments [73, 82]. It was reported that

BoNT/A injections change muscle tone in the active, nonfibrotic and noncontractured sections of muscle and allowed stretching of muscle by decreasing tone, and this in turn was a stimulus for muscle growth. It was indicated that BoNT/A injection decreases agonist activity, supports antagonistic activity and must be combined with therapy to improve function, activity, participation and motor development in children with CP [34].

12. Age range

Spasticity develops in the first few years in children with CP. BoNT/A injections are suggested during 2–6 years of age while walking patterns and motor functions are prone to development [28]. According to a study conducted on 189 children with spastic CP in 2011, it was reported that the increase in dorsiflexion angle following BoNT/A injections made to triceps sure depended on the injected dosage and patient's age. It was reported that the obtained effect was as good as the children was younger [83]. There are limited reports about the usage of BoNT/A injections before 2 years of age. Usage in cases of 1 year 10 months of age was reported as the earliest [35]. BoNT/A was applied in children with CP younger than 2 years of age in very few studies, and in these studies, the effectiveness of the application was not analyzed separately for these children. Information is needed about the potential benefits or reliability in this age group [79].

13. Side effects

There are numerous studies scrutinizing the therapeutic benefits of BoNT/A injections in children with CP; however, there are limited publications about their safety. There were side effects observed depending on the application in 1–2% of children who were applied BoNT/A injections. Some authors consider neutralizing antibodies as responsible for side effects that develop after toxin injection. Formation of these substances increases BoNT/A amount that needs to be applied in the next injection. However, a single injection is not sufficient for many children and the injections need to be repeated in intervals of approximately 6 month intervals. In a research, it was reported that 58% of 4000 injections made during 15 years were first injections, 42% were second and the following [35].

In various researches, side effects of BoNT/A injections were reported as flu-like symptoms, nausea, diplopia, dysphagia, aspiration, respiratory tract infection, bronchitis, pharyngitis, pneumonia, asthma, generalized weakness, muscle weakness, urinary incontinence, falls, seizures, fever and unspecified pain [27, 84]. The start of systemic reactions can vary between the moment right after injection to a few weeks. There are studies reporting that urinary incontinence disappeared within 1–6 weeks. A relationship was found between BoNT/A dosage and hospitalization due to respiratory or urinary problems. It was reported that urinary and pulmonary problems that developed could be caused by systemic spread [35].

General anesthesia can increase side effects because anesthesia is a major risk factor for aspiration and infection. It could be difficult to distinguish whether the side effects occurred from BoNT/A or general anesthesia in the applications made under general anesthesia [35, 85].

It was reported that severity of the side effects related with the toxin was low; however, the number of side effects in children with CP were higher in comparison to other users. There are only a few studies reporting mortality following BoNT/A injections [86]. In literature, there are many studies about the positive effects of injection; however, there is inadequate information about optimal dosage, injection schemes and safety concerns [54].

Although injections generally have a good safety profile in short term, it is not suggested to use high doses in patients who have epilepsy or immune problems. It was reported that the children who were at level IV–V in GMFCS and had laryngeal and pharyngeal dysfunction were under more risk in terms of side effects [35, 85]. Further studies are needed to determine the relationship between especially mortality and epilepsy and BoNT/A injections [84].

The start of systemic reactions can vary between the moment right after injection to a few weeks. General anesthesia can increase side effects because anesthesia is the major risk factor for aspiration and infection. It could be difficult to distinguish whether the side effect stem from BoNT/A or general anesthesia in the applications made under general anesthesia [85].

In this section, it is understood that BoNT/A is a safe tool to decrease muscle tone in children with spastic CP and are effective in improving gross motor functions of children when combined with PT, OT, serial casting and orthesis. The injections have relatively few side effects, caring about patient selection and the dose to be applied should minimize side effects of the application. Further studies are needed to clarify what type of changes the injections cause in the architecture of spastic muscle in children with CP. Children with CP must be treated in a multidisciplinary setting where many specialists work together by combining many treatment approaches.

Author details

Ayse Numanoğlu Akbas

Address all correspondence to: aysenumanoglu@gmail.com

Department of Physical Therapy and Rehabilitation, Abant İzzet Baysal University, Bolu, Turkey

References

[1] Koman, L.A., et al., *Management of cerebral palsy with botulinum-A toxin: preliminary investigation.* Journal of Pediatric Orthopaedics, 1993. **13**(4): pp. 489–495.

[2] Cans, C., *Surveillance of cerebral palsy in Europe: a collaboration of cerebral palsy surveys and registers.* Developmental Medicine & Child Neurology, 2000. **42**(12): pp. 816–824.

[3] Rosenbaum, P., et al., *A report: the definition and classification of cerebral palsy April 2006.* Dev Med Child Neurol Suppl, 2007. **109**(suppl 109): pp. 8–14.

[4] Reddihough, D.S. and K.J. Collins, *The epidemiology and causes of cerebral palsy.* Australian Journal of physiotherapy, 2003. **49**(1): pp. 7–12.

[5] Bax, M.C., *Terminology and classification of cerebral palsy.* Developmental Medicine & Child Neurology, 1964. **6**(3): pp. 295–297.

[6] Ahlin, K., et al., *Cerebral palsy and perinatal infection in children born at term.* Obstetrics & Gynecology, 2013. **122**(1): pp. 41–49.

[7] Krigger, K.W., *Cerebral palsy: an overview.* Am Fam Physician, 2006. **73**(1): pp. 91–100.

[8] Europe, S.o.C.P.i. *CP and CP subtypes.* [cited 2015 29.06.2015]; Available from: http://www.scpenetwork.eu/en/my-scpe/rtm/cp-and-cp-subtypes/.

[9] Shumway-Cook, A. and M.H. Woollacott, *Motor control: theory and practical applications.* 1995: Lippincott Williams & Wilkins.

[10] Miller, F., *Physical therapy of cerebral palsy.* 2007.

[11] Elovic, E.P., L.K. Simone, and R. Zafonte, *Outcome assessment for spasticity management in the patient with traumatic brain injury: the state of the art.* The Journal of Head Trauma Rehabilitation, 2004. **19**(2): pp. 155–177.

[12] Sheean, G., *The pathophysiology of spasticity.* European Journal of Neurology, 2002. **9**(s1): pp. 3–9.

[13] Priori, A., F. Cogiamanian, and S. Mrakic-Sposta, *Pathophysiology of spasticity.* Neurological Sciences, 2006. **27**(4): pp. s307–s309.

[14] Quinby, J.M. and A. Abraham, *Musculoskeletal problems in cerebral palsy.* Current Paediatrics, 2005. **15**(1): pp. 9–14.

[15] Chaturvedi, S.K., et al., *Comparative assessment of therapeutic response to physiotherapy with or without botulinum toxin injection using diffusion tensor tractography and clinical scores in term diplegic cerebral palsy children.* Brain and Development, 2013. **35**(7): pp. 647–653.

[16] Thomas, R.E., et al., *GRIN: "GRoup versus INdividual physiotherapy following lower limb intra-muscular Botulinum Toxin-A injections for ambulant children with cerebral palsy: an assessor-masked randomised comparison trial": study protocol.* BMC Pediatrics, 2014. **14**(1): p. 1.

[17] Jianjun, L., et al., *Botulinum toxin-A with and without rehabilitation for the treatment of spastic cerebral palsy.* Journal of International Medical Research, 2013. **41**(3): pp. 636–641.

[18] Panteliadis, C.P., *Cerebral palsy.* 2004: Dustri-Verlag.

[19] Desloovere, K., et al., *The effect of different physiotherapy interventions in post-BTX-A treatment of children with cerebral palsy.* European Journal of Paediatric Neurology, 2012. **16**(1): pp. 20–28.

[20] Placzek, R., D. Siebold, and J.F. Funk, *Development of treatment concepts for the use of botulinum toxin a in children with cerebral palsy.* Toxins, 2010. **2**(9): pp. 2258–2271.

[21] Speth, L., et al., *Botulinum toxin A and upper limb functional skills in hemiparetic cerebral palsy: a randomized trial in children receiving intensive therapy.* Developmental Medicine & Child Neurology, 2005. **47**(7): pp. 468–473.

[22] Park, E.S., et al., *The effect of botulinum toxin type A injection into the gastrocnemius muscle on sit-to-stand transfer in children with spastic diplegic cerebral palsy.* Clinical Rehabilitation, 2006. **20**(8): pp. 668–674.

[23] Love, S., et al., *The effect of botulinum toxin type A on the functional ability of the child with spastic hemiplegia a randomized controlled trial.* European Journal of Neurology, 2001. **8**(s5): pp. 50–58.

[24] Russo, R.N., et al., *Upper-limb botulinum toxin A injection and occupational therapy in children with hemiplegic cerebral palsy identified from a population register: a single-blind, randomized, controlled trial.* Pediatrics, 2007. **119**(5): pp. e1149–e1158.

[25] Tedroff, K., et al., *Botulinumtoxin A treatment in toddlers with cerebral palsy.* Acta Paediatrica, 2010. **99**(8): pp. 1156–1162.

[26] O'Neil, M.E., M.A. Fragala, and H.M. Dumas, *Physical therapy intervention for children with cerebral palsy who receive botulinum toxin a injections.* Pediatric Physical Therapy, 2003. **15**(4): pp. 204–215.

[27] Love, S., et al., *Botulinum toxin assessment, intervention and after-care for lower limb spasticity in children with cerebral palsy: international consensus statement.* European Journal of Neurology, 2010. **17**(s2): pp. 9–37.

[28] Molenaers, G., et al., *The use of botulinum toxin A in children with cerebral palsy, with a focus on the lower limb.* Journal of Children's Orthopaedics, 2010. **4**(3): pp. 183–195.

[29] English, C.K., et al., *Circuit class therapy versus individual physiotherapy sessions during inpatient stroke rehabilitation: a controlled trial.* Archives of Physical Medicine and Rehabilitation, 2007. **88**(8): pp. 955–963.

[30] Galvin, J., et al., *Does intervention using virtual reality improve upper limb function in children with neurological impairment: a systematic review of the evidence.* Brain Injury, 2011. **25**(5): pp. 435–442.

[31] Novak, I., A. Cusick, and N. Lannin, *Occupational therapy home programs for cerebral palsy: double-blind, randomized, controlled trial.* Pediatrics, 2009. **124**(4): pp. e606–e614.

[32] Palisano, R., et al., *Development and reliability of a system to classify gross motor function in children with cerebral palsy.* Developmental Medicine & Child Neurology, 1997. **39**(4): pp. 214–223.

[33] García Salazar, L.F., et al., *Intrinsic properties and functional changes in spastic muscle after application of BTX-A in children with cerebral palsy: systematic review.* Developmental Neurorehabilitation, 2015. **18**(1): pp. 1–14.

[34] Heinen, F., et al., *The updated European Consensus 2009 on the use of Botulinum toxin for children with cerebral palsy.* European Journal of Paediatric Neurology, 2010. **14**(1): pp. 45–66.

[35] Naidu, K., et al., *Systemic adverse events following botulinum toxin A therapy in children with cerebral palsy.* Developmental Medicine & Child Neurology, 2010. **52**(2): pp. 139–144.

[36] Thorley, M., et al., *Evaluation of the effects of botulinum toxin A injections when used to improve ease of care and comfort in children with cerebral palsy whom are non-ambulant: a double blind randomized controlled trial.* BMC Pediatrics, 2012. **12**(1): p. 120.

[37] Tüzün, E.H., D.K. Guven, and L. Eker, *Pain prevalence and its impact on the quality of life in a sample of Turkish children with cerebral palsy.* Disability and Rehabilitation, 2010. **32**(9): pp. 723–728.

[38] Scholtes, V.A., et al., *The combined effect of lower-limb multilevel botulinum toxin type A and comprehensive rehabilitation on mobility in children with cerebral palsy: a randomized clinical trial.* Archives of Physical Medicine and Rehabilitation, 2006. **87**(12): pp. 1551–1558.

[39] Desloovere, K., et al., *Botulinum toxin type A treatment in children with cerebral palsy: evaluation of treatment success or failure by means of goal attainment scaling.* European Journal of Paediatric Neurology, 2012. **16**(3): pp. 229–236.

[40] Mikov, A., et al., *Use of botulinum toxin type A in children with spastic cerebral palsy.* HealthMED, 2011. **5**: pp. 922–928.

[41] Lee, S.J., et al., *The effect and complication of botulinum toxin type A injection with serial casting for the treatment of spastic equinus foot.* Annals of Rehabilitation Medicine, 2011. **35**(3): pp. 344–353.

[42] Van der Houwen, L., et al., *Botulinum toxin A injections do not improve surface EMG patterns during gait in children with cerebral palsy—A randomized controlled study.* Gait & Posture, 2011. **33**(2): pp. 147–151.

[43] Unlu, E., et al., *Multilevel botulinum toxin type a as a treatment for spasticity in children with cerebral palsy: a retrospective study.* Clinics, 2010. **65**(6): pp. 613–619.

[44] Lukban, M.B., R.L. Rosales, and D. Dressler, *Effectiveness of botulinum toxin A for upper and lower limb spasticity in children with cerebral palsy: a summary of evidence.* Journal of Neural Transmission, 2009. **116**(3): pp. 319–331.

[45] Ryll, U., et al., *Effects of leg muscle botulinum toxin A injections on walking in children with spasticity-related cerebral palsy: a systematic review.* Developmental Medicine & Child Neurology, 2011. **53**(3): pp. 210–216.

[46] Ferrari, A., et al., *A randomized trial of upper limb botulimun toxin versus placebo injection, combined with physiotherapy, in children with hemiplegia.* Research in Developmental Disabilities, 2014. **35**(10): pp. 2505–2513.

[47] Sakzewski, L., J. Ziviani, and R.N. Boyd, *Efficacy of upper limb therapies for unilateral cerebral palsy: a meta-analysis.* Pediatrics, 2013: p. peds. 2013–0675.

[48] Novak, I., et al., *A systematic review of interventions for children with cerebral palsy: state of the evidence.* Developmental Medicine & Child Neurology, 2013. **55**(10): pp. 885–910.

[49] Speth, L., et al., *Effects of botulinum toxin A and/or bimanual task-oriented therapy on upper extremity activities in unilateral Cerebral Palsy: a clinical trial.* BMC Neurology, 2015. **15**(1): p. 1.

[50] Hoare, B.J., et al., *Constraint-induced movement therapy in the treatment of the upper limb in children with hemiplegic cerebral palsy.* Cochrane Database of Systematic Reviews, 2007. **2**.

[51] Hoare, B., et al., *Botulinum toxin A as an adjunct to treatment in the management of the upper limb in children with spastic cerebral palsy (UPDATE)(Review).* Cochrane Database of Systematic Reviews, 2010. **1**: p. CD003469.

[52] Hoare, B., et al., *Intensive therapy following upper limb botulinum toxin A injection in young children with unilateral cerebral palsy: a randomized trial.* Developmental Medicine & Child Neurology, 2013. **55**(3): pp. 238–247.

[53] Lidman, G., et al., *Botulinum toxin A injections and occupational therapy in children with unilateral spastic cerebral palsy: a randomized controlled trial.* Developmental Medicine & Child Neurology, 2015. **57**(8): pp. 754–761.

[54] Friedman, B.-C. and R.D. Goldman, *Use of botulinum toxin A in management of children with cerebral palsy.* Canadian Family Physician, 2011. **57**(9): pp. 1006–1073.

[55] Alhusaini, A.A., et al., *No change in calf muscle passive stiffness after botulinum toxin injection in children with cerebral palsy.* Developmental Medicine & Child Neurology, 2011. **53**(6): pp. 553–558.

[56] Lodha, N., et al., *Force control and degree of motor impairments in chronic stroke.* Clinical Neurophysiology, 2010. **121**(11): pp. 1952–1961.

[57] Bohannon, R.W. and M.B. Smith, *Interrater reliability of a modified Ashworth scale of muscle spasticity.* Physical Therapy, 1987. **67**(2): pp. 206–207.

[58] Haugh, A., A. Pandyan, and G. Johnson, *A systematic review of the Tardieu Scale for the measurement of spasticity.* Disability and Rehabilitation, 2006. **28**(15): pp. 899–907.

[59] Bar-On, L., et al., *Is an instrumented spasticity assessment an improvement over clinical spasticity scales in assessing and predicting the response to integrated botulinum toxin type A treatment in children with cerebral palsy?* Archives of Physical Medicine and Rehabilitation, 2014. **95**(3): pp. 515–523.

[60] Scholtes, V.A., et al., *Clinical assessment of spasticity in children with cerebral palsy: a critical review of available instruments.* Developmental Medicine & Child Neurology, 2006. **48**(1): pp. 64–73.

[61] Flamand, V.H., H. Massé-Alarie, and C. Schneider, *Psychometric evidence of spasticity measurement tools in cerebral palsy children and adolescents: a systematic review.* Journal of Rehabilitation Medicine, 2013. **45**(1): pp. 14–23.

[62] Jethwa, A., et al., *Development of the Hypertonia Assessment Tool (HAT): a discriminative tool for hypertonia in children.* Developmental Medicine & Child Neurology, 2010. **52**(5): pp. e83–e87.

[63] Leonard, C.T., J.U. Stephens, and S.L. Stroppel, *Assessing the spastic condition of individuals with upper motoneuron involvement: validity of the myotonometer.* Archives of Physical Medicine and Rehabilitation, 2001. **82**(10): pp. 1416–1420.

[64] Syczewska, M., M.K. Lebiedowska, and A.D. Pandyan, *Quantifying repeatability of the Wartenberg pendulum test parameters in children with spasticity.* Journal of Neuroscience Methods, 2009. **178**(2): pp. 340–344.

[65] Boiteau, M., F. Malouin, and C.L. Richards, *Use of a hand-held dynamometer and a Kin-Com® dynamometer for evaluating spastic hypertonia in children: a reliability study.* Physical Therapy, 1995. **75**(9): pp. 796–802.

[66] van den Noort, J.C., V.A. Scholtes, and J. Harlaar, *Evaluation of clinical spasticity assessment in cerebral palsy using inertial sensors.* Gait & Posture, 2009. **30**(2): pp. 138–143.

[67] Schmartz, A.C., et al., *Measurement of muscle stiffness using robotic assisted gait orthosis in children with cerebral palsy: a proof of concept.* Disability and Rehabilitation: Assistive Technology, 2011. **6**(1): pp. 29–37.

[68] Kohan, A.H., et al., *Comparison of modified Ashworth scale and Hoffmann reflex in study of spasticity.* Acta Medica Iranica, 2010. **48**(3): pp. 154–157.

[69] Poon, D.M. and C.W. Hui-Chan, *Hyperactive stretch reflexes, co-contraction, and muscle weakness in children with cerebral palsy.* Developmental Medicine & Child Neurology, 2009. **51**(2): pp. 128–135.

[70] Kwon, D.R., G.Y. Park, and J.G. Kwon, *The change of intrinsic stiffness in gastrocnemius after intensive rehabilitation with botulinum toxin A injection in spastic diplegic cerebral palsy.* Annals of Rehabilitation Medicine, 2012. **36**(3): pp. 400–403.

[71] Ackman, J.D., et al., *Comparing botulinum toxin A with casting for treatment of dynamic equinus in children with cerebral palsy.* Developmental Medicine & Child Neurology, 2005. **47**(9): pp. 620–627.

[72] Ubhi, T., et al., *Randomised double blind placebo controlled trial of the effect of botulinum toxin on walking in cerebral palsy.* Archives of Disease in Childhood, 2000. **83**(6): pp. 481–487.

[73] Williams, S.A., et al., *Muscle volume alterations in spastic muscles immediately following botulinum toxin type-A treatment in children with cerebral palsy.* Developmental Medicine & Child Neurology, 2013. **55**(9): pp. 813–820.

[74] El-Etribi, M., et al., *The effect of botulinum toxin type-A injection on spasticity, range of motion and gait patterns in children with spastic diplegic cerebral palsy: an Egyptian study.* International Journal of Rehabilitation Research, 2004. **27**(4): pp. 275–281.

[75] Baird, M.W. and J. Vargus-Adams, *Outcome measures used in studies of botulinum toxin in childhood cerebral palsy: a systematic review.* Journal of Child Neurology, 2010. **25**(6): pp. 721–727.

[76] Sugden, D. and M. Wade, *Typical and atypical motor development.* Adapted Physical Activity Quarterly, 2013. **30**: pp. 387–388.

[77] Park, G.-Y. and D.R. Kwon, *Sonoelastographic evaluation of medial gastrocnemius muscles intrinsic stiffness after rehabilitation therapy with botulinum toxin a injection in spastic cerebral palsy.* Archives of Physical Medicine and Rehabilitation, 2012. **93**(11): pp. 2085–2089.

[78] Cosgrove, A. and H. Graham, *Botulinum toxin A prevents the development of contractures in the hereditary spastc mouse.* Developmental Medicine & Child Neurology, 1994. **36**(5): pp. 379–385.

[79] Bakheit, A.M., *The use of botulinum toxin for the treatment of muscle spasticity in the first 2 years of life.* International Journal of Rehabilitation Research, 2010. **33**(2): pp. 104–108.

[80] Velders, M., et al., *Effect of botulinum toxin A-induced paralysis and exercise training on mechanosensing and signalling gene expression in juvenile rat gastrocnemius muscle.* Experimental Physiology, 2008. **93**(12): pp. 1273–1283.

[81] Chen, C.-M., N.S. Stott, and H.K. Smith, *Effects of botulinum toxin A injection and exercise on the growth of juvenile rat gastrocnemius muscle.* Journal of Applied Physiology, 2002. **93**(4): pp. 1437–1447.

[82] Gough, M., C. Fairhurst, and A. Shortland, *Botulinum toxin and cerebral palsy: time for reflection?* Developmental Medicine & Child Neurology, 2005. **47**(10): pp. 709–712.

[83] Pascual-Pascual, S.I., I. Pascual-Castroviejo, and P.J.G. Ruiz, *Treating spastic equinus foot from cerebral palsy with botulinum toxin type A: what factors influence the results?: an analysis of 189 consecutive cases.* American Journal of Physical Medicine & Rehabilitation, 2011. **90**(7): pp. 554–563.

[84] Albavera-Hernández, C., J.M. Rodríguez, and A.J. Idrovo, *Safety of botulinum toxin type A among children with spasticity secondary to cerebral palsy: a systematic review of randomized clinical trials.* Clinical Rehabilitation, 2009.

[85] Howell, K., et al., *Botulinum neurotoxin A: an unusual systemic effect.* Journal of Paediatrics and Child Health, 2007. **43**(6): pp. 499–501.

[86] Graham, H.K., et al., *Does botulinum toxin A combined with bracing prevent hip displacement in children with cerebral palsy and "hips at risk"?* The Journal of Bone & Joint Surgery, 2008. **90**(1): pp. 23–33.

6

Occupational Therapy's Role in the Treatment of Children with Autism Spectrum Disorders

Bryan M. Gee, Amy Nwora and
Theodore W. Peterson

Abstract

Occupational therapists (OT) offer a wide range of therapies for individuals with ASD on the basis of specific deficits and difficulties. This chapter explores the role that OT plays, and the expertise, in relation to the interdisciplinary team. In addition, it discusses and presents empirical support for several therapeutic approaches commonly used by OTs working with individuals with ASD.

Keywords: occupational therapy, ASD, treatment

1. Learning objectives

After completing this chapter, readers will be able to:

1. Understand and explain the role of occupational therapy in the treatment of autism spectrum disorders.
2. Understand the application occupational therapy interventions to individuals with autism spectrum disorders.
3. Identify and describe a variety of popular therapeutic approaches utilized in occupational therapy for individuals with autism spectrum disorders.
4. Analyze popular therapeutic approaches for treating autism spectrum disorders using an evidence-based practice lens.

2. Occupational therapy

2.1. Introduction

Occupational therapists are part of the rehabilitation team for persons with injury, illness, and/or disability. The primary goal of OT is to promote functional independence.

2.2. Occupational therapy

Occupational therapy has been described as the art and science of helping people do the day-to-day activities that are important and meaningful to their health and well-being through engagement in valued occupations [1]. Occupational therapy draws on the centrality of occupations to daily life. It is concerned with helping clients engage in all the activities that occupy their time, enable them to construct identity through doing, and provide meaning throughout their lives [2]. As a part of the therapy provided, the client, group or population is expected to engage in meaningful occupation(s). Occupational engagement is the capacity to contribute to one's own health and well-being [3].

Ultimately, OT professionals (occupational therapists and occupational therapy assistants) help people of all ages participate in the things they want and need to do through the therapeutic use of everyday activities (occupations). Unlike other professions, occupational therapy helps people function in all of their environments (e.g., home, work, school, community, virtual) and addresses the physical, psychological, and cognitive aspects of their well-being through engagement in occupation(s) [1].

2.3. Occupation

In exploring occupational therapy (OT) and its role in the treatment of individuals with an ASD, time must be spent defining the term occupation. Historically, the term *occupation* was defined as the way in which people use or occupy their time [4]. Yerxa, one of the founders of occupational science, more recently defined occupation as the "specific chunks of activity within an ongoing stream of behavior which are named in the lexicon of the culture.... These daily pursuits are self-initiated, goal directed (purposeful) and socially sanctioned" ([5], p. 5). Other occupational therapy scholars have described occupation as everything people do to occupy themselves, including looking after themselves (self-care), enjoying life (leisure) and contributing to the social and economic fabric of their communities (productivity) [6].

Occupations occur throughout the lifespan, in context, and are influenced by the interplay among client factors (capacities characteristics and beliefs of the person), performance skills (goal directed actions), and performance patterns (habits, routines, and roles). Occupations occur over time; have purpose, meaning, and perceived utility to the individual; and can be observed by others (e.g. writing one's name) or known only to the person involved (e.g. morning grooming routine). Occupations can involve the execution of multiple activities for completion and result in various outcomes. The broad range of occupations are categorized by the American Occupational Therapy Association (AOTA) into activities of daily living

(ADLs), rest and sleep, education, work, play, leisure, and social participation [1]. To understand how these occupational categories are used in therapy, it is important to review the occupational therapy philosophy.

2.4. Occupational therapy philosophy

Hooper and Wood best articulated the philosophical underpinnings of OT, stating that "ever changing humans, interconnected with ever changing environments, occupy time with ever changing occupations, and thereby transform–and are transformed by–their actions, environment and states of health" ([7], p. 38). This philosophy supports the domain, process, and intervention of therapy practice.

2.4.1. Domain

The domain of occupational therapy practice is heavily influenced by AOTA's Occupational Therapy Practice Framework [1] and the World Health Organization's International Classification of Functioning [8]. The domain of occupational therapy includes the areas of occupation: activities of daily living, instrumental activities of daily living, rest and sleep, education, work, play, leisure, and social participation. The domain also encompasses aspects of functioning that impact occupational performance. According to AOTA, these aspects include performance skills (motor skills, process skills, and social interaction skills), performance patterns (habits, routines, rituals, and roles) and context/environment (cultural, personal, physical, social, temporal, and virtual) [1].

2.4.2. Process

The occupational therapy process involves the actions and reasoning of practitioners which are used to provide services that focus on the client's participation and performance in daily occupations. The occupational therapy process is designed to be holistic in nature capturing the client as the individual, his or her family, and other supports, while at the same time taking into consideration the individual's interaction with the physical, social and attitudinal contexts of function [1]. The process may be direct 1:1, group, and/or consultative in delivery, with the aim to create opportunities for optimal health, well-being, and lifelong engagement in occupations [1].

The evaluation aspect of the process includes gathering, interpreting and synthesizing information that is relevant to the client's past and current engagement and performance in meaningful occupations (ADLs, IADLs, play, etc.), in addition to his or her desired goals and priorities for the short and long term future [1]. Furthermore, the evaluating therapist assesses the barriers and supports that impact the client's health, well-being, and participation.

2.4.3. Intervention

The intervention process consists of skilled services provided by occupational therapy practitioners (OTs and occupational therapy assistants) in collaboration with clients to facilitate engagement in occupations related to health, well-being, and participation [1]. The intervention process includes a plan, implementation, and review [9]. The aim of the intervention is to improve the client's desired and expected participation and performance in occupations through the implementation of techniques and procedures that are directed towards the client or towards his or her environment and/or activities [1]. A unique aspect of the intervention process is the standard procedure of practitioners using the collective influence of the client's context and environment, demands of the activity at hand, and the individual characteristics of the client [1]. This procedure is formally characterized as a task analysis [9].

In order to practice occupational therapy, practitioners must first gain an understanding of the domain, process, and intervention utilized in OT while completing their higher education at a school that is accredited by the Accreditation Council for Occupational Therapy Education (ACOTE).

2.5. Education

The current degree required for entry-level occupational therapists is a master's degree. The Occupational Therapy Doctorate (OTD) is also available as an entry level-degree, but is not currently required by ACOTE. Obtaining graduate degree assures that practitioners have the knowledge and skills necessary to fully implement evaluation and intervention to remediate functional deficits.

In addition to occupational therapists, OT personnel are also comprised of occupational therapy assistants (OTAs). OTAs must minimally obtain an associate's degree from an ACOTE accredited institution. OTAs must work under the supervision of an occupational therapist and are generally tasked with implementing intervention and performing other tasks in support of the OT plan of care, which vary depending on the state in which the OTA practices.

After completing their formal education, both occupational therapists and OTAs are required to pass a national registration exam offered by the National Board for Certification in Occupational Therapy. OTs and OTAs who pass the registration exam are then eligible to apply for state licensure and to assume a practice role.

2.6. Occupational therapy roles

Occupational therapists can assume a variety of roles in clinical practice. These roles include, but are not limited to: clinician, manager, case coordinator, policy maker, educator, and advocate. Roles cross a variety of practice settings, such as acute care, subacute care, outpatient care, home care, early intervention, and school-based practice. In a survey study completed by the AOTA, approximately 24% of OT practitioners provide services in school and early intervention based settings while many additional therapists work in freestanding community-based clinics and hospital-based settings that include pediatric services [11, 12].

2.7. Occupational therapy and the treatment of autism spectrum disorders

In the evaluation and treatment of individuals with ASD, OT professionals tend to address ADLs, IADLs, adaptive behavior, rest and sleep, employment/pre-employment, and social participation. Underlying these issues, therapists seek to improve performance with gross motor, fine motor, and visual-motor integration skills; visual perception; sensory processing; and behavioral regulation [1]. Additionally, the evaluation and treatment process of individuals with ASD includes context (conditions within and surrounding the client) and the environment (external physical and social conditions), activity demands (tools, space, action and performance skills needed) and finally client factors (underlying beliefs, abilities and values) [1]. The OT professional takes into account the setting where the services will be provided and the environments where the individual functions and/or plans to function [1]. Caregivers play a significant role in occupational therapy treatment and are recognized as the 'client' while evaluating the child with ASD. Factors such as socio-demographic characteristics, roles, habits, rituals and the occupational balance of caregivers are to be taken into consideration [10, 11].

The specific intervention techniques used in OT with individuals with ASD include; establishing new functional skills, modifying activity demands, creating healthy lifestyles, maintaining existing performance, and preventing future difficulties for clients at risk [12]. One of the hallmark features of individuals with ASD is their tendency towards strong preferences and focused interest. While this tendency may be considered maladaptive for the generation of new skills, the OT may use it to influence the client's self-esteem and motivation to take part in areas of occupation as well as the intervention process through judicious choice of treatment activities that tap into an individual's preferences and interest [1].

3. Treatment approaches for autism spectrum disorders utilized by occupational therapists

With the increase in awareness and identification of children on the autism spectrum, teachers, researchers, clinicians, and families have worked diligently to create programming that can meet the varied and unique needs of this population. Often these approaches are developed for use across all aspects of a child's life, and as such, are intertwined in all services provided. While some approaches are utilized primarily in occupational and physical therapy (e.g. Ayres Sensory Integration), others are used across all disciplines (e.g. Applied Behavior Analysis). Whatever approach is selected, it is important to remember to communicate with the interprofessional team in order to determine best practices with each individual child and that the interventions provide purposeful activity [13, 14]. Occupational therapy professionals place significant value on the individual with autism's community participation and that it can be increased through their participation in meaningful and purposeful activities [15, 16]. The following sections review some of the more commonly used approaches in therapy.

3.1. Sensory processing treatment approaches

Difficulty processing sensory information has been identified as a common feature of ASD. The current best estimates demonstrate that up to 96% of children with ASD demonstrate difficulty with processing sensory information as a part of their daily routines [13, 15, 17]. Restricted, Repetitive Patterns of Behavior, Interest, of Activities" and that one of those 4 has something to do with "sensory features" [18]. The inability to accurately process sensory information impacts all areas of child development, so approaches directed towards remediation of sensory processing deficits are often used by both occupational therapists.

3.2. Ayres sensory integration intervention

3.2.1. Purpose of the technique

Ayers Sensory Integration Intervention® (ASII) is a clinical procedure grounded in sensory integration theory [19]. The intervention focuses on aiding clients to register, process, integrate and adequately respond to internal and external sensations that occur within the clients' daily life, contexts, and relationships. Sensory integration has been defined as "the neurological process that organizes sensations from one's own body and from the environment and makes it possible to use the body effectively in the environment" ([20], p. 11). ASII is aimed at remediating integration disruptions and increasing participation and performance among individuals who experience sensory disturbances or a sensory processing disorder. An internet survey identifying treatments used for children with ASD indicated that Sensory Integration (a broadly used term) was the third most commonly requested intervention requested by caregivers [21].

3.2.2. Overview of the technique

Intervention guided by sensory integration theory [19] has been reported to be commonly used by therapists who work with children with various types of developmental delays and medical and behavioral conditions [22, 23]. ASII includes the following steps within the standardized intervention protocol:

1. ensure physical safety of the client,
2. present active sensory opportunities (tactile, proprioceptive & vestibular),
3. help the client attain and maintain appropriate levels of alertness,
4. challenge postural, ocular, oral and/or bilateral motor control,
5. challenge praxis and organization of behavior,
6. collaborate between the client and the therapist on activity choice,
7. tailor the activities to present a just right challenge for the client,
8. ensure that activities are successful,
9. support the child's intrinsic motivation to play, and
10. establish therapeutic alliance between the client and the therapist [24, 25].

3.2.3. Review of the evidence

Pfeiffer, Koenig, and associates conducted a randomized-control trial with 37 children diagnosed with ASD who were between the ages of 5–12 years of age [26]. Seventeen participants were assigned to a control group focused on fine motor intervention and 20 participants were assigned to the experimental group who received ASII. The study reported no significant differences in the subjective perception of sensory processing difficulties via the Sensory Processing Measure and objective ratings on the Quick Neurological Screening Test, 2nd Edition, between the control and experimental groups. Yet the authors reported a significant difference between groups in the reduction of autistic mannerisms and social responsiveness as measured by the Social Responsiveness Scale. Both groups demonstrated statistically significant improvement with Goal Attainment Scaling (focused on sensory processing, motor skills, & social functioning). However, there was a higher effect size in the ASII group than in the fine motor group.

Another randomized-control trial evaluated the efficacy of ASII among 32 children aged 4–8 years old, diagnosed with ASD [27]. In this trial, the experimental group using ASII ($n = 17$) scored significantly higher at posttest in the areas of self-help skills and socialization, than did the control group ($n = 15$) who received standard care. Additionally, the authors reported that children in the ASII group were better able to reach specific goals than the control group when measured using Goal Attainment Scaling. Children in the ASII group also experienced greater decreases in sensory related behaviors than the control group.

Iwanaga et al. utilized a quasi-experimental design to explore the use of ASII on 20 preschool aged children with high functioning autism [28]. It was reported that the children in the experimental group, who received ASII, demonstrated significantly higher total post test scores on the Miller Assessment of Preschoolers when compared to the control group. Significant improvements were noted specifically in the areas of motor coordination, nonverbal cognitive abilities, and sensory motor abilities following ASII treatment.

Case-Smith et al. conducted a systematic review on sensory integration with standardized administration protocols that occurred in clinics that used sensory-rich, child directed activities to improve a child's adaptive responses to sensory experiences [15]. They found and reviewed two randomized controlled trials, which reported positive effects for ASII on the participants (children with ASD) using Goal Attainment Scaling (with reported effect sizes ranging from .72 to 1.62); the additional studies analyzed included Level III–IV research studies, that reported positive effects on reducing challenging behaviors linked to sensory processing difficulties.

Kashefimehr et al. reported improvement in a sensory integration intervention group ($n = 16$) over a control group ($n = 15$) among children with ASD. The authors reported that the participants in the intervention group demonstrated significant improvements in the subjective measures of the Short Child Occupational Profile and the Sensory Profile. Of significant note the authors reported improvements not only in sensory processing domains (tactile processing, vestibular processing, etc.) but also in occupational performance based upon the Model of Human Occupation [29, 30].

It is important to make a clear distinction between ASII and other sensory-based interventions, as ASII has strict implementation protocol that may not always be followed accurately. In a review of more than 70 published research articles examining the efficacy of ASII, it was found that only three adhered to the theory and intervention protocols [25, 29, 30]. The reason for this disparity is that research conducted (in occupational and speech therapy, special education and psychology) generally did not report if the researchers designed the intervention to represent Ayres' original therapeutic principles. Furthermore, it was not noted if the researchers monitored intervention delivery during the studies to ensure that a high degree of fidelity to the ASII was maintained [30–32]. This is an important notation when evaluating the efficacy of ASII, as the majority of the research claiming to be examining the effects of sensory integration treatment may really be evaluating sensory-based and sensory-motor-based interventions.

3.3. Sound-based interventions

3.3.1. Purpose of the technique

Sound-based interventions (SBIs) are a type of sensory-based intervention used by occupational therapists and some physical therapists with children diagnosed with ASD. SBIs originated from the work of Tomatis [33, 34], whose research on the ear and its connection to the nervous system led to his theory that one's "listening function" affects voice, language, motivation, coordination and learning abilities [35]. The theory that Tomatis postulated was that by listening to certain frequencies, the brain could retrain itself by creating new neural pathways, thereby compensating for dysfunctional brain structures or pathways. Tomatis's ideas led to the development of several SBIs, including the Tomatis Method®, Auditory Integration Training®, Therapeutic Listening®, Integrated Listening Systems® and The Listening Program®.

3.3.2. Overview of the technique

SBIs involve listening to psychoacoustically modified music, yet the manufacture of each SBI differs in the dosage, type of music used, how it is combined with other intervention techniques. In most cases therapists (occupational and some physical therapists) use SBIs as combined modality with other sensory-based treatment or to augment Ayres Sensory Integration Intervention.

3.3.3. Review of the evidence

Because the evidence supporting the use of SBIs with children with ASD is mixed, these techniques are non-reimbursable and should be considered experimental. To date, most research on SBIs has been focused on the Tomatis Method and Auditory Integration Training and has produced mixed empirical results [36, 37]. Some studies have suggested that these interventions may be effective for individuals with ASD, citing improvements in areas such as language, psychomotor skills, personal and social adjustment, non-verbal communication and adaptation to change [38, 39]. However, other research has found little to no significant improvement in individuals who received SBIs as compared to the control groups [40, 41]. Recent single case research indicated that some children with ASD using home-based SBIs demonstrated mild to moderate improvements in behavioral and sensory tolerance [42]. Other case studies observed a reduction in behaviors and scores related to auditory sensory over responsivity, as well as a reduced number and duration of self-stimulatory behaviors after using a SBI in conjunction with occupational therapy [43, 44].

3.4. Weighted blankets

3.4.1. Purpose of the technique

Sleep and rest disturbances are important self-care challenges that are commonly faced by many children with ASD, with 44–83% of individuals reporting some form of sleep disturbances [45]. Humphreys and associates found that children between the ages of 18 months and 11 years with ASD slept 17–43 min less each night than their typically developing matched peers, with decreased sleep patterns found to be most pronounced in children between the ages of 30 and 42 months [46]. Additionally, Malow and associates found that children with ASD who slept poorly showed an average decrease in rapid eye movement sleep, possibly providing a partial explanation for their finding that disordered sleep in children with ASD exacerbates behavioral problems during the day [47].

As sleep is important for overall wellbeing, occupational therapists may work with individuals to establish healthy sleep routines in their clients, commonly including children with ASD and their families. They often assist such children in obtaining adequate sleep by experimenting with different sleep routines, using cognitive and behavioral interventions, and/or implementing sensory-based interventions [48]. Weighted blankets are an example of a sensory-based intervention commonly used in helping children with autism spectrum disorders attain adequate sleep participation. The underlying theory behind their use is that weighted blankets provide deep pressure touch without movement restrictions. This deep pressure, in turn, releases endorphins and serotonin to relax and calm the individual and help the individual to modulate sensory input [49, 50]. These relaxing sensations, it is hypothesized, allow the individual to be better able to fall asleep and stay asleep.

3.4.2. Overview of the technique

Typically, weighted blankets are applied to children during sleep-time activities (nighttime and naps). The weight of the blankets used anecdotally is 10% of the child's body weight. The blankets size is large enough to cover the child's body, not including face and/feet. The intention is that the blanket will remain on top of the child throughout the duration of sleep.

3.4.3. Review of the evidence

The evidence to support the efficacy of using weighted blankets is scarce. Creasey and Finlay were unable to find any relevant primary or secondary evidence exploring the effectiveness of weighted blankets' impact on sleep in children with ASD [51]. Despite this lack of evidence, there is parental/caregiver anecdotal support of use, and as such, many advocate for the use of weighted blankets. One study published after Creasey and Finlay's review studied 73 children, aged 5–16 years, all of whom had an autism spectrum disorder diagnosis and reported sleep disturbances [52]. Using a crossover design, study participants were given a weighed blanket to sleep with for 2 weeks, followed by a period during which they slept with a non-weighted blanket that was provided by the researchers. The core findings were that weighted blankets were no more effective than a typical blanket in helping children with ASD improve their total sleep time or other qualitative and quantitative sleep measures. Parents of the children in the study, however, reported an improvement in next-day behaviors, a finding that the authors hypothesized might have been due to improved bedtime behaviors, improved parent/child interactions, or inflated reports by parents wishing to please the study team.

Gee and associates conducted a study to explore the efficacy of weighted blankets with children with an ASD and sleep disturbances using a single case, multiple baseline design [44]. This study focused on two children with an ASD and sensory over-responsivity. The authors found that there were minimal changes reported via caregivers after 14 nights of use, yet they indicated improvement in the areas of time to fall asleep, number of wakings in the night, duration of sleep and behavior in the morning. Gee and associates, utilizing a similar demographic, sample size, and measures, reported that children with ASD and sensory over-responsivity demonstrated a correlation between their morning mood and the number of hours slept the previous night [53]. Furthermore, it was reported that morning mood of the participants improved during the intervention phase of the ABA design.

Overall, the evidence supporting the use of weighted blankets continues to be weak, as such, this technique is considered experimental and should be used with caution.

3.5. Weighted vests

3.5.1. Purpose of the technique

Weighted vests have been used for individuals with ASD presumably to influence their somatosensory systems [54]. Specifically, weighted vests are often used to provide deep pressure for individuals who demonstrate sensory over-responsiveness, and resistance to those with sensory under-responsiveness/seeking behaviors. However, the use of weighted vests has become popular with children with ASD in hopes of increasing attention, on-task behaviors, and social engagement [55], while decreasing stereotypical behaviors [56].

3.5.2. Overview of the technique

A weighted vest is a type of sensory-based intervention. A weighted vest is a garment that typically has 1–4 lbs. (approximately 10% of the child's total body weight) of total weight evenly distributed across it [56]. These vests are primarily applied to preschool and elementary school-aged children with the diagnoses of ASD or attention deficit disorder [56]. The weighted vest is worn according to a pre-determined schedule at certain times of the day, including during everyday activities and for specified tasks at home, in the classroom, or in the community. The vest is typically applied for less than 1 h, one to two times per day during tabletop type tasks [56]. These are general intervention recommendations, but not a manualized approach. Lacking a standardized protocol for the weighted vest, most occupational therapists rely on clinical reasoning in devising an appropriate wearing schedule [57].

3.5.3. Review of the evidence

According to reviews, studies regarding the use of weighted vests are limited in size, scope, and quality. In a meta-analysis study of single subject designs, Stephenson and Carter reported that using weighted vests among young children was on the ineffective side, partially due to small sample sizes and poor methodology within the literature [58]. In another meta-synthesis by Losinski and associates, the research studies included were found to be of low quality, with the effects of deep pressure via weighted vests for individuals with disabilities (including ASD) were small among the variables of attention, disruptive behavior, self-injury, and stereotypy [59].

Small scale studies offer mixed results of the use of weighted vests. McGinnis and associates, reported that young children with ASD actual enjoy using weighted vests, and the application of these vests may serve as positive reinforcement, rather than bringing about changes in sensory processing [60]. Another study using an AB single subject design, found that weighted vests did not decrease problem behaviors (distraction, emotional reaction, withdrawal, escape/avoid, etc.) nor facilitate joint attention with primary caregivers among four toddlers with ASD and sensory processing difficulties [55].

The evidence in support of using weighted vests to address challenging behaviors rooted in sensory processing is almost absent, with additional research exploring the intervention with more typical behaviors among individuals with ASD. As such, AOTA does not include the use of weighted vests as a therapeutic technique in its publications. This is exemplified in two recent seminal works that therapists rely upon to guide practice: *Autism: A Comprehensive Occupational Therapy Approach* [61] and *Occupational Therapy Practice Guidelines for Individuals with Autism Spectrum Disorder* [62]. Due to the lack of evidence, weighted vests should be used with caution. Any use of weighted vests should be aligned with strong diagnostics related to sensory processing behaviors, deficits, and outcomes.

3.6. Task-oriented treatment approaches

Task-oriented treatment approaches assist children with ASD to develop the skills necessary to complete a particular task. Children with ASD often have difficulty completing tasks due to a variety of difficulties in communication, socialization, motor skills, and sensory processing. Task-oriented approaches consider the task to be completed and ways in which to accomplish the goal. Task-oriented approaches are utilized by both occupational and physical therapists to teach functional skills.

3.7. Treatment and Education of Autistic and Related Communication-Handicapped Children (TEACCH)

3.7.1. Purpose of the technique

The Treatment and Education of Autistic and Communication-Handicapped Children (TEACCH) program is intended to assist children in completing daily tasks by providing instructions that are clear and understandable in an environment that is highly structured and supportive [63]. TEACCH is considered a structured teaching program that recognizes the characteristics commonly associated with autism spectrum disorder, specifically communication problems, preference for visual information, sensory-related difficulties, attention variability, intense interests/impulses, and time management issues [64]. By offering a highly structured teaching environment focused on each child's individual ASD characteristics and the task at hand, learning development can occur. TEACCH is considered to be a multi-disciplinary approach, focused on collaboration between a variety of service providers, including teachers, therapists, family, and community [65].

3.7.2. Overview of the technique

The TEACCH program was developed in 1972 by Eric Schopler, Ph.D. at the University of North Carolina at Chapel Hill [66]. The program focuses on utilizing structure in a manner that encourages learning. According to Mesibov and Shea, structure in TEACCH comprises four components: physical structure, timing structure, task structure, and work/activity system structure [66]. Physical structure requires that the environment be set up in order to focus learning. This includes offering visual cues in the environment. Timing structure incorporates the use of a schedule, including scheduling cues. Organizing the task into manageable chunks is part of the task structure, this includes offering explicit directions. Finally, work/activity system structure involves synthesizing smaller tasks into a complete activity. By controlling these four structural elements, care providers can create an environment that maximizes functional capabilities of the child with ASD.

Along with utilizing TEACCH in a school or clinic setting, it is recommended that a home TEACCH program be developed for carry-over by parents/caregivers [67]. Ideally, the home TEACCH program would provide training and clinician supervision to parents/caregivers to assist them in structuring the home environment in order to support teaching skills in self-care, academics, and communication [67].

3.7.3. Review of literature

As TEACCH was developed and has training facilities housed within the University of North Carolina at Chapel Hill, there are researchers embedded in the program who have worked to establish a strong research base. When analyzing efficacy, it is important to identify potential bias that might occur by reviewing studies conducted only by researchers working where the technique was developed. To avoid that bias, a number of studies from within and outside the University of North Carolina at Chapel Hill were reviewed.

A meta-analysis of intervention studies using TEACCH (level 1 evidence) was conducted by Virues-Ortega, Julio, and Pastor-Barriuso in 2013 [68]. This meta-analysis utilized 13 studies, with a combined sample of 172 children diagnosed with ASD, assessing perceptual and motor skills, adaptive behaviors, and language and cognition. Results indicated that TEACCH had a small magnitude impact on perceptual, motor, verbal and cognitive skills, a negligible impact on communication, activities of daily living, and motor functioning, and moderate to large gains in social behavior and maladaptive behavior. The overall effect of the TEACCH program on all the outcomes measured in the meta-analysis was moderate, with effects in older children being higher than those in younger children. The authors cautioned that while these findings indicate success with TEACCH, the small number of studies and sample size should be considered.

D'Elia and associates conducted a longitudinal study of low-intensity TEACCH in preschool aged children [65]. The study followed a sample of 30 children, aged 2–6.11 years, diagnosed with autistic disorder or pervasive developmental disorder – not otherwise specified over a 2 year period. The group was split evenly into a control group that did not receive TEACCH and an experimental group that received the TEACCH intervention 2 h per week at school and 2 h per week at home. Results for the main outcome indicators of severity of autism, language, and adaptive functioning showed no significant difference between the control group and the experimental group. Results for the secondary outcomes of parental stress and psychopathological comorbidity indicated significant differences between the control group and the experimental group. Both secondary outcomes indicated greater improvement in the experimental group. The authors indicate that the lack of significance in primary outcomes could possibly be attributed to the low intensity of the TEACCH intervention, which is not standard protocol. The positive secondary outcomes indicate potential of the TEACCH program in decreasing parental stress and child behavioral/emotional problems.

With home-based TEACCH being a major component of the program, it is important to determine the efficacy of that particular approach. Weterlin and associates conducted a study on the efficacy of the Home-TEACCHing Program (HTP) on toddlers with ASD [67]. The sample included twenty 2–3 year old children and their parents. Children and their parents were randomly assigned to either the treatment (HTP) group or the waitlist (WL) group. WL group members were informed that they would receive the treatment at the conclusion of a 12 week wait period. This study yielded three major findings: (1) HTP improved children's independent work skills; (2) Parents were able to structure the physical environment to improve child outcomes; (3) Parents improved their effective prompting, including using visual prompts. Although the sample size was small, findings demonstrate support for the use of the Home-TEACCHing Program.

Overall, research to date on effectiveness of the TEACCH program is very encouraging. Therapists use the components of TEACCH to assist children with ASD in learning tasks. Specifically, therapists using this technique will structure the physical environment (including visual cues), and organize the task with explicit directions in order to assist the child in learning new skills that aid in improved functional outcomes.

3.8. Cognitive orientation to occupational performance (CO-OP)

3.8.1. Purpose of the technique

The Cognitive Orientation to Occupational Performance (CO-OP) is a task-oriented, problem-solving approach that uses cognitive skills to improve occupational performance. It is typically a verbally based approach that emphasizes teaching clients to incorporate self-talk and problem-solving to address difficulty with the execution of various motor skills [69]. According to Missiuna and associates, elements of CO-OP include concepts related to problem-solving, learning theory, motor learning theory, cognitive strategies, client-centered practice, goal setting, and motivation [69]. CO-OP has been observed to be highly individualized, starting with clinician generated verbal guidance, followed by the development of client internal self-dialog, and finally independent application of problem-solving strategies ([70], p. 190).

Missuana and associates identified that the three main objectives addressed by CO-OP are: (1) skill acquisition in client-chosen goals/tasks, (2) cognitive strategy development, and (3) generalization of subsequently learned skills and strategies to a variety of contexts. Specifically, in the CO-OP process the client is learning a new motor skill or improving performance on one that has not yet developed sufficiently to be functional [69].

In CO-OP, a client-centered approach is used to encourage clients to select their own goals for the intervention plan. The CO-OP cognitive strategies are used to influence skill acquisition. Generalization and transfer of skills is supported through the use of an executive, or problem-solving, strategy that trains the child to monitor his performance and self-evaluate the outcome [69].

Rodger et al. have argued that in order for clients with ASD to be successful in taking part in CO-OP, therapists need to ensure they have accommodated the language and communication needs of the clients, given that the technique relies heavily on language and communication [71]. The goal of CO-OP is to create a process to teach clients how to think, instead of what to think.

3.8.2. Overview of the technique

According to Polatajko and Mandich, during CO-OP, clients are instructed on a global cognitive strategy and are then guided in the process of discovering other cognitive strategies that are relevant to their chosen goals. The global strategy used in CO-OP is "the goal, plan, do, check" [70]. Specifically, this foundational strategy involves working with the client to identify "what needs to be done, planning how to achieve this, carrying out the plan and then evaluating its effectiveness" ([72], p. 184).

Domain specific strategies (DSS) are specific cognitive strategies that are task, child or situation specific and focus on facilitating or improving performance [69]. The child is guided to develop his/her own strategies based on the problems encountered during tasks [72].

3.8.3. Review of the evidence

CO-OP has been evaluated across diverse populations (pediatric and adult) and conditions (ASD, cerebral palsy, developmental coordination disorder, cerebral vascular accident, traumatic brain injury) [73–76]. The current research of CO-OP among children and adolescents diagnosed with high functioning and/or mild ASD have emerged using case studies/series approaches.

Several case studies (Level IV-V) have been conducted among diverse segments of the spectrum of children/adolescents with autism. Phelan and associates reported general improvement on the Canadian Occupational Performance Measure and the Performance Quality Rating Scale among two children with ASD [77]. Visual analysis indicated consistent increase in performance on both subjective scales and across the three client-centered goals across a 10 session plan of care.

In another case study of two participants with ASD, Rodger and Brandenburg found that after 10 weekly sessions using CO-OP, the participants demonstrated improvements on the pre and post-intervention assessment [78]. Specifically, moderate to significant improvement was noted on the caregiver subjective scale using the Canadian Occupational Performance Measure, Performance Quality Rating Scales and the Vineland Adaptive Behavior Scales.

Overall, the CO-OP approach for children and adolescents with ASD has yielded positive findings, enhancing function and participation in meaningful activities as a part of activities of daily living and instrumental activities of daily living and supports its use in clinical practice, yet more research needs to be conducted using more robust designs.

3.9. Behavioral treatment approaches

Behavioral treatment approaches to ASD incorporate components of operant conditioning in order to manipulate behavior to create positive outcomes. When considering ASD, the primary behavioral treatment approach used is Applied Behavior Analysis (ABA), which is applied in a variety of forms (school-based, clinic-based, home-based, discrete trial training, Lovaas therapy, inclusive programs). Generally, occupational and physical therapists will follow an ABA approach if the child is currently enrolled in a program that specifically uses ABA, or if the child is learning a discrete skill that would benefit from an ABA approach (e.g. toileting, shoe-tying).

3.10. Applied behavior analysis (ABA)

3.10.1. Purpose of the technique

The purpose of Applied Behavior Analysis (ABA) is to teach discrete skills by modifying the environment in order to manipulate behavior [79]. To teach these skills, therapists utilize the "ABC technique" to determine why a behavior is occurring: *antecedent, behavior, consequence* [63]. Antecedent refers to what is happening prior to the behavior. The *antecedent* prompts the behavior to occur. The *behavior* is what the child does in response to a stimulus (antecedent). Finally, the *consequence* is what the child receives as a response to the behavior. The consequence can perpetuate or extinguish the behavior. Once therapists have determined the "ABC," then they can create a structured plan that addresses each component to create an optimal outcome.

3.10.2. Overview of the technique

Based on principles developed by B.F. Skinner in the 1950s, Clinical Psychologist O. Ivar Lovaas created ABA as a behavior modification program for use in children with ASD [63]. The program is intended for use across a variety of instructional formats, including both group and individual sessions, which allows for independent and observational learning [80].

In ABA programming, once a functional behavior assessment has determined the ABC (antecedent, behavior, consequence), the therapist will determine the target behavior and how the environment will be modified to achieve that behavior. Additionally, the therapist will determine what reinforcement to use and the reinforcement schedule. Reinforcement is a critical component of ABA, and determining appropriate reinforcers is crucial for program success. Often people are tempted to use edible reinforcers (candy, chips). This practice is highly discouraged, as it can lead to unhealthy eating habits and an inability to develop other motivating reinforcers [80].

Therapists using ABA must be cognizant of their surroundings and the influence of all types of reinforcement, applying a variety of positive reinforcement to keep the child focused and on track. Knowledge of what may reinforce poor behavior is as important as knowing what impacts pro-social behavior. For example, if a child seeks attention and receives it every time he or she acts out, then the attention serves to positively reinforce the acting out behavior. Therapists need to be aware of this and modify reinforcement accordingly.

Once the reinforcement is determined, ABA can begin. A commonly used form of ABA is called Discrete Trial Training (DTT). DTT identifies a specific task, then teaches the task by breaking it into its component parts and repeatedly presenting it to the child until mastery is achieved [63]. This is a repetitive process that often involves multiple presentations over days or weeks. Reinforcement occurs each time the child correctly responds, or in the case of a developing skill, when the response approximates the skill.

3.10.3. Review of literature

The seminal research for the use of ABA for children with ASD was conducted by Lovaas in 1987. This study specifically investigated DTT on a group of 4 year olds over the course of 2–3 years. Lovaas found that 47% of the children in the ABA demonstrated functional improvements, compared to only 2% in the control group. This study has been replicated numerous times across the years, with similar results, indicating that DTT improves IQ, communication, and socialization in children under 4 years old with ASD [63].

A systematic review of behavioral and developmental interventions for children with ASD was conducted by Ospina and associates [81]. In regard to ABA, this review specifically examined 31 studies with a total sample of 770 subjects. Findings related to DTT were inconsistent, with motor and functional outcomes trending positively, while speech outcomes trended negatively. High intensity Lovaas therapy was found to be superior to low intensity programming, and treatment was consistently found to be better than standard care.

Virues-Ortega conducted a meta-analysis of ABA and autism in 2010 [82]. The review analyzed results from 22 studies that included a total of 323 subjects in intervention groups that ranged in age from 22.6 to 66.3 months old. Results indicated positive effects in IQ (18 studies), receptive language (11 studies), expressive language (10 studies), and adaptive behaviors (communication, daily living skills, and socialization, 11 studies). The author did note that analysis was difficult due to the varying methodology used, but indicated overall that ABA intervention is associated with medium to large positive effects in IQ, language, and adaptive behavior.

Overall, research has demonstrated that ABA can be an effective therapeutic technique to teach children with ASD specific skills. Therapists utilize this technique in a variety of formats in order to help improve functional outcomes.

3.11. Social-emotional treatment approaches

Social-emotional treatment approaches are gaining in popularity with children with ASD as research reveals the impact of social/emotional development on all other functional areas.

Embodied cognition is created only when an individual can actively engage in his or her environment [83], which requires social interaction with objects and others. To encourage these interactions and relationships, the Developmental, Individual Difference, Relationship-Based Model (DIR®/Floortime™) was created. This treatment approach is used by both occupational and physical therapists to encourage participation in therapy for children with ASD.

3.12. Developmental, individual difference, relationship-based model (DIR®/Floortime™)

3.12.1. Purpose of the technique

DIR®/Floortime™ is a framework for assessment and intervention that focuses on building social, emotional, and intellectual abilities [84]. This framework seeks to assist children in creating an emotional foundation on which other skills can be encouraged to grow and develop. An important concept of this framework is that is does not seek to teach individual skills in isolation, but rather focuses on the child with ASD as a unique being that is capable of growth by establishing relationships and circles of communication within the environment [84].

3.12.2. Overview of the technique

According to Greenspan and Wieder [84], the DIR® Model was created by Dr. Stanley Greenspan in the 1980s. The model highlights the developmental, individual differences, and relationship-based components of emotional development in children. The developmental part of the model focuses specifically on the six identified developmental levels that are required for emotional health. These hierarchical levels include: (1) self-regulation and interest in the world, (2) engaging and relating, (3) purposeful two-way communication, (4) complex communication and problem-solving, (5) using symbols and creating emotional ideas, and (6) logical thinking and building bridges between ideas.

Individual differences in the DIR® Model refer to the child-specific ways that information can be taken in and processed [84]. It is commonly understood that children with ASD are unique; with each child demonstrating individualized ways of responding to sensory input. These individual differences need to be considered when attempting to factiliate in social–emotional development.

The relationship-based component of the DIR® model refers to the use of emotional connection to foster development. Clinicians utilizing a DIR® approach need to purposefully tailor their actions and communication to engage the child in an emotional relationship [84].

Clinical application of the DIR® model occurs in what is called Floortime™. Therapists engaging in Floortime™ techniques demonstrate skills in getting to the child's level and allowing the child's actions and communications to lead the emotional relationship [84]. By engaging in the child's world, this technique postulates that you can then bring the child into a "shared world" [85]. These techniques, when employed correctly, can help the child with ASD progress through the levels of emotional development.

3.12.3. Review of literature

Research regarding DIR®/Floortime™ appears to be somewhat limited in both scope and vigor, although the research base is expanding. A pilot randomized controlled trial was completed in 2011 by Pajareya and Nopmaneejumruslers in Thailand [86]. This study utilized 32 participants that were 2–6 years old and were diagnosed with autistic disorder according to the DSM-IV. Participants were randomly assigned to the typical treatment group, or the DIR®/Floortime™—supplemented treatment group. Findings from the study revealed that DIR®/Floortime™ helped children with autism to better engage with caregivers. Additionally, the study found that engagement in DIR/Floortime™ helped parents to better play with their children with autism.

Liao and associates completed a study involving the use of DIR®/Floortime™ at home on preschool-aged children [87]. The study had a sample of 11 young boys and their mothers. Results of the study indicated that the use of DIR®/Floortime™ significantly improved two-way communication, relationship formation, problem solving, and behavioral organization, and adaptive skills. Additionally, mothers who utilized the intervention felt that their parent–child interactions improved.

A randomized controlled trial regarding ASD and DIR®/Floortime™ was conducted by Lal and Chhabria in 2013 [88]. This study utilized a sample of 26 children aged 3–6 who were diagnosed with ASD. These children were randomly assigned to treatment and control groups, with 13 participants in each group. The treatment group received 20 sessions of DIR®/Floortime™ that lasted 30 min each, while the control group received typical early intervention services. Results of this study indicated that all children who received DIR®/Floortime™ demonstrated improved social behavior from pre-test to post-test. Comparison between the control group and treatment group from pre to post-test indicated significant differences, with the DIR®/Floortime™ group showing greater improvement.

These positive results suggest that DIR®/Floortime™ does help in promoting social–emotional growth, which can improve functional outcomes. While the evidence is positive, scope is limited, which suggests caution in application until further studies regarding efficacy can be completed.

4. Conclusion

Occupational therapy is a rehabilitation specialty that facilitates the development of functional skills in children with ASD. Occupational therapists often work as part of an interdisciplinary treatment team. In this capacity, it is important for therapists to communicate across disciplines to be sure that treatment is carried over from one area to another.

There are many therapeutic approaches that occupational therapists can use to encourage growth and development in children with ASD. These treatment approaches have varying levels of evidence supporting their efficacy. Clinicians need to be mindful of the current evidence and use their knowledge of the child and the treatment, along with their clinical judgment, to create effective interventions.

Author details

Bryan M. Gee[1]*, Amy Nwora[2] and Theodore W. Peterson[1]

*Address all correspondence to: geebrya@isu.edu

1 Idaho State University, Pocatello, ID, USA

2 D'Youville College, Buffalo, NY, USA

References

[1] American Occupational Therapy Association. Occupational therapy practice framework: Domain and process, 3rd ed. The American Journal of Occupational Therapy 2014;**68**(Suppl 1):S1-S48

[2] Christiansen CH. Defining lives: Occupation as identity: An essay on competence, coherence, and the creation of meaning. The American Journal of Occupational Therapy. 1999;**53**(6):547-558

[3] Clark F, Azen SP, Zemke R, et al. Occupational therapy for independent-living older adults: A randomized controlled trial. Journal of the American Medical Association. 1997;**278**(16):1321-1326

[4] Boyt Schell BA, Gillen G, Scaffa M, Cohn E, et al. Willard and Spackman's Occupational Therapy. 12th ed. Philadelphia, PA: Wolters Kluwer Lippincott Williams & Wilkins; 2014

[5] Yerxa EJ. An introduction to occupational science, a foundation for occupational therapy in the 21st century. Occupational Therapy in Health Care. 1990;**6**(4):1-17

[6] Law M, Steinwender S, Leclair L. Occupation, health and well-being. Canadian Journal of Occupational Therapy. 1998;**65**(2):81-91

[7] Hooper B, Wood W. The philosophy of occupational therapy: A framework for practice. In: Boyt Schell BA, Gillen G, Scaffa M, Cohn E, editors. Willard and Spackman's Occupational Therapy. 12th ed. Philadelphia, PA: Wolters Kluwer Lippincott Williams & Wilkins; 2014. pp. 35-46

[8] World Health Organization. International Classification of Functioning, Disability and Health: ICF. Geneva, Switzerland: World Health Organization; 2001

[9] Fisher AG, Griswold LA. Performance skills: Implementing performance analyses to evaluate quality of occupational performance. In: Boyt Schell BA, Gillen G, Scaffa M, Cohn E, editors. Willard and Spackman's Occupational Therapy. 12th ed. Philadelphia, PA: Wolters Kluwer Lippincott Williams & Wilkins; 2014. pp. 249-264

[10] Akdem F, Akel BS. Otizmli Bireylerin Bakım Verenlerinin Yaşam Kalitesi ve Zaman Yönetimini Etkileyen Faktörlerin İncelenmesi. Ergoterapi ve Rehabilitasyon Dergisi. 2014;**2**(3):121-129

[11] American Occupational Therapy Association. 2015 AOTA Salary and Workforce Survey. Bethesda, MD: American Occupational Therapy Association; 2015

[12] Dunn W. Ecology of human performance model. In: Dunbar SB, editor. Occupational Therapy Models for Intervention with Children and Families. Thorofare, NJ: Slack; 2007. pp. 127-155

[13] Pekçetin S, Günal A. Early Intervention in Pediatric Occupational Therapy, Occupational Therapy Meral Huri. IntechOpen; July 5th 2017. DOI: 10.5772/intechopen.68316

[14] Ben-Sasson A, Hen L, Fluss R, Cermak SA, Engel-Yeger B, Gal E. A meta-analysis of sensory modulation symptoms in individuals with autism spectrum disorders. Journal of Autism and Developmental Disorders. 2009;**39**(1):1-11

[15] Bumin G, Huri M, Salar S, Kayihan H. Occupational therapy in autism. In: Autism Spectrum Disorder Michael Fitzgerald. IntechOpen; April 2nd 2015. DOI: 10.5772/59168

[16] Case-Smith J, Weaver LL, Fristad MA. A systematic review of sensory processing interventions for children with autism spectrum disorders. Autism. 2014;**19**(2):133-148

[17] Lane AE, Young RL, Baker AE, Angley MT. Sensory processing subtypes in autism: Association with adaptive behavior. Journal of Autism and Developmental Disorders. 2010;**40**(1):112-122

[18] American Psychiatric Association. Diagnostic and Statistical Manual of Mental Disorders. 5th ed. Washington, DC: American Psychiatric Association; 2013

[19] Ayres AJ. Sensory Integration and Learning Disorders. Los Angeles: Western Psychological Services; 1972

[20] Ayres AJ. Sensory Integration and Praxis Tests (SIPT). Los Angeles: Western Psychological Services; 1989

[21] Green VA, Pituch KA, Itchon J, Choi A, O'Reilly M, Sigafoos J. Internet survey of treatments used by parents of children with autism. Research in Developmental Disabilities. 2006;**27**(1):70-84

[22] Case-Smith J, Miller H. Occupational therapy with children with pervasive developmental disorders. The American Journal of Occupational Therapy. 1999;**53**(5):506-513

[23] Roley SS, Blanche EI, Schaaf RC. Understanding the Nature of Sensory Integration with Diverse Populations. San Antonio, TX: Therapy Skill Builders; 2001

[24] Schaaf R, Mallioux Z. Clincians Guide to Ayres Sensory Integration Intervention: Promoting Participation for Children with Autism. Bethesda, MD: AOTA Press; 2015

[25] Parham LD, Roley SS, May-Benson TA, et al. Development of a fidelity measure for research on the effectiveness of the Ayres sensory integration® intervention. The American Journal of Occupational Therapy. 2011;**65**(2):133-142

[26] Pfeiffer BA, Koenig K, Kinnealey M, Sheppard M, Henderson L. Effectiveness of sensory integration interventions in children with autism spectrum disorders: A pilot study. The American Journal of Occupational Therapy. 2011;**65**(1):76-85

[27] Schaaf RC, Benevides T, Mailloux Z, et al. An intervention for sensory difficulties in children with autism: A randomized trial. Journal of Autism and Developmental Disorders. 2014;**44**(7):1493-1506

[28] Iwanaga R, Honda S, Nakane H, Tanaka K, Toeda H, Tanaka G. Pilot study: Efficacy of sensory integration therapy for Japanese children with high-functioning autism Spectrum disorder. Occupational Therapy International. 2014;**21**(1):4-11

[29] Kashefimehr B, Kayihan H, Huri M. The effect of sensory integration therapy on occupational performance in children with autism. Occupation, Participation and Health. 2017;**38**(2):75-83

[30] Miller LJ, Coll JR, Schoen SA. A randomized controlled pilot study of the effectiveness of occupational therapy for children with sensory modulation disorder. The American Journal of Occupational Therapy. 2007;**61**(2):228-238

[31] Parham LD, Cohn ES, Spitzer S, et al. Fidelity in sensory integration intervention research. The American Journal of Occupational Therapy. 2007;**61**(2):216-227

[32] May-Benson T, Koomar J. Systematic review of the research evidence examining the effectiveness of interventions using a sensory integrative approach for children. The American Journal of Occupational Therapy. 2010;**64**(3):403-414

[33] Hall L, Case-Smith J. The effect of sound-based intervention on children with sensory processing disorders and visual-motor delays. The American Journal of Occupational Therapy. 2007;**61**(2):209-215

[34] Bazyk S, Cimino J, Hayes K, Goodman G, Farrell P. The use of therapeutic listening with preschoolers with developmental disabilities: A look at the outcomes. Journal of Occupational Therapy, Schools, and Early Intervention. 2010;**3**(2):124-138

[35] Thompson B, Andrews S. An historical commentary on the physiological effects of music: Tomatis, Mozart and neuropsychology. Integrative Psychological & Behavioral Science. 2000;**35**(3):174-188

[36] Spencer KC, Turkett A, Vaughan R, Koenig S. School-based practice patterns: A survey of occupational therapists in Colorado. The American Journal of Occupational Therapy. 2006;**60**(1):81-91

[37] Case-Smith J, Arbesman M. Evidence-based review of interventions for autism used in or of relevance to occupational therapy. The American Journal of Occupational Therapy. 2008;**62**(4):416-429

[38] Gilmor T. The efficacy of the Tomatis method for children with learning and communication disorders: A meta-analysis. International Journal of Listening. 1999;**13**(1):12-23

[39] Neysmith-Roy JM. The Tomatis method with severely autistic boys: Individual case studies of behavioral changes. South Africa Journal of Psychology. 2001;**31**(1):19-28

[40] Corbett BA, Shickman K, Ferrer E. Brief report: The effects of Tomatis sound therapy on language in children with autism. Journal of Autism and Developmental Disorders. 2008;**38**(3):562-566

[41] Sinha SY, Silove N, Wheeler DM, Williams KJ. Auditory integration training and other sound therapies for autism spectrum disorders. Cochrane Library. 2009;**2009**(1):1-24

[42] Nwora A, Gee B. A case study of a five-year old child with pervasive developmental disorder-not otherwise specified using sound-based interventions. Occupational Therapy International. 2009;**16**(1):25-43

[43] Gee BM, Thompson K, St. John H. Efficacy of a sound-based intervention with a child with an autism spectrum disorder and auditory sensory over-responsivity. Occupational Therapy International. 2014;**21**(1):12-20

[44] Gee BM, Peterson TW, Buck A, Lloyd K. Improving sleep quality using weighted blankets among young children with an autism spectrum disorder: A single case design. International Journal of Therapy and Rehabilitation. 2016;**23**(4):173-181

[45] Tumiran MA, Mohamad SP, Saat RM, Yusoff MYZM, Rahman NNA, Adli DSH. Addressing sleep disorder of autistic children with Qur'anic sound therapy. Health. 2013;**5**(8B):73-79

[46] Humphreys JS, Gringras P, Blair PS, et al. Sleep patterns in children with autistic spectrum disorders: A prospective cohort study. Archives of Disease in Childhood. 2014; **99**(2):114-118

[47] Malow BA, Marzec ML, McGrew SG, Wang L, Henderson LM, Stone WL. Characterizing sleep in children with autism spectrum disorders: A multidimensional approach. Sleep. 2006;**29**(12):1563-1571

[48] Picard MM. Occupational Therapy's Role in Sleep. 2012. http://www.aota.org/en/About-Occupational-Therapy/Professionals/HW/Sleep.aspx. [Accessed: 18 February 2017]

[49] Mullen B, Champagne T, Krishnamurty S, Dickson D, Gao RX. Exploring the safety and therapeutic effects of deep pressure stimulation using a weighted blanket. Occupational Therapy in Mental Health. 2008;**24**(1):65-88

[50] Mosiac Weighted Blankets. How Do Weighted Blankets Work? 2014. http://www.mosaicweightedblankets.com/how-doweighted-blankets-work. [Accessed: 18 February 2017]

[51] Creasey N, Finlay F. Question 2: Do weighted blankets improve sleep in children with an autistic spectrum disorder? Archives of Disease in Childhood. 2013;**98**(11):919-920

[52] Gringas P, Green D, Wright B, et al. Weighted blankets and sleep in autistic children—A randomized controlled trial. Pediatrics. 2014;**134**(2):298-306

[53] Gee B, McOmber T, Sutton J, Lloyd K. Improving sleep quality using weighted blankets among young children with an autism spectrum disorder: A single case design. Paper presentation at the American Occupational Therapy Association National Conference; Philadelphia, PA. 2017

[54] Kane A, Luiselli SD, Dearborn S, Young N. Wearing a weighted vest as intervention for children with autism/pervasive developmental disorder: Behavioral assessment of stereotypy and attention to task. The Scientific Review of Mental Health Practice. 2005;**3**(2):19-24

[55] Leew SV, Stein NG, Gibbard WB. Weighted vests' effect on social attention for toddlers with autism spectrum disorders. Canadian Journal of Occupational Therapy. 2010; **77**(2):113-124

[56] Olson LJ, Moulton HJ. Occupational therapists' reported experiences using weighted vests with children with specific developmental disorders. Occupational Therapy International. 2004;**11**(1):52-66

[57] Morrison EE. A review of research on the use of weighted vests with children on the autism spectrum. Education. 2007;**127**(3):323

[58] Stephenson J, Carter M. The use of weighted vests with children with autism spectrum disorders and other disabilities. Journal of Autism and Developmental Disorders. 2009;**39**(1):105-114

[59] Losinski M, Sanders SA, Wiseman NM. Examining the use of deep touch pressure to improve the educational performance of students with disabilities: A meta-analysis. Research and Practice for Persons with Severe Disabilities. 2016;**41**(1):3-18

[60] McGinnis AA, Blakely EQ, Harvey AC, Hodges AC, Rickards JB. The behavioral effects of a procedure used by pediatric occupational therapists. Behavioral Interventions. 2013;**28**(1):48-57

[61] Kuhaneck H, Watling R. Autism: A Comprehensive Occupational Therapy Approach. 3rd ed. Bethesda, MD: AOTA Press; 2014

[62] Tomchek SD, Koenig KP. Occupational Therapy Practice Guidelines for Individuals with Autism Spectrum Disorder. AOTA Press, The American Occupational Therapy Association, Incorporated; 2016

[63] Ryan JB, Hughes EM, Katsiyannis A, McDaniel M, Sprinkle C. Research-based educational practices for students with autism spectrum disorders. Teaching Exceptional Children. 2011;**43**(3):56-64

[64] Mesibov GB, Shea V, Schopler E. The TEACCH Approach to Autism Spectrum Disorders. New York, NY: Springer; 2005

[65] D'Elia L, Valeri G, Sonnino F, Fontana I, Mammone A, Vicari S. A longitudinal study of the teacch program in different settings: The potential benefits of low intensity intervention in preschool children with autism spectrum disorder. Journal of Autism and Developmental Disorders. 2014;**44**(3):615-626

[66] Mesibov GB, Shea V. The TEACCH program in the era of evidence-based practice. Journal of Autism and Developmental Disorders. 2010;**40**(5):570-579

[67] Weterlin A, Turner-Brown LM, Harris S, Mesibov G, Delmolino L. The home TEACCHing program for toddlers with autism. Journal of Autism and Developmental Disorders. 2012;**42**(9):1827-1835

[68] Virues-Ortega J, Julio F, Pastor-Barriuso R. The TEACCH program for children and adults with autism: A meta-analysis of intervention studies. Clinical Psychology Review. 2013;**33**(8):940-953

[69] Missiuna C, Mandich AD, Polatajko HJ, Malloy-Miller T. Cognitive orientation to daily occupational performance (CO-OP) part I–Theoretical foundations. Physical & Occupational Therapy in Pediatrics. 2001;**20**(2-3):69-81

[70] Polatajko HJ, Mandich A. Enabling Occupation in Children: The Cognitive Orientation to Daily Occupational Performance (CO-OP) Approach. Ottawa, ON: CAOT Publications ACE; 2004

[71] Rodger S, Ireland S, Vun M. Can cognitive orientation to daily occupational performance (CO-OP) help children with Asperger's syndrome to master social and organisational goals? British Journal of Occupational Therapy. 2008;**71**(1):23-32

[72] Miller LT, Polatajko HJ, Missiuna C, Mandich AD, Macnab JJ. A pilot trial of a cognitive treatment for children with developmental coordination disorder. Human Movement Science. 2001;**20**(1-2):183-210

[73] Ward A, Rodger S. The application of cognitive orientation to daily occupational performance (CO-OP) with children 5-7 years with developmental coordination disorder. British Journal of Occupational Therapy. 2004;**67**(6):256-264

[74] Chan DY. The application of cognitive orientation to daily occupational performance (CO-OP) in children with developmental coordination disorder (DCD) in Hong Kong: A pilot study. Hong Kong Journal of Occupational Therapy. 2007;**17**(2):39-44

[75] Dawson DR, Gaya A, Hunt A, Levine B, Lemsky C, Polatajko HJ. Using the cognitive orientation to occupational performance (CO-OP) with adults with executive dysfunction following traumatic brain injury. Canadian Journal of Occupational Therapy. 2009;**76**(2):115-127

[76] Polatajko HJ, McEwen SE, Ryan JD, Baum CM. Pilot randomized controlled trial investigating cognitive strategy use to improve goal performance after stroke. The American Journal of Occupational Therapy. 2012;**66**(1):104-109

[77] Phelan S, Steinke L, Mandich A. Exploring a cognitive intervention for children with pervasive developmental disorder. Canadian Journal of Occupational Therapy. 2009; **76**(1):23-28

[78] Rodger S, Brandenburg J. Cognitive orientation to (daily) occupational performance (CO-OP) with children with Asperger's syndrome who have motor-based occupational performance goals. Australian Occupational Therapy Journal. 2009;**56**(1):41-50

[79] Chiesa M. Radical Behaviorism: The Philosophy and the Science. Boston, MA: Authors Cooperative; 2004

[80] Leaf JB, Leaf R, McEachin J, et al. Applied behavior analysis is a science and, therefore, progressive. Journal of Autism and Developmental Disorders. 2016;**46**:720-731

[81] Ospina MB, Seida JK, Clark B, et al. Behavioural and developmental interventions for autism spectrum disorder: A clinical systematic review. PLoS One. 2008;**3**(11):e3755

[82] Virues-Ortega J. Applied behavior analytic intervention for autism in early childhood: Meta-analysis, meta-regression and dose-response meta-analysis of multiple outcomes. Clinical Psychology Review. 2010;**30**(4):387-399

[83] Hellendoorn A, Wijnroks L, vanDaalen E, Dietz C, Buitelaar JK, Leseman P. Motor functioning, exploration, visuospatial cognition and language development in preschool children with autism. Research in Developmental Disabilities. 2015;**39**:32-42

[84] Greenspan SI, Wieder S. Engaging Autism: The Floortime Approach to Helping Children Relate, Communicate and Think. Philadelphia, PA: Perseus Books; 2006

[85] Hess E. DIR/Floortime: Evidence based practice towards the treatment of autism and sensory processing disorder in children and adolescents. The International Journal of Child Health and Human Development. 2013;**6**(3):267-274

[86] Pajareya K, Nopmaneejumruslers K. A pilot randomized controlled trial of DIR/Floortime parent training intervention for pre-school children with autistic spectrum disorders. Autism. 2011;**15**(5):563-577. DOI: 10.1177/1362361310386502

[87] Liao ST, Hwang YS, Chen YJ, Lee P, Chen SJ, Lin LY. Home-based DIR/Floortime intervention program for preschool children with autism spectrum disorders: Preliminary findings. Physical & Occupational Therapy in Pediatrics. 2014;**34**(4):356-367. DOI: 10.3109/01942638.2014.918074

[88] Lal R, Chhabria R. Early intervention of autism: A case for floor time approach. Recent Advances in Autism Spectrum Disorders. 2013;**1**(29):691-717. DOI: 10.5772/54378

7

Executive Functions and Neurology in Children and Adolescents

Gokcen Akyurek

Abstract

This chapter discusses the theoretical and methodological issues of creating a developmental perspective on executive function (EF) in childhood and adolescence. Focusing on school periods, this section outlines the development of the basic components of EF—inhibition, working memory, and attention. Cognitive and neurophysiological evaluations show that despite the emergence of EF in the first few years of life, it continues to grow significantly in childhood and adolescence. The components vary slightly according to their developmental sequence. The chapter links findings to long-standing developmental issues (i.e. developmental sequences and processes) and suggests the necessary research to establish a developmental framework covering early childhood throughout adolescence.

Keywords: executive function, executive control, prefrontal cortex, children, adolescent behavior

1. Introduction

Coordination of the executive functions (EFs) with the frontal lobe is seen in all mammalian species. Executive functions are not specific to people and their need of advanced information computing, but it is an integral part of the mammalian brain development that emerges over time to facilitate a more complex problem-solving and goal-oriented behavior [1]. The basic function of the developing nervous system is revealing the efforts that are necessary for effective learning and successful adaptation. Vertical and horizontal development processes of brain development and the accompanying age and experience make control and communication more automatic and effective [2, 3]. This is a demonstration of the skills and adaptation that we have developed over time while allowing us to understand what managing means in childhood and adolescence. We acquire mastery of having and using cognitive controls with maturation. However, although the system is more effective at the beginning of maturation in parallel with increasing needs, it may provide less support afterward [4].

1.1. Basics of executive functions

The cognitive capacity of an individual increases with the executive functions being involved in many different aspects of information processing and behavior over time. The emergence of basic skills such as orientation and attention is followed by strategy determination, implementation, and then problem-solving. Executive functions change from a developmental perspective to multiple creative cognitive skills. Understanding what executive mean requires you to understand how each ability develops over time [5].

1.1.1. Attention

The attention system is a basic and supporting component of the execution system. It is a tool that guards learning for the developing individual and directs interaction with the environment, especially from birth [6, 7]. Throughout childhood, the child increasingly masters in creating schemas and representations by taking information about the environment. This supports the child's adaptation and learning of the demands and challenges of the community. For this reason, attention, regulation, and maintaining attention interact neurodevelopmentally with memory processes and constitute cognitive structures necessary for executive and behavioral control. As a result, attention during infancy and crawling period emerges as targeted behavior and serves to develop executive function skills over time [7, 8].

The infant begins to see the effects of his growing awareness with the events and experiences surrounding him over his perceived knowledge. This encourages cognitive and behavioral dialog through direct and indirect interactions with objects and people. The motor functions, senses, and cognitive functions interact to create the connection between the baby and the environment, which facilitates the infant's experience with the surroundings. This increases the infant's control over the interaction with the environment. This is initially a passive response to the environment but then it turns into an environment research process. Then, the quest for increased ties and interaction becomes an active process. As people, events, and experiences increase, babies carefully separate events and experiences that they find stimulating or uncomfortable and seek support through behavior or voice responses [9]. In the game period, the child begins to realize that they are influencing their environment and surroundings through mechanisms such as attention, reaching a target, and exploring. This awareness turns into realizing goals and desires and improves early problem-solving skills.

1.1.2. Behavioral and emotional regulation

Self-regulation develops throughout the age of infancy, walking, and primary education period. Guiding parenting initially directs this development capacity, but the baby and then the child develops his own reactions on how he behaves [7, 10]. In "real" experience, the child reacts to events through observation and imitation. By actively recalling these experiences, the child makes behavioral choices. The strategy begins to play a greater role in their behavior so that during late infancy examples of purposeful actions or even "secret" behaviors (i.e. game hiding, early denial of responsibilities) are observed [11]. These efforts are examples of executive functions that arise such as problem-solving, self-monitoring, strategy definition and implementation, and even primitive flexibility. Memory is the basis for the development of many basic executive functions; the information processed and stored in the working memory governs attention, and constant impulse control arises and evolves. As a response to the child's efforts to guide and shape experience, orientation and engagement occur.

1.2. Executive functions in childhood

Middle childhood is one of the basic periods in which executive functions are necessary to support successful learning and the development of academic skills [8]. With executive functions in the first three grades, children can identify what's important and integrate new information with the existing information. However, from the fourth-grade onward, the learners who are expected to manage integrated academic requirements more competently and strategically have considerable demands on working memory, impulse control, self-monitoring, and intent to facilitate independent problem-solving and productivity [12]. For the typically developing middle school child while learning success proceeds in a forward line which indicates a growing capacity for independence, demands are met via variable engagement of EF skills. For example, impulse control develops completely between 10 and 12 years old [13, 14]. Similar speed in organizational skills with the speed of processing, verbal fluency, multidimensional transition, and planning usually occurs during middle childhood [14].

Middle childhood is a time period in which attention and motivation are necessary and a child should be under observation. For successful learning, behavioral regulation must increase [15]. Children who are 6 years old start to make tasks more successfully that require impulse control, and at age 9, most children can self-monitor and correct their behavior moderately [16]. Children who manage the tasks of increased attention and regulation effectively are more resistant to situations such as blocking, dissatisfaction, insistence, and self-control. Emotional regulation should be underlined with increasing daily demands and challenges, especially in terms of disappointment, anxiety, and anger. However, the difficulties associated with attention and behavior control, which are frequently seen with attention deficit and hyperactivity disorder (ADHD) and disruptive behavior disorders (DBD), emphasize that there is a major hurdle in the development of executive functions. As difficulties arise such as inefficiency, carelessness, and poor self-control, executive dysfunction manifests itself [17].

The enhanced self-control capacity in this period is necessary to meet additional demands, especially in social areas. Young people in this age start to establish stronger ties with their peers, and the opportunities in playing and learning reinforce belonging. This social inclusion increases opportunities by providing a wider range of participation and influence across all aspects of executive control. Especially, trying to solve problems together gives children the opportunity to accept and consider the opinions of others in situations where they can develop and change their ideas and goals [18].

Cooperation and reconciliation-related activities help the child struggle on his/her own and master on these skills. A child who is weak about understanding society and solving problems in society also faces difficulties in social participation. A child who is not able to observe the wide range of perspectives, or a wide range of options offered during a group event, is usually incomplete in executive functions, and it is possible to observe that a child with faults on executive functions is affected by more than one area of socialization and academic skills [18, 19].

1.3. Executive functions in adolescents

Adolescence, in other words, upper cognitive access, is an important period in which an individual is able to make a strategic choice to increase learning capacity, evaluate options, and meet that demand. Ongoing development of the executive neural network (frontal lobe) explains the inconsistencies of high-level skills of adolescence [20]. Frontal functions, especially the dorsolateral prefrontal cortex and the orbitofrontal cortex areas, gradually begin to engage. In addition, there is a marked decrease in the gray matter of the cortex and an increase in white matter during this period [21]. While these important changes in brain structure change social awareness and expectations in this period, hormonal and physical changes improve the interaction between the individual and the environment [22]. For this reason, adolescents' capacities of awareness, decision-making, and problem-solving, which are highly affected by cognitive skills and emotional, social, and physical situations, also vary [23]. As a result, it is theorized that the development of executive functions in adolescence may be modulated in an emotional or social context. Luna and Sweeney also described adolescence as a "transition to an effective working relationship with the brain." During the adult period, executive networks become more consolidated and refined. Actions are more in sync with behaviors and interact more with others with better behavioral and emotional control [24].

Increasing independence and its capacity and managing multidimensional learning and behavioral demands develop during this period. This is a reflection of progress in the areas of attention control, flexibility and processing speed, capacity and working memory, planning, and problem-solving in conjunction with the increase in frontal cortex pruning and myelinization that occurs during adolescence [25].

While Anderson believes that cognitive flexibility and target-setting capacity mature up to the age of 12, some researchers later argue that executive functioning, memory, impulse control, and planning continue to evolve considerably in adolescence and early adulthood [26]. This theory was more widely accepted because of the proliferation of synapses at the beginning of adolescence. These developments turn into emotional decision-making and less responsive reactions to the will of the environment, and this is an appropriate response to the theory of self-control and social rules [27].

Disorder in the development of executive control during adolescence is present in psychopathology. The capacity to think before moving, to assess the appropriateness of one's answer, and to determine the most effective action that gives the desired result often varies in adolescence. However, in a typically developing young person, these skills become increasingly more effective over time [27]. Young people with impaired executive functions cannot make effective choices and cannot reach the result. In fact, while adolescents are more conscious at the beginning of pubertal maturation, they then enter into risky and sometimes reckless behavior and become more sensitive to others' views and assessments. This can make their relationships difficult with peers and adults [20].

2. Executive functions and its neurology

2.1. Executive functions and prefrontal cortex

Executive functions are interdependent and progressively acquired; high-level cognitive skills that occur in conjunction with the expansion and integration of cerebellar, subcortical, and prefrontal nerve networks during early childhood and adolescence until early adulthood. Because the development of nervous systems that support executive functions lasts too long, they are vulnerable to changes that occur during development, which can lead to multiple executive dysfunctions [20].

The prefrontal cortex has an important role in the development of executive functions. The prefrontal cortex is located in the anterior part of the premotor cortex and constitutes approximately one-third of the cortex (**Figure 1**). The neural connections between the prefrontal cortex, motor and sensory cortices, and the brain's subcortical structures are carefully regulated and are responsible for controlling, influencing, and regulating behavioral goals and behaviors. As the individuals mature, large neural networks that are responsible for learning and behavior become increasingly integrated and coordinated with prefrontal cortex-related networks. As a result, the regulation of high skill levels that lead to many behaviors is related to the neurodevelopmental processes of the mature brain. This contributes to the enhancement of coordination of communication and behavioral regulation related to executive functions [21].

At the beginning of life, subcortically managed neural processing is the primary ability to interact and understand sensory input, to interact more extensively with the environment, and to reinforce and remember these experiences over time. These experiences reinforce the link between more integrated sources of knowledge that are better understood by the ongoing myelination of the more integrated and mature brain (**Figure 2**). As the connections between the subcortical structures and the prefrontal cortex increase, attention and memory control increases. In infants and children who begun to walk, growth episodes are associated with increases in attention control and working memory capacity. Subsequent brain growth episodes occur at 6–8, 10–12, and 14–16 years of age. Coordination between the prefrontal cortex and regulatory and executive networks improves the communication further [22].

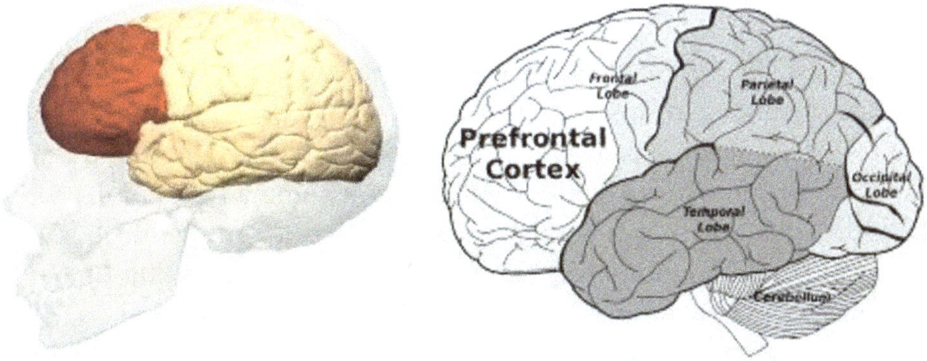

Figure 1. Prefrontal cortex.

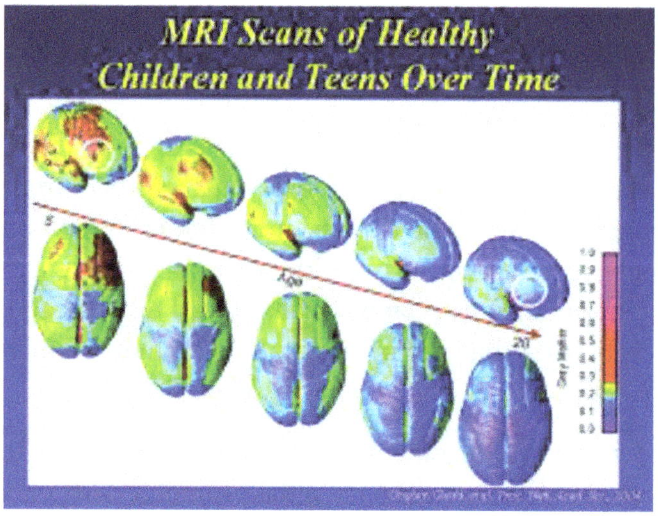

Figure 2. Development of the dorsolateral prefrontal cortex.

In the first years of life, the prefrontal cortex grows with its expanding nets which leads to the development of facilitation and memory increase. As the child progresses toward middle childhood, connections related to prefrontal cortex and communication develop. The development of the prefrontal cortex accelerates the development of information processing and cognitive flexibility between the ages of 7 and 9 years. These developments in the frontal system and related networks encourage the analysis and integration of complex information and the communication needed for effective decision-making. The prefrontal cortex is especially involved in impulse control and the following strategy development and self-monitoring [23].

Given the central role of the prefrontal cortex in the successful development of executive functions, lesions of this critical region have been associated with memory weakness, impulsivity, attention problems, and disorganization. It is known that the damage of the left dominant prefrontal cortex causes particularly the impairment of the divided attention. Contrary to the lateral prefrontal cortex, regions associated with the ventral and medial prefrontal cortex show strong neural connections toward the limbic system and amygdala and are therefore responsible for the integration of mainly emotional and nonemotional information. Given the nature of this relationship, damage to the medial prefrontal cortex means impaired activity initiation, and individuals with lesions in this region are typically irrelevant, flat, and unmotivated [24–26].

It is difficult to determine the contribution of a particular cortical area over the executive functions. Although studies to this date have indicated that the main area control is related to the prefrontal cortex and the component structures, it is seen that the indefinite variability persists. Although some investigations suggest that some aspects of executive functions may be related to certain subregions of the prefrontal cortex, much of this work has been completed with adult and nonhuman specimens [28]. For this reason, the age in which brainstem connections of executive functions are established and whether these distinctions are appropriate for children or not are yet unknown. Preliminary studies, however, show that children have larger and less specific work in brain regions during executive functions. For example, when children and adults were assessed for "Go/No-Go" tasks, while both groups showed functional magnetic resonance imaging (fMRI) activation in the anterior cingulate cortex, orbitofrontal cortex, and lower and middle frontal glands (**Figure 3**), children showed more activation on the anterior cingulate cortex and prefrontal cortex than adults [29]. These findings suggest that children work in wider areas of the prefrontal cortex during inhibitor tasks compared to adults. In a similar study, the increase in cortical activation on the left inferior frontal gyrus and orbitofrontal cortex due to the age is further emphasized; also it was shown that the activation of the left upper and middle frontal gyrus and anterior cingulate cortex decreased with age.

Another study that tackles the relationship between conflict resolution and cortical activation in children and adults, using event-related potentials, supports that executive functions become more productive as the brain signals become more mature [30].

Functions of the prefrontal cortex: *Inhibitory control* is described as the basis of the executive functions. Anterior prefrontal cortex is defined as the responsible area for impulse control in walking children and adolescence [31]. Impulse control processes are lateralized in the right hemisphere and are connected to the parietal lobes via ventral prefrontal cortex. At the same time, orbitofrontal cortex, anterior cingulate cortex, parietal and temporal cortex, and gyrus rectus are responsible for the impulse control [32]. A group of children with normal development, the ages between 4 years, 4 months, and 6 years, 8 months is the highest age for the cortex activation level with the working memory task [33]. This suggests that important morphological and structural changes affecting impulse control occur in the prefrontal cortex and the connected brain regions during childhood and adolescence.

Working memory depends on the prefrontal cortex activation, and tasks related to working memory development are age-related (especially during childhood) [32]. In the prefrontal cortex, in particular, the left middle frontal gyrus and the lower frontal gyrus are associated with working memory. The mid-frontal gyrus also plays a role in the control of automatic behaviors and competing answers and in responding to conflicting emotional intelligence. The right middle frontal gyrus is associated with judgmental response and the organization of the activity used to reach a goal [34].

The shifting, interaction with the prefrontal cortex, and its activation is a common finding with the adult period. The prefrontal cortex produces a strategy against the surrounding

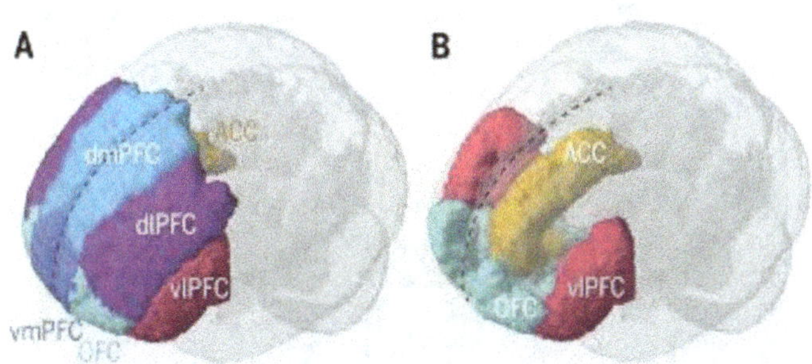

Figure 3. Dorsolateral prefrontal cortex, orbitofrontal cortex and anterior cingulate cortex.

information. This situation changes with regional activation differences, intelligence, and age. An event-related fMRI study investigated the performance of young adults and adults in the task of shifting attention using intelligence quotient (IQ) as a covariant and found that the average IQ individuals showed a higher activation of both prefrontal cortex and anterior cingulate cortex during the activation of response [35]. During the feedback, participants in the high IQ group showed a more complex relationship, including parietal, caudate, fusiform, and occipital regions. The authors reported that the feedback of high IQ people may be more strategic and they may experience less response overlap in the choice of responses for the task.

The prefrontal cortex is also associated with multitasking ability. The prefrontal cortex plays a role in the ability to hold knowledge as well. This feature is unique, prefrontal cortex neurons do not interrupt firing against a new stimulus [36]. This response pattern is useful in terms of showing maturity when individuals are forced to interfere independently with an increasingly complex and changing environment. Blakemore and Choudhury suggest that adult's multitasking skills are better than children or adolescents. Adolescents (aged 11–14) and children (aged 6–10) completed a number of tasks related to prospective memory with an adult group (mean age 25); results showed that adults use more effective strategies than adolescents or children. Thus, the prefrontal cortex also allows us to recall our daily life and the necessary information to achieve its mission despite disturbing stimuli [37].

2.2. Executive functions and limbic system

Regarding executive functions, the limbic system and prefrontal cortex, especially the anterior cingulate cortex are related to emotional regulation and processing, impulse control, and directing attention (**Figure 4**). An error monitoring task study on early adolescence, late adolescence, and adult performance revealed that the error rates were 11% in young adolescents, 7% in late adolescence, and in adulthood, it was even lower [38]. Potential related to the events during the mission localized on the anterior cingulate cortex or on its surroundings, which suggests that the difference in age-related task performance may be due to the maturation of the anterior cingulate cortex. Adults with good performance in an impulse control task were found to have larger anterior cingulate cortexes on magnetic resonance imaging (MRI) [39].

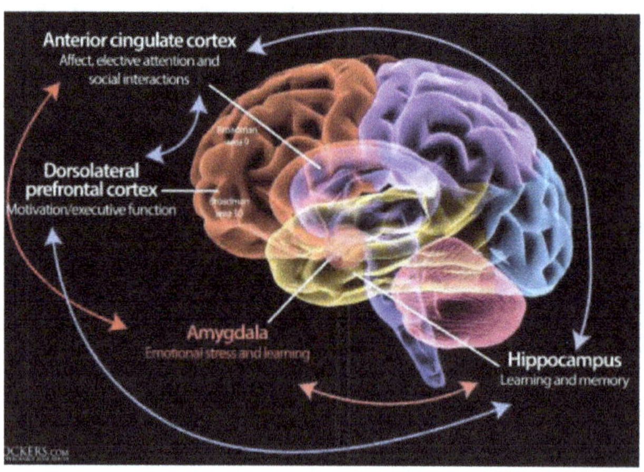

Figure 4. ACC with limbic system.

In addition, the relationship between anterior cingulate cortex and attention maintenance control is supported. According to Rueda and colleagues, the anterior cingulate cortex is a kind of "control rod" that allows the attention system to be arbitrary [40]. A group to define the relationship between anterior cingulate cortex and lateral prefrontal cortex during direct attention tasks showed that the anterior cingulate cortex takes place during tasks requiring continuous attention control and performance monitoring [41]. Another study examined the reciprocal relationship between emotional control and effort; hence, the anterior cingulate cortex has a proximity to emotional processing regions. Accordingly, the anterior cingulate cortex is associated with the cognitive evaluation of distressing photographs, thereby reducing the negative effect [42].

2.3. Parietal and temporal cortexes

Temporal and parietal cortexes are also important components of the executive net at the same time. Both temporal cortex and parietal cortex are associated with inhibitory control, set shifting, initiation, goal-directed behavior, and working memory (**Figure 5**). The upper parietal cortex plays a primary role in task change, regardless of whether the task involves verbal, visual, or spatial knowledge or not. Other areas of the parietal cortex are primarily responsible for initiating and completing targeted activities. It appears that the parietal cortex regions are also involved in updating the working memory. Especially, the upper left parietal region is linked to the current tasks of ongoing activity [43].

2.4. Executive functions and cerebellum

The cerebellum is a major but often a less well-understood component of the executive functions system. Cerebellum reaches its size at about 11 years for girls and 15 years for boys and is as important as regions that control executive function in early childhood [44]. Cerebellum gains maturity during motor control, emotional processing, and adolescence period and plays a central role in high cognitive functions. The cortico-ponto-cerebellar network works intensively in the timing and ordering of requests such as verbal working memory and executive aspects of visual and verbal analysis (**Figure 6**) [45]. In addition, it is also known

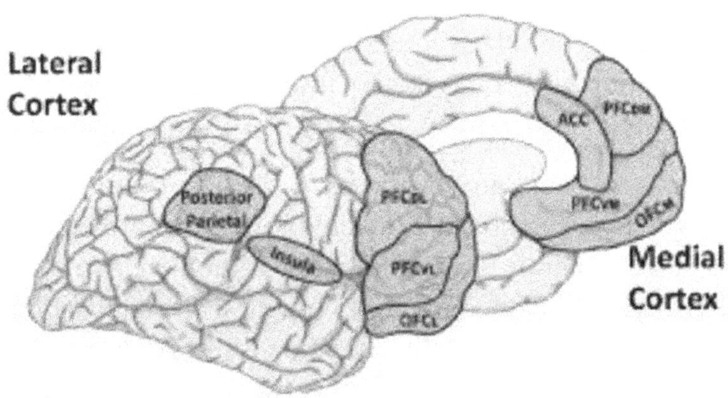

Figure 5. Prefrontal cortex and parietal cortex.

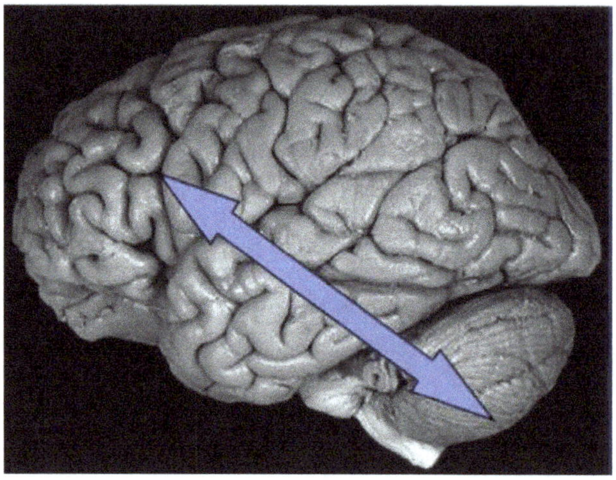

Figure 6. Prefrontal cortex and cerebellum.

that cerebellum has a modulating effect on emotional, cognitive, and regulatory capacities. However, cerebellar lesions do not appear to explain the impairment executive functions alone. It is thought that when executive dysfunctions are accompanied by cerebellar dysfunction, executive functions are impacted [46].

3. Dyslexia and executive functions

Evidence supports that executive functions are accompanied by learning difficulties (commonly known as learning disorder [LD]). In general, the first indicator of learning difficulty is the low rate of academic achievement in reading, mathematics, or writing [47–50].

Students with learning disabilities who have difficulty in planning, initiating activity, organizing thoughts and materials, self-monitoring and progression, impulse control, or attention shifting cannot learn as effectively as those who master these executive function skills [49]. While executive dysfunctions and learning disabilities often coexist, the relationship between executive dysfunctions and learning disability is still not fully established. A fundamental question is whether the specific characteristics of a particular academic field challenge are executive function difficulties or not. Even if there are no academic weaknesses, it is a bigger question to consider the difficulties of executive functioning as a learning disadvantage.

Phonological difficulties are seen as the greatest cause of reading difficulty, but the difficulty of executive functioning presents an additional difficulty in reading. A recent study has shown that children with dyslexia produce fewer words and complete fewer categorical tasks than typical readers in the semantic fluency task. In addition, in learning disorders, the meta-analyses of executive functions show that children with learning disabilities typically cannot achieve their peers' performance in executive function tests [51]. For example, a meta-analysis involving 48 studies, typically comparing the difficulties of executive functions on developing children with learning disability, attributed moderate (0.56) effect dimension on executive functions [52]. Wechsler intelligence scale for children- fourth edition (WISC-IV) Coding has distinguished and identified the participants with learning disability the most accurately from their typically developing peers. Similarly, the meta-analysis of 13 researchers comparing children with learning disorder and children with typical development has shown that the overall impact dimension which was measured by planning, organizing, strategy development, attention to detail, and recall tests for executive functions is moderate. Although verbal and visual working memory seems to be effective, verbal working memory has been shown to be more effective than visual working memory [53–56]. It is seen that the difference between the subjects with reading difficulty and typical readers increases with age. Overall, findings suggest a strong association between learning disability and executive functions [49, 57, 58].

Some studies have investigated the difficulties of executive functioning in subtypes of reading disorders. In particular, researchers compared the difficulty of reading a word with the difficulty of understanding reading. For example, in one study, adolescents were categorized as difficulty in reading a word, difficulty in isolated understanding, or typical reading achievement. Working memory and planning (when controlling attention, coding, fluency, and vocabulary) make a meaningful contribution to understanding what is being read but not word recognition. Findings of difficulty in planning have continued in adolescents who had difficulty understanding the reading even after controlling the accompanying ADHD and phonological processing ability. Although reading disorders are often accompanied by ADHD, these studies show that executive functioning difficulties may also occur in individuals without ADHD but reading-comprehension difficulties, and that the difficulties of strategic planning are closely related to the difficulties of understanding [58–60].

4. Evaluation of executive functions

During the individual assessment, a child's approach to a mission can reveal the strengths and weaknesses of executive functions. While some tests are designed to evaluate executive functions, each component of the evaluation process may provide different information about executive functions and disorders.

4.1. Key issues in evaluating executive functions

1. Almost every test contains executive functions. The executive function is related to many things, and it is impossible to draw conclusions from an evaluation alone. For example, even completing the most standard scales requires some planning, strategy, or impulse control. The opposite is also true; most of the tests described as primary "executive functioning evaluation tool" include other cognitive processes. This is called "task impurity" [61]. As a result, other tests (including intellectual work and academic achievement) and behavioral observations also provide information about executive functions. It is important to be aware of these elements and their role in evaluation and definition.
2. Standardization can remove features of executive functions. The structure of an ironically standardized test may reduce the requirements of some of the aspects of executive functions [62, 63]. Most of the standardized tests contain clear instructions and scoring. This

reduces the chances of the person who applies the test to observe executive dysfunctions that are more likely to appear in uncertain situations. Some uncommonly used tests due to difficulties in standardization include open-ended scenarios. A person can gather enough cognitive resources to perform executive functions tasks for a short period of time [64].

3. It is difficult to isolate the skills of a single executive function. Each aspect of the executive functions is intertwined, which makes it difficult to assess a single executive skill. For example, self-monitoring is part of impulse control or vice versa. These skills are different from each other, but it is difficult to distinguish them because they usually occur at the same time and affect each other. A low score on a test aiming to measure the performance of an executive function may reflect the difficulty in a different execution process.

4. The executive functions may vary depending on the environment. Unfortunately, when evaluating executive functions, a child can perform differently in different environments. This can be clearly seen even when comparing home and school, different classes or everyday challenges. In such cases, it is important to examine the people, circumstances, and all sources of information that would lead to confusion regarding the child's functions.

   For a child with executive dysfunction, some environments may have their own advantages (such as getting immediate, specific, explicit feedback from the teacher and learning in a highly structured classroom). The support and coherence of some people according to the nature of the child can intuitively increase this advantage. During interactive games, the success of the activity can be improved by providing clear, consistent, and clear results or awards for the child's actions. In such cases, it is important to include environmental factors in the developed treatment plan for the person and the activity success. It is important to gather information not only about the most challenging environment of the child's executive function but also in the environments that the child is successful at the same time. These exceptions may provide the data needed to describe the executive functioning difficulties and possible remediation strategies. It is important to assess the performance of the child in different environments (home/school and daily/laboratory).

5. Some factors can worsen (or heal) executive functions. These include self-care factors such as fatigue [65, 66], hunger [65], pain [67], stress [68], mood (positive or negative) [69], or lack of exercise [70]. Excessive stimulation with multiple sensory inputs (e.g. auditory, visual, and tactile) and multiple cognitive demands are also significant exacerbations [71, 72]. The sudden change of the surrounding and people around, a new teacher, new classroom, or new school may cause the difficulties in temporary executive functions occurrence. However, a child who is already struggling with compensation for executive function difficulties typically has less cognitive reserves [73]. The child is more vulnerable to the occurrence of any of these factors, and as soon as the effect of these factors accumulates, they become choked. For this reason, it is important to keep them under control. Teachers or their families can be informed of this by creating a checklist for various skills, such as self-care in children.

6. It is difficult to define appropriate peer comparison. It is important to identify the appropriate peer group when evaluating the executive functions. This allows you to make a

direct comparison. Given the "typical" expectations and differences, it provides an important contrast point. However, it is not easy to determine the best comparison group, as the appropriate comparison group can be chosen by age, gender, intellectual ability, school grade, or other factors.

7. A statistically significant inconsistency between average executive functions and a high IQ is not necessarily a clinical deficit [74, 75]. Compared to IQ scores, there are a number of factors that can lead to lower executive function scores. A person's low motor performance can cause average executive functions.

8. Disability is an important aspect of executive dysfunction. As in any circumstance, assessing the existence and degree of disability is also a necessary condition for examining executive functions. In cases where the child interferes with daily life, it will be difficult to provide parental, teacher, or student care. It is important to remember that even when there is an inconsistency between skill and executive function scores, there may be also a difficulty in obtaining or expecting developmentally expected benefits.

Executive function causes challenges in a range of areas including academic [76–79], emotional [16], behavioral [16], social [16, 79, 80], and adaptive functions [81]. When we think about many aspects of functioning, such as social interactions, family relationships, family responsibilities, and community involvement, and employment for adolescents and young adults, the success of the individual is greatly influenced by adaptation via limiting the actual independence of executive dysfunction [81].

It is also important to assess the effect of executive dysfunction on the functional and emotional well-being of the person. For example, a teenage girl in class may have difficulty in integrating and expressing emotional and social life-related feelings and thoughts. In addition, the struggle with the school can increase her anxiety by reducing its prosperity and self-confidence. These issues can further aggravate her executive functioning difficulty.

4.2. Rating scales

In its simplest form, the assessment scale is a list of items that are evaluated to identify the presence, frequency, and/or severity of a behavior, emotion, or thought. A number of evaluation scales have been developed over the past decade to help to define executive functions. In general, such assessment scales are thought to be more predictive of executive dysfunctions than laboratory tests [82]. This difference can be attributed to the contextual factors (clinic/home, school, community). This difficulty in assessing highlights the fact that it is important to understand the story of the assessed child.

When evaluating children, it is important to have age-based normative data. Smaller age groups allow the child's symptoms to be assessed more accurately in terms of appropriate development or consistent with a psychopathology. Many studies have shown a change in executive function performance during childhood and adolescence. Most of the statistical analyses for the assessment scales also show significant gender effects, against men in executive function ratings [83, 84].

Behavioral Rating Inventory of Executive Function, which is available for parents and teachers to complete developed to evaluate executive functions—for preschoolers (2–5 years old, BRIEF-P) and for school age children (aged 6–18 years). There is a self-report form for completion by youth 11– 18 years old (BRIEF-SR), as well as a group of forms for adults 18–90 years old (BRIEF-A). BRIEF was developed by a group of pediatric neuropsychologists who are collecting data on real-life executive function in the home and school environment. For this reason, expectations of daily adaptive needs and academic achievement provide reasonable information to parents and teachers. Normative data for BRIEF is somewhat restrictive because it is collected from a limited geographical area, and therefore may not represent the general population. EFBAI scores provide summaries of various aspects of executive functions (e.g. impulse, working memory, self-monitoring, etc.), and a clinician tells where and why a student struggles. It has been found that executive functions of BRIEF have a greater correlation with the descriptions of parents and teachers than the performance on laboratory tests and therefore considered to be a good standard tool for executive functions of the person.

Clearly, although executive functions are a tool for assessment. The Brown Attention Deficit Disorder Scales for Children and Adolescents (Brown ADD Scales) are based on the theory that attention deficit represents a developmental disorder of executive functioning. These assessment scales include organizing, prioritizing/activating, focusing/sustaining/recording attention, and executive functioning.

Conners 3 is another attention deficit and hyperactivity disorder (ADHD)-based assessment scale that includes executive functional aspects of the assessed areas. "Executive Functionality" includes the scale, initiation, time management, planning, prioritization, and organization concepts. Other scales in Conners 3 can also reflect executive functions such as attention/focus and self-control. The information obtained with Conners 3, such as the Brown ADD scale and BRIEF, can help identify the areas that require more focus and evaluation which leads to intervention initiatives [85].

Assessment scales such as the Behavior Assessment System for Children, Second Edition (BACS-2), the Conners Comprehensive Behavior Rating Scales (Conners CBRS), and the Achenbach System of Empirically Based Assessment (ASEBA) do not explicitly refer to executive functions, but they can provide information about executive functions. Comprehensive assessment scales such as these can help gathering relevant information in a broader context of issues beyond executive functions.

5. Conclusions

Unlike previous exams focusing on pre-school EF, this focus on EF focuses on a much larger age range. This view allows the study of the developmental form of EF, the gains in EF development, to be examined in the light of developments in behavioral and neural levels. Based on the developmental problems, the following research bases can be established: (1) to compare developmental progress of each EF component with a sample of a wide range of age and (2) to evaluate the developmental sequence of the EF component. Thus, cognitive neuroscience can provide a developmental theoretical focus on EFs for children with/without dyslexia.

Acknowledgements

Author thank to Gonca Bumin Prof PhD for useful feedback.

Conflict of interest

No conflicts of interest.

Author details

Gokcen Akyurek

Address all correspondence to: gkcnakyrk@gmail.com

Department of Occupational Therapy, Faculty of Health Science, Hacettepe University, Ankara, Turkey

References

[1] Jerison HJ. Evolution of prefrontal cortex. In: Krasnegor NA, Lyon GR, Rakic G, editors. Development of the Prefrontal Cortex. Baltimore, MD: Brookes; 1997. pp. 9-26

[2] Williamson J. A lifespan review of developmental neuroanatomy. In: Donders J, Hunter SJ, editors. Principles and Practice of Lifespan Developmental Neuropsychology. Cambridge, UK: Cambridge University Press; 2010. pp. 3-16

[3] Best JR, Miller PH. A developmental perspective on executive function. Child Development. 2010;**81**(6):1641-1660

[4] Diamond A, Barnett WS, Thomas J, Munro S. Preschool program improves cognitive control. Science. 2007;**318**(5855):1387-1388

[5] Hunter SJ, Edidin JP, Hinkle CD. The developmental neuropsychology of executive function. In: Hunter SJ, Sparrow EP, editors. Executive Function and Dysfunction İdentification, Assessment and Treatment. Cambridge, UK: Cambridge University Press; 2012. pp. 17-36

[6] Courage ML, Reynolds GD, Richards JE. Infants' attention of patterned stimuli: Developmental change from 3 to 12 months of age. Child Development. 2006;**77**(3):680-695

[7] Posner MI, Rothbart MK. Educating the Human Brain. Washington, DC: American Psychological Association; 2007

[8] Anderson V, Anderson PJ, Jacobs R, Smith MS. Development and assessment of executive function: From preschool to adolescence. In: Anderson V, Jacobs R, Anderson P, editors.

Executive Functions and the Frontal Lobes: A Lifespan Perspective. Philadelphia, PA: Taylor & Francis; 2008. pp. 123-154

[9] Sheese BE, Rothbart MK, Posner MI, White LK, Fraundorf SH. Executive attention and self-regulation in infancy. Infant Behavior & Development. 2008;**31**(3):501-510

[10] Bernier A, Carlson SM, Whipple N. From external regulation to self-regulation: Early parenting precursors to young children's executive functioning. Child Development. 2010;**81**(1):326-339

[11] Calkins SD. The emergence of self- regulation: Biological and behavioral control mechanisms supporting toddler competencies. In: Brownell CA, Kopp CB, editors. Socioemotional Development in the Toddler Years: Transitions and Transformations. New York, NY: Guilford Press; 2007. pp. 1-45

[12] Denckla MB. Introduction: ADHD and modifiers of the syndrome: Influences on educational outcomes. Developmental Disabilities Research Reviews. 2008;**14**(4):259-260

[13] Brocki K, Fan J, Fossella J. Placing neuroanatomical models of executive function in a developmental context: Imaging and imaging-genetic strategies. In: Pfaff DW, Kieffer BL, editors. Molecular and Biophysical Mechanisms of Arousal, Alertness, and Attention. Boston, MA: Blackwell Publishing; 2008. pp. 246-255

[14] Brocki KC, Bohlin G. Executive functions in children aged 6 to 13: A dimensional and developmental study. Developmental Neuropsychology. 2004;**26**(2):571-593

[15] Valiente C, Lemery-Chalfant K, Castro KS. Children's effortful control and academic competence mediation through school liking. Science. 2007;**53**(1):1-25

[16] Anderson P. Assessment and development of executive function (EF) during childhood. Child Neuropsychology. 2002;**8**(2):71-82

[17] Geurts HM, Verté S, Oosterlaan J, Roeyers H, Sergeant JA. ADHD subtypes: Do they differ in their executive functioning profile? Archives of Clinical Neuropsychology. 2005;**20**(4): 457-477

[18] Fahie CM, Symons DK. Executive functioning and theory of mind in children clinically referred for attention and behavior problems. Journal of Applied Developmental Psychology. 2003;**24**(1):51-73

[19] Luciana M, Conklin HM, Hooper CJ, Yarger RS. The development of nonverbal working memory and executive control processes in adolescents. Child Development. 2005;**76**: 697-712

[20] Pharo H, Sim C, Graham M, Gross J, Hayne H. Risky business: Executive function, personality, and reckless behavior during adolescence and emerging adulthood. Behavioral Neuroscience. 2011;**125**(6):970-978

[21] Giedd JN, Blumenthal J, Jeffries NO, et al. Brain development during childhood and adolescence: A longitudinal MRI study. Nature Neuroscience. 1999;**2**(1):861-863

[22] Steinberg L. Cognitive and affective development in adolescence. Trends in Cognitive Sciences. 2005;**9**(2):69-74

[23] De Luca CR, Leventer RJ. Developmental trajectories of executive functions across the lifespan. In: Anderson V, Jacobs R, Anderson P, editors. Executive Functions and the Frontal Lobes: A Lifespan Perspective. Philadelphia, PA: Taylor & Francis; 2008. pp. 23-56

[24] Luna B, Sweeney JA. The emergence of collaborative brain function: fMRI studies of the development of response inhibition. In: Dahl RE, Spear LP, editors. Adolescent Brain Development: Vulnerabilities and Opportunities. New York, NY: New York Academy of Sciences; 2004. pp. 296-309

[25] Blakemore S, Choudhury S. Development of the adolescent brain: Implications for executive function and social cognition. Journal of Child Psychology and Psychiatry. 2006;**47**(3-4):296-312

[26] Anderson PJ. Towards a developmental model of executive function. In: Anderson V, Jacobs R, Anderson P, editors. Executive Functions and the Frontal Lobes: A Lifespan Perspective. Philadelphia, PA: Taylor & Francis; 2008. pp. 3-21

[27] Smith DG, Xiao L, Bechara A. Decision making in children and adolescents: Impaired Iowa gambling task performance in early adolescence. Developmental Psychology;**2011**:1-8. DOI: 10.1037/a0026342

[28] Morton JB. Understanding genetic, neurophysiological, and experiential influences on the development of executive functioning: The need for developmental models. WIREs Cognitive Science. 2010;**1**(5):709-723

[29] Cragg L, Nation K. Go or no-go? Developmental improvements in the efficiency of response inhibition in mid-childhood. Developmental Science. 2008;**11**:819-827

[30] Rueda MR, Posner MI, Rothbart MK. The development of executive attention: Contributions to the emergence of self- regulation. Developmental Neuropsychology. 2005; **28**(2):573-594

[31] Diamond A. The early development of executive functions. In: Bialystok E, Craik FIM, editors. Lifespan Cognition: Mechanisms of Change. New York, NY: Oxford University Press; 2006. pp. 70-95

[32] Tamnes CK, stby Y, Walhovd KB, Westlye LT, Due-Tønnessen P, Fjell AM. Neuroanatomical correlates of executive functions in children and adolescents: A magnetic resonance imaging (MRI) study of cortical thickness. Neuropsychologia. 2010;**48**(9): 2496-2508

[33] Tsujimoto S, Yamamoto T, Kawaguchi H, Koizumi H, Sawaguchi T. Functional Maturation of the Prefrontal Cortex in Preschool Children Measured by Optical Topography. Program No. 196.15. 2003 Abstract Viewer/Itinerary Planner. Washington, DC: Society for Neuroscience; 2003

[34] Spielberg JM, Miller GA, Engels AS, et al. Trait approach and avoidance motivation: Lateralized neural activity associated with executive function. NeuroImage. 2011;**54**(1): 661-670

[35] Graham S, Jiang J, Manning V, et al. IQ- related fMRI differences during cognitive set shifting. Cerebral Cortex. 2010;**20**(3):641-649

[36] Arnsten AFT, Bao-Ming L. Neurobiology of executive functions: Catecholamine influences on prefrontal cortical functions. Biological Psychiatry. 2005;**57**(11):1377-1384

[37] Mackinlay R, Charman T, Karmiloff- Smith A. Remembering to Remember: A Developmental Study of Prospective Memory in a Multitasking Paradigm: Biennial Meeting of the Society for Research in Child Development; 2003 Apr 24-27; Tampa, FL

[38] LaDouceur CD, Dahl RE, Carter CS. Development of action monitoring through adolescence into adulthood: ERP and source localization. Developmental Science. 2007; **10**(6):874-891

[39] Brocki K, Clerkin SM, Guise KG, Fan J, Fossella JA. Assessing the molecular genetics of the development of executive attention in children: Focus on genetic pathways related to the anterior cingulate cortex and dopamine. Neuroscience. 2009;**164**(1):241-246

[40] Fan J, McCandliss BD, Sommer T, Raz A, Posner MI. Testing the efficiency and independence of attentional networks. Journal of Cognitive Neuroscience. 2002;**14**(3):340-347

[41] Osaka N, Osaka M, Kondo H, Morishita M, Fukuyama H, Shibasaki H. The neural basis of executive function in working memory: An fMRI study based on individual differences. NeuroImage. 2004;**21**:623-631

[42] Ochsner KN, Bunge SA, Gross JJ, Gabrieli JDE. Rethinking feelings: An fMRI study of the cognitive regulation of emotion. Journal of Cognitive Neuroscience. 2002;**14**(8):1215-1229

[43] Collette F, Hogge M, Salmon E, van der Linden M. Exploration of the neural substrates of executive functioning by functional neuroimaging. Neuroscience. 2006;**139**(1):209-221

[44] Giedd JN, Stockman M, Weddle C, et al. Anatomic magnetic resonance imaging of the developing child and adolescent brain and effects of genetic variation. Neuropsychology Review. 2010;**20**(4):349-361

[45] Ramnani N, Behrens TE, Johansen-Berg H, et al. The evolution of prefrontal inputs to the cortico-pontine system: Diffusion imaging evidence from macaque monkeys and humans. Cerebral Cortex. 2006;**16**(6):811-818

[46] Steinlin M. Cerebellar disorders in childhood: Cognitive problems. Cerebellum. 2008;**7**(4): 607-610

[47] Fuchs D, Compton DL, Fuchs LS, Bryant J, Davis GN. Making "secondary intervention" work in a three-tier responsiveness-to-intervention model: Findings from the first-grade longitudinal reading study of the National Research Center on learning disabilities. Reading and Writing. 2008;**21**:413-436

[48] McMaster KL, Fuchs D, Fuchs LS, Compton DL. Responding to nonresponders: An experimental field trial of identification and intervention methods. Exceptional Children. 2005;(4):445-463

[49] Johnson ES, Humphrey M, Mellard DF, Woods K, Swanson HL. Cognitive processing deficits and students with specific learning disabilities: A selective meta-analysis of the literature. Learning Disability Quarterly. 2010;**33**:3-18

[50] Kavale KA. Identifying specific learning disability: Is responsiveness to intervention the answer? Journal of Learning Disabilities. 2005;**38**:553-562

[51] Borella E, Carretti B, Pelegrina S. The specific role of inhibition in reading comprehension in good and poor comprehenders. Journal of Learning Disabilities. 2010;**43**:541-551

[52] Booth JN, Boyle JME, Kelly SW. Do tasks make a difference? Accounting for heterogeneity of performance of children with reading difficulties on tasks of executive function: Findings from a meta- analysis. The British Journal of Developmental Psychology. 2010;**28**:133-176

[53] Fletcher JM, Francis DJ, Rourke BP, Shaywitz SE, Shaywitz BA. The validity of discrepancy-based definitions of reading disabilities. Journal of Learning Disabilities. 1992;**25**:555-561

[54] Vellutino FR, Scanlon DM, Lyon GR. Differentiating between difficult-to- remediate and readily remediated poor readers: More evidence against the IQ- achievement discrepancy definition of reading disability. Journal of Learning Disabilities. 2000;**33**:223-238

[55] Siegel LS. IQ is irrelevant to the definition of learning disabilities. Journal of Learning Disabilities. 1989;**22**:469-479

[56] Stuebing K, Fletcher JM, LeDoux JM, Lyon GR, Shaywitz SE, Shaywitz BA. Validity of IQ-discrepancy classification of reading difficulties: A meta-analysis. American Educational Research Journal. 2002;**39**:469-518

[57] Swanson HL, Sachse-Lee C. Mathematical problem solving and working memory in children with learning disabilities: Both executive and phonological processes are important. Journal of Experimental Child Psychology. 2001;**79**:294-321

[58] Gathercole SE, Alloway TP, Willis C, Adams A-M. Working memory in children with reading disabilities. Journal of Experimental Child Psychology. 2006;**93**:265-281

[59] Locascio G, Mahone EM, Eason SH, Cutting LE. Executive dysfunction among children with reading comprehension deficits. Journal of Learning Disabilities. 2010;**43**:441-454

[60] Cutting LE, Materek A, Cole CAS, Levine TM, Mahone EM. Effects of fluency, oral language, and executive function on reading comprehension performance. Annals of Dyslexia. 2009;**59**:34-54

[61] Burgess PW. Theory and methodology in executive function research. In: Rabbitt P, editor. Methodology of Frontal and Executive Function. Hove, England: Psychology Press; 1997. pp. 81-116

[62] Lezak MD. The problem of assessing executive functions. International Journal of Psychology. 1982;**17**:281-297

[63] Bernstein J, Waber D. Developmental neuropsychological assessment: The systemic approach. In: Boulton A, Baker G, Hiscock M, editors. Neuromethods: Neuropsychology. Clifton, NJ: Humana Press; 1990. pp. 311-371

[64] Barkley R, Murphy K. The nature of executive function (EF) deficits in daily life activities in adults with ADHD and their relationship to performance on EF tests. Journal of Psychopathology and Behavioral Assessment. 2011;**33**(2):137-135

[65] Ståhle L, Ståhle EL, Granström E, Isaksson S, Annas P, Sepp H. Effects of sleep or food deprivation during civilian survival training on cognition, blood glucose and 3-OH-butyrate. Wilderness & Environmental Medicine. 2011;**22**(3):202-210

[66] Waters F, Bucks RS. Neuropsychological effects of sleep loss: Implication for neuropsychologists. Journal of the International Neuropsychological Society. 2011;**4**:571-586

[67] Abeare CA, Cohen JL, Axelrod BN, Leisen JC, Mosley-Williams A, Lumley MA. Pain, executive functioning, and affect in patients with rheumatoid arthritis. The Clinical Journal of Pain. 2010;**26**(8):683-689

[68] Arnsten AF. The biology of being frazzled. Science. 1998;**280**(5370):1711-1712

[69] Mitchell RL, Phillips LH. The psychological, neurochemical and functional neuroanatomical mediators of the effects of positive and negative mood on executive functions. Neuropsychologia. 2007;**45**(4):617-629

[70] Chaddock L, Pontifex MB, Hillman CH, Kramer AF. A review of the relation of aerobic fitness and physical activity to brain structure and function in children. Journal of the International Neuropsychological Society. 2011;**17**(6):975-985

[71] Rogers SJ, Ozonoff S. Annotation: What do we know about sensory dysfunction in autism? A critical review of the empirical evidence. Journal of Child Psychology and Psychiatry. 2005;**46**(12):1255-1268

[72] Iarocci G, McDonald J. Sensory integration and the perceptual experience of persons with autism. Journal of Autism and Developmental Disorders. 2006;**36**(1):77-90

[73] Suchy Y. Executive functioning: Overview, assessment, and research issues for non-neuropsychologists. Annals of Behavioral Medicine. 2009;**37**(2):106-116

[74] Dodrill CB. Myths of neuropsychology. The Clinical Neuropsychologist. 1997;**11**(1):1-17

[75] Dodrill CB. Myths of neuropsychology: Further considerations. The Clinical Neuropsychologist. 1999;**13**(4):562-572

[76] Rabin LA, Fogel J, Nutter-Upham KE. Academic procrastination in college students: The role of self-reported executive function. Journal of Clinical and Experimental Neuropsychology. 2011;**33**(3):344-357

[77] Bull R, Espy KA, Wiebe SA. Short-term memory, working memory, and executive functioning in preschoolers: Longitudinal predictors of mathematical achievement at age 7 years. Developmental Neuropsychology. 2008;**33**(3):205-228

[78] Johnson S, Wolke D, Hennessy E, Marlow N. Educational outcomes in extremely preterm children: Neuropsychological correlates and predictors of attainment. Developmental Neuropsychology. 2011;**36**(1):74-95

[79] Miller M, Hinshaw SP. Does childhood executive function predict adolescent functional outcomes in girls with ADHD? Journal of Abnormal Child Psychology. 2010;**38**(3):315-326

[80] Rinsky JR, Hinshaw SP. Linkages between childhood executive functioning and adolescent social functioning and psychopathology in girls with ADHD. Child Neuropsychology. 2011;**17**(4):368-390

[81] Harrison PL, Oakland T. Adaptive Behavior Assessment System, 2nd EDN (ABAS-II) Manual. San Antonio, Texas: The Psychological Corporation; 2003

[82] Barkley RA, Murphy KR. Impairment in occupational functioning and adult ADHD: The predictive utility of executive function (EF) ratings versus EF tests. Archives of Clinical Neuropsychology. 2010;**25**(3):157-173

[83] Conners CK. Conners 3rd Edition (Conners 3) Manual. Toronto, ON, Canada: Multi-Health Systems, Inc; 2008

[84] Gioia GA, Isquith PK, Guy SC, Kenworthy L. Test review behavior rating inventory of executive function. Child Neuropsychology. 2000;**6**(3):235-238

[85] McAuley T, Chen S, Goos L, Schachar R, Crosbie J. Is the behavior rating inventory of executive function more strongly associated with measures of impairment or executive function? Journal of the International Neuropsychological Society. 2010;**16**:495-505

8

Occupational Therapy in Forensic Settings

Esma Ozkan, Sümeyye Belhan, Mahmut Yaran and
Meral Zarif

Abstract

It is necessary for a person to comply with the expectations of society and the rules of law to which these expectations are secured. Offenders turn back to the community after the penalty was executed by isolating from society and some occupations. An occupational imbalance is seen in the individuals, during this penalty period and afterward, because of limited occupational participation. As an occupational being, this affects their physical, mental and psychological well-being. Imprisonment is an important practice in criminal law to punish criminals. This may be necessary for the protection of society from criminals, but successful integration into a community after exiting the prison is the most important factor in preventing recidivism. Occupational therapy focuses on health and well-being by using meaningful and purposeful occupations. Occupation involves any activity that people perform or participate in, such as giving care to themselves or others, working, learning, playing games, and interacting with others. From this perspective, the role of occupational therapists in forensic settings is to determine the abilities of these individuals to congregate their deprived freedoms and use them to train them for an independent and autonomous life; to provide a professional orientation, career counseling, and self-esteem; to gain some habits for physical, spiritual and moral life and to reinforce.

Keywords: forensic setting, occupational therapy, recidivism, offender, intervention

1. Introduction

Human is a social being, which occupies in different ways to survive. Occupations are all of the daily activities in one's life that make him who he is. Occupations are formed by cultural backgrounds and include all the tasks performed to fulfill the time and give life meaning. Occupational therapy is a treatment option for individuals with physical, mental or developmental conditions that focus on health and well-being by using meaningful and purposeful occupations for individuals for the development, improvement or maintenance of the essential skills needed to be successful in their environment [1].

Forensic occupational therapy refers the occupational therapy service that assesses and makes interventions to the individuals with occupational problems in the criminal justice system [2]. The forensic settings can be variable and be challenging, but the main point here to pay attention is the holistic and humanistic view of occupational therapy which says that occupation is vital for human and is essential for health and well-being. From this view, forensic occupational therapy is the same as the mental health occupational therapy practice in some ways [3]. The main difference is the legal context and the restrictive correctional environment. The legal context is usually built upon deprivation of some occupations, and this alienates the individual to the occupation. Also, labeling and stigma affect reintegration to the community [4].

In terms of the individual, occupational therapy is an important necessity for occupational participation and occupational balance. With these, occupational therapy prepares the person for community life and protects the individual from recidivism [5]. This is not the sole benefit of occupational therapy. Also, there are benefits for the community; reducing crime provides social well-being and also increases social welfare by contributing to the individual's productivity activities, so that, forensic occupational therapy has dual aim both for the individual and the community.

The forensic population is growing all over the world and brings challenges with this growing population [5–8]. These challenges can depend on the person, environment and/or activity. The thing that should never be ignored is the legal context, and the therapists must consider the needs of individuals in the legal context [9].

Offenders' rehabilitation is a multidisciplinary teamwork, and occupational therapy is a key part of the treatment and rehabilitation. The methods are similar to other mental health settings. The key focuses for the occupational therapists working in forensic settings are assessment, prevention of occupational deprivation, development of occupations to prevent recidivism, preparation for discharge and activities of daily living (ADLs), preparation to community and the vocational rehabilitation.

This chapter describes the occupational therapy in forensic settings such as prisons, secure hospitals and community reintegration services. The chapter also discusses the assessments, models that can be used in forensic settings, interventions and challenges in forensic settings.

2. Forensic settings

Correctional administration is the reinstatement and retraining of a person's antisocial behavior and feelings through confinement for treatment purposes. Correctional settings regulate the individual's psychosocial status and provide health care service for the prisoners [10].

Correctional settings are a way to facilitate the mental health recovery of the inmates. Since, many of the inmates have serious mental disorders, the forensic unit, of the correctional facility, plays an important part in their recovery. The unit reduces the risk associated with the inmates and facilitates their transition into the community or less restricted settings. However, the same results could be achieved with occupational therapists. The two main methods that are adopted by occupational therapists (OTs) are the reduction of occupation deprivation and increasing skills by occupational participation. Hence, the inmates are provided with an opportunity to play a purposeful and meaningful occupation in society [3].

Patients, who are admitted to the forensic units and get in contact with the criminal justice system as a consequence of their committed crimes, are detained in accordance with the country-specific mental health legislation. However, some patients are admitted due to severe behavioral issues.

There are several types of correctional settings where charged offenders are held. The main institutions are forensic mental health settings, jails and prisons. Forensic mental health settings include the following: high secure units, medium secure units, low secure units, psychiatric/acute mental health units, community, forensic hostel, special hospital, acute unit of a forensic hospital, high-security section of a forensic hospital, sub-acute unit of a forensic hospital, consultation/liaison position in the community sector, tertiary mental health facility, extended forensic/psychiatric safe care and medium to high secure unit [11].

Jails and prisons are the main correctional facilities since they are able to hold the greatest number of people. There are approximately 12 million jail admissions, which is approximately 19 times that of state and federal prisons [12].

Jails and prisons served for different purposes; have restricted opportunities for rehabilitation; offer a similar grade of occupational deprivation, inadequate access to health services and poorly planned methods; are temporary in nature and lack systematic regulation and resources [13].

Jails and prisons provide care for mentally disturbed offenders in ill-equipped correctional institutions. In particular, jails are used for temporary confinement and are usually lacking in mental health screenings and treatment received by inmates in jails is more limited. Prisons, however, might offer inmates the opportunity to access consulting service for substance abuse treatment even though the service delivery is generally insufficient [14].

2.1. Jails

Jails serve as an introduction to the incarceration system. They are local correctional facilities operated by a city or country instead of the federal or state government. The main purpose of jails and prisoner distribution centers is to confine a person before and after court judgments and to filter prisoners to and from courts and other correctional facilities. Some people in jails have been sentenced, while others might be waiting to be convicted. Many individuals receive an imprisonment of less than 2 years [3].

Judgment is mostly a complex process of sentencing. In this respect, inmates in forensic settings might either be arraigned or experiencing the trial process.

2.2. Prisons

Prisons are classified as high, medium and low security institutions that are typically used for convicted criminals who have been sentenced to at least a year of imprisonment in U.S. Federal Bureau of Prisons. In addition, depending on the severity of the crime, some individuals are sentenced to either state or federal prisons. However, compared to jails, prisons offer a far more stable environment for the inmates and restrict their interaction with society for longer periods of time [3].

The primary purpose of prisons is to ensure public safety and the security of inmates. In addition to incarcerating criminals, prisons offer them programs to address their criminogenic needs related to education, substance abuse, employment and transition to the community.

Basic services in prisons involve intake and screening of psychotropic medicines and to provide occupational therapy services. Those services are substantially provided for prisoners to decrease their social isolation and increase their problem solving and adaptation skills, self-efficacy and self-esteem. The occupational therapy services also promote emotional regulation abilities and social and emotional skills in order for the inmate to deal with prison life and take this opportunity to improve on self-efficacy and occupational engagement [15].

1. High-security units: Individuals classified as high risk to public safety have been sentenced to life imprisonment and are receiving long term treatment, are housed in high-security prisons. The physical environment in these facilities consists of a number of physical and structural barriers between the facilities and the external environment of the institution.

   In high-security prisons with highest number of staff, and both multiple and single cells, criminals remain in their cells or in an outer cage in the facilities' yard. Each cell is equipped with a toilet, screwed to its floor, and prisoners are permitted up to three 10-min showers per week. Movement is firmly restricted and activity within the cellblock does not occur without other constraints, such as handcuffs, leg irons and corrective officer escorts [3]. Orientation can be considered as essential because it gives the staff the chance to be acquainted with the prisoners. The ward program focus areas, such as improving awareness of self, others and the environment; orientation to time, place and situation; probing cognitive abilities and teaching of new skills to improve leisure time use and psychomotor activation, should be maintained after discharge [16].

2. Medium-security prisons: Those institutions house individuals with a criminal background and requiring 2–5 years of treatment [17]. Medium-security prisons, where prisoners' accessibility to prison gardens and exercise areas, libraries, showers and health services are high, offer far more opportunities in terms of interaction, movement and activity in-between prisoners [3]. Medium-security prisons usually have a wide diversity of work-oriented and treatment programs. Parole is more frequently granted in medium-security prisons and may be classified as supervised (always less than 1 h), limited (sent to wards for only 1 or 2 h), occupational therapy parole (join structured activities or subcontract work) and unlimited parole (mostly on weekends and during the week when they do not join specific rehabilitation activities).

Patients included in the rehabilitation process are integrated into community life by developing intellectual and emotional insight, self-care and self-expression skills and general work abilities. Furthermore, providing stress and anger management, psychoeducation and prevention programs for substance abuse in psychoeducation groups facilitates the patients/inmates return to society [16].

3. Low-security prisons: These facilities have windows and open spaces that allow the prisoners to move and interact freely within the environment. Even though low-security prisons are surrounded by double-rings, they have no prison fences or other secured perimeter and are often unpatrolled by armed guards. Since the inmates might work on agriculture, transport or conservation projects, they can provide training to the prison's staff; in addition to meeting the labor force needs of other institutions [3].

   In open wards (low or minimum-security prisons), during the therapeutic leave and discharge periods, greater priority is given to preparation of patient participation. Patients are expected to adhere to hospital rules and regulations, but are allowed to freely leave their wards and take the opportunity to practice skills acquired in the medium secure wards and joining educational training programs outside the health services [3].

The intensive life skills training program is comprised of communication, conflict management and criticism handling, problem-solving, money handling (budgeting, current price trends) and work-related skills (job seeking, application for a job, writing of curriculum vitae, work interviews through the use of role play). In addition, recreational activity program, and specific work skills-related programs are implemented to enhance psychosocial interactions [15, 16].

2.3. Forensic hospitals

Forensic psychiatric settings are generally located in secure units that rehabilitate individuals deemed unfit to stand trial or not criminally responsible. Those inmates pose a serious threat to either themselves or others because of severe mental illness. A forensic psychiatric setting provides treatment-based approaches with a view to rehabilitating patients while keeping the public safe. Patients, temporarily transferred from correctional facilities or incarcerated environment, are assessed and treated for mental illness in the facility that consists of secure, closed and open common units [17].

Forensic psychiatric hospitals reintegrate patients systematically into the community with well-equipped and specialized clinical services, as well as an exhaustive range of vocational and rehabilitative programs. Treatment is typically long-term, in order to improve and safely stabilize patients' mental well-being.

2.4. Community reentry centers

Reentry centers are facilities that help inmates by offering structured and supervised residential settings just before or after their release. In addition to providing a permanent residence to the individuals, assistance in financial management and facilitating, their return to the society is also arranged. These centers might be especially useful, because the psychological adaptation required for offenders, with expansive criminal histories, returning to the community after a long period of imprisonment, can be particularly demanding.

A crucial component of community reentry centers is substance abuse management and mental health treatment and counseling. Growing prison populations are largely due to drug-related crime and drug abuse, but relatively few prisoners receive the appropriate treatment. In this respect, community-based correctional settings have launched out prison-based drug treatment programs during the past few years [3].

2.5. Psychological models in forensic rehabilitation

There are two main models of psychology about correctional treatment. The risk, need and responsivity model (RNR model) was built up by Andrews and Bonta, and they describe the criminal risk variables named 'central eight' (**Tables 1**) [18]. Good lives model (GLM) is the other model which claims, that rather than addressing criminogenic needs, the focus of treatment should be on the enhancement offenders' abilities to obtain primary human goods [19]. Purvis describes 11 primary human goods (**Tables 2**) [20].

If it is examined the models, both are similar, but RNR Model is based on cognitive-behavioral and the GLM is based on humanistic philosophy. The GLM identifies 11 'primary human goods' and RNR identifies 'central eight' which are inverse overlap. It can be said that GLM 'primary human goods' are inverse restatements of the 'central eight' risk factors, viewed from the lens of humanistic psychology [19]. Depending on these criminal risk factors, it is argued that the criminal procedure of the individual can be predicted and therefore the criminal procedure can be prevented by taking the necessary precautions. However, the RNR model is not compatible with occupational therapy outlook in the view of the possibility of irreversible risk factors and bias holding against the individual.

1. History of antisocial behavior: If there is an early involvement in antisocial acts and if they are still continuing, it is a big risk variable.

2. Antisocial personality: Adventurous, pleasure-seeking, poor self-control personality pattern are other risk factors.

3. Antisocial cognition: Attitudes, values and beliefs supporting crime cause a personal identity favorable to crime.

4. Antisocial associates: Quality of relationship affects the behavior. So that, having close association with criminal peers and relative isolation from prosocial others because of either the individual or the community affects the criminal behavior.

5. Family/marital: Problematic circumstances of home, lack of nurturing relationship and/or poor monitoring behavior.

6. School/work: Circumstances such as low levels of performance and satisfaction in school or work

7. Leisure/recreation: Low levels of involvement and satisfaction in prosocial activities such as leisure time activities

8. Substance abuse: Abuse of alcohol or drugs affects the criminal behaviors.

Table 1. The 'central eight' criminal risk variables.

1. **Life** (including healthy living and optimal physical functioning, sexual satisfaction)
2. **Knowledge**(how well informed one feels about things that are important to them)
3. **Excellence in work** (including mastery experiences)
4. **Excellence in play** (hobbies and recreational pursuits)
5. **Excellence in agency** (autonomy and self-directedness)
6. **Inner peace** (freedom from emotional turmoil and stress)
7. **Relatedness** (including intimate, romantic and family relationships)
8. **Community** (connection to wider social groups)
9. **Spirituality** (in the broad sense of finding meaning and purpose in life)
10. **Pleasure** (feeling good in the here and now)
11. **Creativity** (expressing oneself through alternative forms)

Table 2. The 'primary human goods'.

3. Occupational therapy models in forensic rehabilitation

The use of occupational therapy models in forensic rehabilitation focus on client-centered, holistic and occupation-focused practice with the approach of clinical reasoning based on individual preferences and needs. Normally, individuals engage in occupations which they prefer or want throughout their life; however, in secure environment situations, this ability of the individual can be limited or can be restricted by the individual's mental health/disorder/learning disability, their perceived and their actual risks to themselves or others and institutional regulations, policies or legal restrictions. Individuals who need forensic rehabilitation face some participation limitations to all or a combination of activities and this can cause occupational deprivation additionally to the sense of hopelessness and poor mental health [6, 11, 15]. Moreover, community life skills and performing daily living activities and interaction with the environment of the individual can be limited. Therefore, group or individual occupational therapy programs often target basic living skills, self-care, vocational skills, adaptive coping strategies, creative arts and anger or stress management. The general aim of occupational therapy is to enable individual to experience occupational enrichment and achieve optimal occupational functioning. Occupational enrichment in forensic settings can be considered as both the goal and process of occupational therapy interventions, so evidence-based practice is very important [15].

Occupational therapy guideline recommendations show that Model of Human Occupation (MOHO) and its associated assessments are the most used occupational therapy model in forensic occupational therapy. The model was developed in the 1980s by Professor Gary Kielhofner and has had some revisions and collaborations until now. MOHO supports that human occupation is motivated, patterned and performed. Humans are conceptualized as three interrelated components: volition, habituation and performance capacity [16]. Also, environmental considerations are very important to increase the occupational participation of the individual having forensic occupational therapy and rehabilitation [15].

Volition presents the individual's motivation for occupation and relates to individual's motivation to participate to occupations combined with their self-belief and capacity to succeed which means personal causation. Motivation and personal causation can be affected by the individual's mental health (such as depression, schizophrenia, personality disorder) or their perception of the reason and need for their admission. Therefore, the literature supports that it is important to establish the individual's own goals to ensure treatment readiness. Some individuals can have complex occupational histories, which are situated within social tensions related to their antisocial or criminal occupations present lack of motivation to engage and participate activities they want and these individuals can view the environment as a barrier to participation in usual activities which can impact the individual's mental health and well-being negatively. It is supported that volitional problems are likely to be highly relevant in the secure setting which can cause decrease in personal causation, difficulty in identifying or having unrealistic goals and an inability to and meaning or interest in activities [15, 16].

Occupational therapists have the skills and expertise to assess and engage people in those occupations which are meaningful and motivating. This requires a careful understanding and appreciation of what underlies the motivation and creating occupational opportunities like self-care, productivity and recreational activities. Occupational therapists also help people to identify and achieve their own hopes and aspirations such as vocational rehabilitation and work skills [15, 16].

Habituation refers the individual's roles and behavior patterns consistent with his/her lifestyle. It presents automatically and effectively doing routine tasks related to their environment. Roles of the individual are responsibilities of the individual associated with personal identity, occupations and activities of daily life and extraordinary occupations. Individual with criminal lifestyles can have problems on participating prosocial roles with their daily routines and occupations [15, 16].

Occupational therapy interventions in secure environments help individual to participate in prosocial roles and occupations in an effort to live within society without resorting to previous criminal or new antisocial behaviors. The imposed legal and security restrictions in secure environments can mean that patients are unable to participate in their habitual or chosen occupations; this may be because such occupations are antisocial, or due to lack of resources, facilities or particular environments being available in secure settings. Often patients benefit from the structure, stability and consistency of admission [19].

For occupational therapy interventions age, ethnicity and culture, finding the 'right' occupations that are culturally relevant, risk-managed and appropriate to the 'typical' forensic population can be challenging. The literature supports that not only redesigning lifestyle but also technological advances have an impact on the range of occupations that occupational therapist is able to offer to extend the inclusion level of the individual such as contemporary videogames and Nintendo® WiiTM additionally to participating actual sports and recreation activities [16].

According to the Model of Human Occupation, performance capacity is related to an individual's adaptive interaction with the environment, and the ability to do activities provided by physical and mental components and the associated subjective experience. Occupationally restricted individuals have problems with occupational performance skills for independence in daily living. Moreover, performance skills may not be acquired or learned during transition from child to adult. Occupational therapists in secure environments have a major role to play in helping patients to develop, maintain or acquire new skills for successful community reintegration or transition to less secure settings, for example in the area of vocational rehabilitation. Occupational therapists can guide individuals to identify possible vocational areas such as study/education, voluntary or paid employment [16, 20, 21].

Occupational therapy interventions should help the individual to identify prevocational needs and sometimes individuals have not been or will not have a productive activity like working again and therefore the therapists need to help them to establish different prosocial, productive and meaningful occupations to increase health, wellbeing, occupational performance and general quality of life. For these reasons, it is important for occupational therapists to measure and follow the progress of the individual with outcome measures during daily living activities [17, 18, 21].

Social and physical isolation of the individuals can cause problems to access their own complex occupational and environmental worlds. Being cut from own life can cause limitations over occupational choices and experience, so environmental changes and supports during activity performance can provide opportunities, constraints and demands to the individual. The literature supports that individuals in secure environments spend much of their time in passive leisure, personal care and rest occupations and occupational therapists are one of the core elements in increasing activity participation of the individual and develop occupations of their choice [15, 16]. Also, occupational therapists can facilitate the exploration of new or unknown occupations to increase positive life experiences of the individual.

As it is given earlier, there is a great model need to understand the volition, habituation, performance skills, physical and social environments in which an individual's occupation takes place. MOHO assists the understanding of occupation(s) and problems of occupation that occur in terms of volition, habituation, performance capacity and environmental context. This system-based model includes well-designed assessments, observational, self-report and interview schedules. One of the advantages of this model is that because of its extensive use in mental health settings; a forensic version of an assessment tool 'Occupational Circumstances Assessment and Interview and Rating Scale' was designed. But, the literature also supports that this tool is not the only one for the use of occupational therapists, and occupational therapists may find any particular model, or standardized assessment/outcome measures to support their interventions [4, 15, 16, 21, 22].The literature supports that the use of occupational therapy models in forensic mental health may increase evidence-based practice and help the professionals to show the effect of occupational therapy. As Model of Human Occupation is seen to be the most used occupational therapy model, models including environmental and individual issues such as psychological issues, desires, wants, activity performance and satisfaction from the activity performance can help the occupational therapist to plan more effective assessments and interventions. Although the literature is still limited; different occupational models such as KAWA model, creative ability model, PEOP (Person, environment, occupation, performance), the Canadian model of occupational performance and engagement and the individual placement and support model with can be effectively used with standardized assessments and outcome measures in various individuals, situations, cultures and environments in provision of occupational therapy services in a cost-effective way [6, 15, 16].

4. Assessment in forensic occupational therapy services

Occupational therapy process commences with contiguity between the offender and occupational therapy service. Collecting information about the person and making special evaluations is the first step in this process. Gathering information about the individual and special assessments helps to determine the problems and needs, as well as the reason for the intervention. It also allows for the setting of intervention targets and the determination of the intervention plan. In the process of occupational therapy, the intervention plan is followed by the implementation of the intervention. The intermediate evaluation may be needed to determine the effectiveness of the intervention or to reveal new intervention goals and plans. After intervention plans that have been modified or reorganized after the interim evaluation are applied, the intervention is assessed. As seen in the abovementioned occupational therapies process, information gathering and evaluation also play an important role in the intervention for forensic occupational therapy applications. In summary, an occupational therapist working with prisoners should use a three-stage assessment of initial assessment, interim evaluation and outcome measurement during the occupational therapy intervention process [15, 21].

Occupational therapy sees people as active and social entities and treats the person, his occupations and the environment holistically in order for the individual to achieve or regain well-being. It is also important to assess the individual as a whole in the information gathering and evaluation process for the creation of a suitable intervention plan [15] . According to the occupational therapy reference frame written by AOTA [15], personal factors include the individual's values, interests, and spirituality as well as body structure and functions. Having knowledge about the boundaries and areas of internal energy in prisoners' participation in occupations can be useful to guide activity preferences and motivation processes. The things that constitute the meaning of prisoners' lives are values and beliefs they believe to be worth trying and taking the time. The occupational therapist in forensic setting desires recreates occupational identification of offenders who lose their roles by being isolated from the social environment. For this reason, it is very important to understand the value, relevance, strengths and limitations of the individual [4, 16, 22].

It is also necessary to assess the sensory, motor and cognitive skills involved in the body structure and functions of the person in need to meet the occupation requirements they wish to perform. These skills can make or break an individual's daily life. One point that should not be overlooked here is that during the process of occupational therapy collecting and evaluating information, the prisoner does not play a passive role, so the occupational therapist does not seem to be running a process alone. The occupational therapist and the prisoner are in the business association during the presentation of information, evaluation and outcome measures, and the prisoner is actively involved in this process.

Occupational therapists are aware that the occupational performance of an individual is influenced by factors related to the individual as well as by the performance patterns and the environment. Roles, routines, rituals, and habits constitute performance patterns [15]. Routines and habits allow the individual to perform his/her daily activities without thinking about how to move, without trying to remember. Occupational therapists working in forensic health services care about whether the prisoner has useful habits and routines for him. It is necessary to know how individuals spend their days and which routines they create from day to guide to get new routines and habits to use the time and energy more efficiently when the living conditions change [11]. Roles are the whole of the behaviors that an individual imposes on his/her responsibility, which is imposed by the environment and culture. Rituals are symbolic behaviors that are understood by social, cultural and spiritual values that shape the occupational identity of the individual. During the evaluations, the roles of the prisoner and the importance of these roles and the determination of meaningful rituals in the individual's life provide significant benefits for the therapist's intervention plan. Changes in location and time can also cause changes in the roles and rituals of individuals. The change in the role and ritual of the individual after conviction can cause occupational alienation in the individual. In the context of a forensic health service, acquisition of the prisoner's new skills and habits, and the new roles and rituals that are well integrated with the environment make an important contribution to the occupational balance of the individual [3, 16, 23].

Understanding the environments in which occupational performance takes place, it is important for occupational therapists to understand the underlying effects of occupational participation. The environment includes dimensions related to physical, social (including individuals in the individual's life) and policies, and at the same time creates a supportive or restrictive effect for the occupational adaptation of the individual. Situations such as an absence of freedom for the individual, individual secrecy, and the meaningful and socially acceptable occupations constitute a barrier to prisoners' participation in their environment and occupation [15, 24]. Occupational therapists should also be thoroughly evaluating the environment of individuals who are establishing an intervention plan with prisoners applying to the occupational therapy service.

We have already mentioned the preferred models for forensic occupational therapy applications. MOHO, one of these theories, includes structured and unstructured assessment and information gathering tools [3, 4, 11] for collecting and evaluating information about offenders. Some of those:

- Occupational performance history interview (OPHI II)—A semi-structured measure of self-care and information about the individual's life history;
- Assessment of communication and interaction skills (ACIS)—evaluates three subdomain individuals, including the physical dimension of communication, information exchange, and relationships, in an occupational pattern or in a social group [25];

- The Model of Human Occupation Screening Tool (MOHOST)—gives the client a holistic view of his or her motivation to achieve occupation, communication and interaction skills, occupation patterns and the individual's process and motor skills as well as the environment. MOHOST also allows a highly effective assessment of the effectiveness of occupational therapy interventions [26];
- Occupational Self-Assessment (OSA)—a method of assessment that reveals how the individual focuses on the occupational competence of the individual about his/her occupational adaptation, helping to shape the needs and values of the individual. OSA is a highly recommended assessment tool for evaluating forensic occupational therapy. Individuals are given a very wide list of daily occupations, individualists are asked to evaluate the occupations in their own eyes and the level of their own performance [26];
- Occupational circumstances assessment interview and rating scale (OCAIRS-Forensic Mental Health Version)—the therapist has extensive content to get detailed information about the offender. It gives the individual an accurate and holistic view of occupational functionality. If the more fully involved the offender is in the evaluation process, the higher the participation in intervention practices [27, 28].

Evaluations such as Canadian occupational performance measurement, assessment of motor and process skill, independent living scale, and the role checklist are other measures preferred by occupational therapists [3, 24].

Another assessment heading in the forensic occupational therapy process is risk assessment. When considering the evaluation processes mentioned earlier, a prisoner who has forensic settings should be considered as a means of risk assessment to determine the potential for another crime or previous crime. Occupational therapists take into account the risk assessment and management of risks posed by each client and to increase the occupational involvement of individuals by taking environmental precautions and managing them to manage risks in environments such as high-risk kitchens and workshops to improve individual skills as well as providing positive risk-taking opportunities to enhance the capabilities of both individuals.

Current risk factors such as age and gender, substance use status, criminal history and potential risk factors such as marital status, occupational participation level in the forensic setting, family support should be considered in the risk assessment. Occupational therapists pay attention to the influence of the person-environment-occupation interaction on the occupational adaptation of the individual. Occupational therapists can estimate the effects of individual's personality and sociodemographic characteristics (physical, cognitive and psychological), their level of skill and the environmental risk factors, including interpersonal interaction, social support network, hospice environment, social security status on the possible risk factors. For this reason, they may play an active role in providing counseling to minimize the risks faced by prisoners and these risks' adverse effects on occupational adaptation [3, 21].

5. Interventions in offenders rehabilitation

As already mentioned, offender rehabilitation in forensic settings is not different from other mental services. Intervention methods used by occupational therapists must include life skills development (such as ADLs, IADLs, and health management), occupational development, awareness (such as self-awareness and social awareness), self-management, skill-building (such as social, relationship, vocational skills), education etc.

The GLM is a model that overlaps the humanistic point of view of occupational therapy. Although the GLM is a psychology-based model, it supports occupational therapies' application models such as PEO, MOHO, CMOP and role acquisition model. Occupational therapists may develop interventions taking into account the GLM's the primary human goods components. Some intervention recommendations based on the 'primary human goods' are given in **Table 3**.

The 'primary human goods'	**Intervention recommendations**
1. Life (including healthy living and optimal physical functioning, sexual satisfaction)	**Aim:** Understand themselves, reach personal satisfaction, live life better and achieve their goals **Occupational strategies:** Functional life skills Role development Independent living skills Literacy and education ADLs IADLs Health management Gender-specific issues Money management
2. Knowledge (how well informed one feels about things that are important to them)	**Aim:** Identify one's emotions, thoughts, interests, and values; understand how internal characteristics influence actions; maintain a sense of self-confidence and self-efficacy **Occupational strategies:** Self-awareness Drug and alcohol awareness
3. Excellence in work (including mastery experiences)	**Aim:** To keep the physical, psychological and social needs of the individual together, to increase the independence of the individual and to work with a holistic and customer-centric approach in the role of the worker. **Occupational strategies:** Prevocational training Job search skills Work-related practice Vocational rehabilitation: work preparation, voluntary and paid work Work hardening
4. Excellence in play (hobbies and recreational pursuits)	**Aim:** To build up hobbies, recreational pursuits **Occupational strategies:** Recreational skills Time management

The 'primary human goods'	Intervention recommendations
5. Excellence in agency (autonomy and self-directedness)	**Aim:** To organize and adapt a behavior to achieve individually selected goals and values **Occupational strategies:** Anger management Stress management Problem solving skills Motivation
6. Inner peace (freedom from emotional turmoil and stress)	**Aim:** Regulate emotions, thoughts and behaviors across contexts; cope with stress and manage impulses; set goals **Occupational strategies:** Self-management Increase self-esteem and confidence by promoting personal responsibility
7. Relatedness (including intimate, romantic and family relationships)	**Aim:** Establishing and maintaining relationships with others; resisting inappropriate social pressure; working in cooperation; preventing and resolving interpersonal conflict; asking for help when necessary [29]. **Occupational strategies:** Relationship skills Complex relationship building Facilitating development of supportive relationships Social skills
8. Community (connection to wider social groups)	**Aim:** Being active in social groups **Occupational strategies:** Social skills Social awareness Responsible decision-making Graded community engagement and one-to-one goal planning Empathy
9. Spirituality (in the broad sense of finding meaning and purpose in life)	**Aim:** To find meaning and purpose of life **Occupational strategies:** Motivation
10. Pleasure (feeling good in the here and now)	**Aim:** Feeling good, loving life **Occupational strategies:** Motivation Increase self-esteem and confidence
11. Creativity (expressing oneself through alternative forms).	**Aim:** Knowing himself about what he can do **Occupational strategies:** Skills development Vocational activities include such as woodwork, crafts, graphics, horticulture

Table 3. Intervention recommendations in offender's rehabilitation from the view of occupational therapy.

1. Life: Life skills training is a commonly used occupational therapy intervention in mental health [30]. Offenders are at a higher risk for poverty, unemployment and difficulties in relationships. The life skills training interventions can focus on self-care, self-maintenance, intrinsic gratification, social contribution and interpersonal relatedness skills. The interventions must be client centered and the context must be well evaluated. While working with an offender, the balance of daily occupations should be kept in mind for a healthy lifestyle.
2. Knowledge: The development of interventions for improving self-awareness is very important in offenders' rehabilitation. Self-awareness is the ability to recognize him/herself as an individual who is different from other individuals. Self-awareness is having a clear perception of personality, including strengths, weaknesses, thoughts, beliefs, motivation and emotions. The aim of the interventions is to gain a sense of self-worth. Facilitatory interventions, such as education, feedback, behavior therapy and psychotherapy have been recommended to a greater extent than compensatory interventions.
3. Excellence in work: The main problem of ex-offenders is employment to maintain their lives [31]. Unemployment concerns begin to increase still they are in prison. They face substantial barriers to many types of legal employment [32]. These barriers are poor basic skills, low self-esteem, a lack of recent work experience, employer discrimination, behavioral and health problems. Interventions must include prevocational training, job search skills, work-related practice and also work hardening.
4. Excellence in play: Recreational activities and hobbies are the enjoyable, activities that are restorative in which the clients' choice and control often associated with leisure time. Recreational pursuits and hobbies are the power of life. The main aim of the therapeutic recreation is to enhance the patient's quality of life and ability to participate in leisure and/or play. Also, it can improve social participation and social skills which is very important for the offenders.
5. Excellence in agency: Self-directedness is the ability to organize and adapt a behavior to achieve individual selected goals and values. Self-directedness includes the concept of an autonomous individual and concepts of personal integrity, self-respect, dignity, efficacy and feelings about one's life [33].
6. Inner peace: Anger management problems affect all parts of a persons' life. The goals of treatment are to increase the client's resources for coping with stress and try to decrease the demands made on the client. Treatment is first achieved by increasing awareness of the client about the relationship between anger and stress and then increasing the effective use of the stress management techniques that the client is able to cope with [11, 34]. Anger management interventions begin with recognizing the triggers of anger. The client must take responsibility for his/her own change so that the problem can be solved. The second stage of the intervention is the awareness of the behaviors when the client is angry, such as, shouting, swearing, treating verbal, postural or gestures, abusive behaviors such as phone calls, messaging or other communication ways, harassments, emotional abuses or violent. Also in this stage, the therapist must help the client to identify times when his/her thoughts do not lead to logical or rational conclusions. The third stage is teaching specific skills to help the client to manage triggers for anger effectively, such as relaxation techniques, mindfulness and assertiveness.

7. Relatedness: Group interventions in which the family members and friends are engaged are suitable for relatedness [35]. The aim of the interventions must be establishing and maintaining relationships with others, resisting inappropriate social pressure, working in cooperation, preventing and resolving interpersonal conflict, asking for help when necessary [29].

8. Community: Deficits in social skills are often seen in forensic groups. Social skills training is the main intervention method for being active in a group [36]. For being in a group, it is also important to make responsible decision to identify and evaluate the problems correctly, making decisions based on ethical and social norms, to evaluate decisions in context, contribute to the welfare of society, accurately identify and evaluate problems, make decisions based on ethical and social norms, consider context in decisions, contribute to well-being of community [29]. Social skills training consists of learning activities that use behavioral techniques that enable individuals to acquire independent life skills for better functioning in their communities. Direct teaching, modeling, role playing, behavior rehearsal, and social reinforcement can be used during the interventions.

9. Spirituality: The spirituality is the 'meaning and purpose in life, the life force or integrating aspect of the person and transcendence or connectedness unrelated to belief in a higher being' in occupational therapy perspective [37] . The meaning of spirituality is different for everyone, can be participating a religion, visiting religious places (such as churches, mosques, synagogues etc.) regularly and can be different for some praying alone, yoga, meditation, being in the nature, walking and so on. There can be challenges about talking about the beliefs and spirituality with the client and that much of spiritual experience can be culturally influenced [37]. Motivation techniques can be used to find meaning and purpose in life.

10. Pleasure: Pleasure is one of the subjective experiences of the human need-based experiences to engage in occupations [38]. It influences productivity, restoration and being active to engage occupations [39]. Motivational and increasing self-esteem and confidence interventions can be used to improve pleasure.

11. Creativity: It is stated that 'creativity is part of everyday practice; the use of creativity as a conscious approach; creativity involves risk-taking; creativity needs a supportive environment; and creativity is the use of expressive arts in therapy' [40]. Especially creative arts increase the capacities of offenders, help to explore their own resources, assist them to locate hope and motivation, recognize their interconnectedness with others without external pressure to comply [41].

6. Challenges in forensic occupational therapy

The main challenge is the context because of the complexity of the rules affecting the freedom of the offender and the occupational opportunities [7]. The heterogeneous client population is another challenging condition with in the context. Restricted daily living activities cause the loss of control and autonomy. Time use is another challenging factor, the lack of structured time use besides the loss of control and autonomy affects the client's volitions, habits, and routines. Also, lack of opportunities for meaningful, individualized career choices for patients affects the client.

Also, change, itself is a challenging condition. There are many factors that affect the daily living activities that are the volitions, habits of the individual and the environment. Therefore, it is not possible to catch the change in every environment. Even in a prison or in a secure hospital or a probation service, the offender has always an obligation and mostly a restricted occupational choice. Motivation or perceived lack of choice is an important challenge. Another challenge is the obligations dictate some occupations and this is not the individual's choice. Occupational therapy is client-centered, but freedom deprivation is a challenge to make interventions. Occupational therapy is client-centered but freedom deprivation is a challenge to make interventions. Labeling and stigma are other challenging parts of the offenders' participation in the occupations and the community.

Keeping the three justices—criminal justice, occupational justice and social justice—in a balance is the main aim of the offender's rehabilitation and the most challenging part of the rehabilitation.

Author details

Esma Ozkan[1], Sümeyye Belhan[1], Mahmut Yaran[2]* and Meral Zarif[3]

*Address all correspondence to: mahmut.yaran@omu.edu.tr

1 Department of Occupational Therapy, Faculty of Health Sciences, Sağlık Bilimleri University, Istanbul, Turkey

2 Department of Therapy and Rehabilitation, Havza Vocational School, Ondokuz Mayıs University, Samsun, Turkey

3 Department of Occupational Therapy, Faculty of Health Sciences, Hacettepe University, Ankara, Turkey

References

[1] Townsend E, Polatajko HJ. Enabling Occupation II: Advancing an Occupational Therapy Vision for Health, Well-Being & Justice through Occupation. Ottawa: Canadian Association of Occupational Therapists; 2007

[2] Hitch D, Hii QK, Davey I. Occupational therapy in forensic psychiatry: Recent developments in our understandings (2007-2013). British Journal of Occupational Therapy. 2016;**79**(4):197-205

[3] Munoz J. Mental Health Practice in Forensic Settings. Philedelphia: F.A. Davis Company; 2011

[4] McNeill S, Bannigan K. Forensic and prison services. In: Bryant W, Fieldhouse J, Bannigan K, editors. Creek's Occupational Therapy and Mental Health. 5th ed. Edinburgh: Churchill Livingstone Elsevier; 2014. pp. 424-437

[5] Lindstedt H, Grann M, Söderlund A. Mentally disordered offenders' daily occupations after one year of forensic care. Scandinavian Journal of Occupational Therapy. 2011;**18**:302-311

[6] Munoz J, Farnworth L, Dieleman C. Harnessing the power of occupation to meet the needs of people in criminal justice settings. Occupational Therapy International. 2016;**23**:221-228

[7] Chiu L, Wong CI, Maraj SA, Fry D, Jecker J, Jung B. Forensic occupational therapy in Canada: The current state of practice. Occupational Therapy International. 2016;**23**: 229-240

[8] Tan B, Kumar VR, Deveraj P. Development of a new occupational therapy service in a Singapore prison. British Journal of Occupational Therapy. 2015;**78**(8):525-529

[9] Lylods C. Trends in forensic psychiatry. British Journal of Occupational Therapy. 1995;**58**(5):209-213

[10] Srivastava S. The nature of crisis of correction. Indian Journal of Criminology. 1981;**9**(1):23

[11] RCoO Therapists. Occupational Therapists' Use of Occupation-Focused Practice in Secure Hospitals Practice Guideline. 2nd ed. Davis J, Sainty, M., editor. London: Royal College of Occupational Therapists; 2017

[12] Subramanian R, Delaney R, Roberts S, Fishman N, McGarry P. Incarceration's Front Door: The Misuse of Jails in America. New York: Vera Institute of Justice; 2015

[13] Bradbury R. The Role of Occupational Therapy in Corrections Settings. New York: Ithaca College; 2015

[14] Abramsky S, Fellner J. Ill-Equipped: U.S. Prisons and Offenders with Mental Illness. New York: Human Rights Watch; 2003

[15] AOT Association. Occupational therapy practice framework: Domain and process. In: Association AOT, editor. American Journal of Occupational Therapy. 3 ed. 2014

[16] Moore M. Forensic psychiatry and occupational therapy. In: Crouch R, Alers V, editors. Occupational Therapy in Psychiatry and Mental Health. 5th ed. India: John Wiley & Sons; 2014. pp. 106-114

[17] O'Connell M, Farnworth L, Hanson EC. Time use in forensic psychiatry: A naturalistic inquiry into two forensic patients in Australia. International Journal of Forensic Mental Health. 2010;**9**:101-109

[18] Andrews D, Bonta J. The Psychology of Criminal Conduct. 5th ed. New Providence, NJ: LexiNexis Group; 2010

[19] Looman J, Abracen J. The risk need responsivity model of offender rehabilitation: Is there really need for a paradigm shift? International Journal of Behavioral Consultation and Therapy. 2013;**8**(3-4):30-36

[20] Purvis M. Seeking a Good Life: Human Goods and Sexual Offending. Germany: Lambert Academic Press; 2010. 353 p

[21] Bullock A. Assessment and outcome measurement. In: Ryant W, Fieldhouse J, Bannigan K, editors. Creek's Occupational Therapy and Mental Health. 5th ed. Edinburg: Churchill Livingstone Elsevier; 2014. pp. 72-85

[22] Mccullough S. Planning and implementing interventions. In: Bryant W, Fieldhouse J, Bannigan K, editors. Creek's Occupational Therapy and Mental Health. Edinburgh: Churchill Livingstone Elsevier; 2014. pp. 86-102

[23] Hunter E, McKay EA. 'Doing' in secure settings. In: Mckay E, Kee CC, Lim H, Richards G, editors. Advancing Occupational Therapy in Mental Health Practice. 1st ed. Singapore: Blackwell. pp. 76-89

[24] Hatton J. The Profile and Work Practices of Occupational Therapists Working in Forensic Mental Health and Prison Settings in Australia and New Zealand. Townsville: James Cook University; 2004

[25] Forsyth K, Marclle S, Simon S, Kielhofner G. The Assessment of Communication and Interaction Skills (ACIS): (A Userś Guide to.) (Version 4.0). Chicago: University of Illinois; 1998

[26] Keilhofner G. Model of Human Occupation: Theory and Application. Philadelphia: Lippincott, Williams & Wilkins; 2008

[27] Forsyth K, Deshpande S, Kielhofner G, Henriksson C, Haglund L, Olson L, Skinner S, Kulkarni S. The Occupational Circumstances Assessment Interview and Rating Scale (OCAIRS) (Version 4.0). Chicago: MOHO Clearinghouse; 2005

[28] Withers P, Boulton N, Morrison J, Jones A. Occupational therapy in a medium secure intellectual disability and personality disorder service. Journal of Learning Disabilities and Offending Behaviour. 2012;**3**(4):206-218

[29] AOTA. Social and Emotional Learning (SEL). Maryland: AOTA; 2018

[30] Ammeraal M, Coppers J. Understanding living skills: First steps to evidence based practice. Lessons learned from a practice-based journey in the Netherlands. Occupational Therapy International. 2012;**19**:45-53

[31] Bilgiç S. Mahkûmların Suç Algısı. KMÜ Sosyal ve Ekonomık Arastırmalar Dergisi. 2014;**16**(1):8-17

[32] Visher C, Winterfield L, Coggeshall MB. Ex-offender employment programs and recidivism: A meta-analysis. Journal of Experimental Criminology. 2005;**1**(3):295-316

[33] Nilsson T, Falk Ö, Billstedt E, Kerekes N, Anckarsäter H, Wallinius M, Hofvander B. Aggressive antisocial behaviors are related to character maturity in young Swedish violent offenders independent of ADHD. Frontiers in Psychiatry. 2016;**7**:1-12

[34] Taylor E. Anger intervention. American Journal of Occupational Therapy. 1988;**42**(3): 147-155

[35] Brown C. Motivation. In: Brown C, Stoffel VC, editors. Occupational Therapy in Mental Health: A Vision for Participation. Philadelphia: F.A Davis Company; 2011. pp. 330-344

[36] Henderson M, Hollin C. A critical review of social skills training with young offenders. Criminal Justice and Behavior. 1983;**10**(3):316-341

[37] Unruh A, Versnel J, Kerr N. Spirituality unplugged: A review of commonalities and contentions, and a resolution. Canadian Journal of Occupational Therapy. 2002;**69**(1):5-19

[38] Atler K, Barney L, Moravec A, Sample PL, Fruhauf CA. The daily experiences of pleasure, productivity, and restoration profile: A case study. Canadian Journal of Occupational Therapy. 2017;**84**(4-5):262-272

[39] Atler K. The daily experiences of pleasure, productivity and restoration profile: A measure of subjective experiences. In: Pierce D, editor. Occupational Science for Occupational Therapy. Thorofare, NJ: Slack; 2014. pp. 187-199

[40] Schmid T. Meanings of creativity within occupational therapy practice. Australian Occupational Therapy Journal. 2004;**51**(2)

[41] Albertson K. Creativity, self-exploration and change: Creative-arts based activities and transformational identity desistance narratives. The Howard Journal Of Criminal Justice. 2015;**54**(3):277-291

9

Employment of People with Disabilities and Ergonomic Risk Factors at Workplace

Beliz Belgen Kaygisiz

Abstract

The importance of employment to people with disabilities has been increasing in recent years. Participation in working life as active producers has been the main factor in community integration of people with disabilities. It has been proven that if people with disabilities are given the opportunity to develop and use their working capacity, they can be as successful as those who do not have any disabilities, and nowadays the most rational way of helping people with disabilities is to provide them with profession and work. Vocational rehabilitation is a process that helps someone to overcome the barriers when beginning to work, continuing to work, or returning to work after any accident, illness, or disorder. Although the employee is selected according to his/her ability according to the work to be done, it is very important that the place to work matches the physical and psychological characteristics of the employee. Ergonomics is important at working life as it affects productivity. Many different ergonomic risk factors are available to affect the quality of life of a person at workplace. This chapter focuses on the employment of people with disabilities, the risk factors they may face at workplace and assessment of risk factors.

Keywords: employment, disability, workplace, ergonomics, risk factors

1. Introduction

Participation of people with disabilities in business life has been increasing in many countries in recent years [1–3]. The use of rehabilitation services and the participation in working life as active producers have been the main factors in community integration of people with disabilities [2–4]. Developed countries make legal arrangements in this area to enable people with disabilities to gain profession. The Americans with Disabilities Act (ADA) emphasizes that work for people with disabilities is a right, not just a social participation. The United Nations has also taken a major step in recent years, placing 'work' in the basic rights of people with disabilities and obliging employer to prepare accommodation that is compatible with the employee's needs [5].

The International Labour Organization (ILO) states that all persons with disabilities are entitled to vocational rehabilitation, employment and progress at work, regardless of the type of disability and the level of disability [6, 7]. It has been scientifically proven that if people with disabilities are given the opportunity to develop and use their working capacity, they can be as successful as those who do not have any disabilities, and nowadays the most rational way of helping people with disabilities is to provide them with profession and work [1, 4, 6, 8, 9]. Thus, instead of being dependent on others, they will be able to earn an income and perceive themselves as persons who are productive, efficient and economic contributors [2, 3, 6].

The chance of a permanent or temporary physical or psychological discomfort during the life of an employee is 20% [9]. This disturbance can change the functional capacity of the person [9]. An acquired physical disability may cause a person to change jobs or to continue existing work with assistive devices and adaptations [10]. However, it may not always be enough to find a suitable workplace and to adapt the individual to work independently [1]. It is necessary to evaluate the person's ability to continue to work over a long period of time [1]. Some jobs can cause a person's physical condition to deteriorate, which leads to an increase the level of disability both at work and during daily life [1].

People who are permanently or temporarily disappeared from work after a disease or accident can receive financial support for a period of time [9]. Social security institutions, health councils and insurers evaluate the person's functional capacity to determine the person's ability to return to work [9–11]. Job losses due to the loss of working capacity of individuals cause social and economic consequences for both the person and the society [1, 6, 11]. Especially, long-term job losses are costly for countries [1]. Therefore, efforts are being made to minimize the loss of work that can occur through the provision of work security and the measurement of risks [1]. Many countries work on the vocational rehabilitation programs for workers who have lost their working capacity irreversibly, making them to enter the economic arena again [11].

The criteria for returning to work for an employee established by a rehabilitation team in the case of an accident or illness are as follows [9]:

1. Comparison of physical/cognitive requirements of work with function
2. Possible requirements for job modification and settlement
3. Adaptive device or assistive technology requirement
4. Permission for body mechanic training or treatment
5. The need to return to part-time or gradually work within a limited time

The above factors are agreed with the employer and the employee to form the action plan. This is a dynamic planner that can be changed according to the progress. The plan can continue until he or she returns to work [9].

2. Employment of people with disabilities

2.1. Barriers to employment of people with disabilities

There are personal and programmed facilitators and barriers in the participation of people with disabilities in their working life [12, 13]. The interaction between these facilitators and barriers constitutes the personal economy of energy and resource [12, 13]. As the barriers increase, the resources within the personal economy decrease [12]. The person should either give decreasing personal source to work or transfer the source into family and social life [12, 13].

The personal factors that are barriers to the working life of people with disabilities are secondary conditions such as pain, fatigue, mobility change, depression, change in perception [12, 14], change in vision, change in bowel and bladder control [12]. Personal factors which are related to disability or not, such as education level, social support status and self-esteem, may also be barriers [6, 13, 14]. People with disabilities who return home without working have stated that secondary conditions have worsened; that no energy is left to participate in the family and social life; that they are stuck between work, financial income and health status; and that they lose from non-work-related quality of life [13, 15, 16]. As a result, the interaction of these secondary conditions with social and environmental barriers negatively affects the economy.

Social and environmental factors alone can also be barriers to the working lives of people with disabilities [6, 12]. Factors such as the lack of a general healthcare coverage and the inability to transfer one's health coverage when going into another work are social barriers [12]. As environmental factors, we can count the barriers when reaching the workplace and all the barriers that prevent mobility at workplace [13]. Inaccessible toilets, pavements and unreachable computer tables are among the environmental barriers [6, 12–14].

It is very important that a person with a disability is able to continue to work or to arrange a suitable place for a new job. In each country, compulsory laws must be enforced to plan and implement a suitable settlement for the employee's needs. Thus, the barriers that may arise in the working life should be tried to be reduced to a minimum. Such problems in the employment of people with disabilities are accompanied by the risk of social exclusion and poverty [6]. Resolving the problems in employment helps participation of disabled people and their families in productive life, as well as it is the only way to increase independence and quality of life [6].

2.2. The importance of vocational rehabilitation in people with disabilities

Vocational rehabilitation is a process that helps someone to overcome the barriers when beginning to work, continuing to work, or returning to work after any accident, illness, or disorder [6, 11]. This process consists of a flexible set of applications that takes shape from one step to the next according to the needs of the individual [12]. These practices are a very important step for participation in social life again for people with disabilities who have not been able to enter the education system for various reasons; who are disconnected from this system at any stage, disabled while working; or who want to change their occupation [6]. Vocational rehabilitation practices involving individuals who lose their jobs, employers, family members and related persons cover procedures that can help them to easily reach and continue these programs.

In vocational rehabilitation, the person's disability, cause, nature and age do not matter [6]. What is important is whether the disability situation creates a barrier from a professional point of view [6]. If the present obstacle situation is a real problem for the present or future work, it indicates the need for vocational rehabilitation [6].

2.3. The scope of vocational rehabilitation

Like all other rehabilitation services, vocational rehabilitation will continue to be a developing field based on the evidence gained through research. Described by H. Kayıhan in 2009 [17], vocational rehabilitation includes steps of assessment, guidance, training, placement, protection and monitoring. In the assessment, an analysis of the physical, mental and vocational abilities of a person who is injured or remains after the disease is made. During this analysis, it is very important for the evaluator to evaluate the findings effectively and efficiently and to know that the findings can vary according to personality traits during this process [11]. Proposals are made in the field of guidance for vocational education and employment opportunities. In the training section, the person is trained and prepared for the job. The next step is to help the person find a suitable job. Special arrangements make it easier for the recruited person to work. In the last step, the person is followed until the full adaptation to the job is secured [17].

In vocational rehabilitation, the cause of disability, the nature of disability and the age of the disabled person do not matter. The important thing is whether there is an obstacle to work. If the physical and/or mental disability of the person is an obstacle to the current or future work, then professional rehabilitation is needed [18, 19]. People with disabilities should be assessed on the basis of their capacities, competencies, potential and relevance before starting vocational training. Akel et al. [19] reported that even adolescents with chronic diseases should be educated about possible future occupations. Functional and work capacity of the people is investigated. Parallel to the results obtained, training is provided to increase the work potential of the person and to prepare him to the activities. Vocational rehabilitation team includes people from professional groups such as doctors, physiotherapists, occupational therapists/ergotherapists, psychiatrists, psychologists, course teachers, social workers, professional advisers and some other professionals as architects or engineers [17].

The 'International Classification of Functioning, Disability and Health' (ICF), created by the World Health Organization in 2002, classifies health and health-related areas by defining body functions and structure, activities and participation [11, 20]. These areas are categorized by physical, personal and social aspects. Since the function and disability of the subject are in the same context, ICF also includes environmental factors [11]. The social model and ICF are the models that professional rehabilitation practitioners can use. Even if the content of the models is not fully used, general order and principles can be used, while vocational rehabilitation programs are being created [11, 21]. In a study published in 2011 by Escorpizo et al., relevant results were found between assessment methods used in vocational rehabilitation and some ICF categories and pointed out the importance of using this model in vocational rehabilitation [21]. In another study in the United States, it was argued that the ICF model is a new turning point in understanding and addressing health and health problems [22]. It has been determined that this method may assist in occupational rehabilitation team, determine the necessary treatments, develop effective placement strategies and evaluate outcomes [22]. The ICF's core set for vocational rehabilitation has been formed to serve as an international standard and to measure and/or report concerning functioning of individuals at vocational rehabilitation programs [23].

2.4. Importance of functional capacity evaluations in vocational rehabilitation

Functional capacity evaluations are an objective measurement method that evaluates the activity status, activity limitations, physical requirements of the work and the general work situation of people with disabilities and those who have experienced work injury and gives suggestions for ultimately taking part in the job-related and participatory role [24–27]. These assessment methods have been used in North America since the early 1980s [13]. This term coincides with the time when ergotherapy is developing rapidly. The desire to find valid data in order to increase the return of persons to safe work has increased the importance of functional capacity evaluations. For the last 40 years, with the development of technology, more objective and computerized measures began to be used, resulting in healthier work choices and successful job placements [27–29]. Functional capacity evaluations are implemented by physiotherapists, occupational therapists, physicians, occupational rehabilitation consultants and many other professional occupations [9]. It is stated that the person who made the measurement should be trained in this subject [9, 11].

For people with physical disabilities to be employed, functional capacity needs to be evaluated first and then placed in appropriate jobs [8, 9, 30, 31]. Functional capacity evaluations can be made from medical, functional, psychological, physical and occupational aspects. Following the determination of the functional capacity, it is stated that the work analysis should be carried out at a later stage to assess the requirements of the work and the functional capacity should be adjusted to meet the needs of the job [4]. The decision should be made to place the person with disabilities in the work course or job [4]. As a result of the functional capacity evaluations, it is aimed to determine the capacity of the person to meet the demands of the job and the appropriate jobs [8–10]. If there is a problem to continue to work, an action plan should be made [10]. This plan should be to place the person in a modified job, to train the person about job demands, to direct the person to a treatment center when there is a medical problem, or to prepare the person for a new job with vocational rehabilitation if it is not possible to return to the previous job [10].

The purpose is very important when choosing a functional capacity evaluation method [24, 31]. If it is the intention to return to the old job, job requirements should be determined by job analysis [24]. Functional capacity evaluation results should be compared with the physical requirements of the job [24]. A more general and comprehensive assessment should be done if the person is to be placed in a new job [24]. The physical condition is investigated from many directions and the most appropriate ones are identified from the various types of job opportunities available [24]. If the objective assessment of the functional capacity is to determine the disability status, then an evaluation method should be chosen where the evaluator can collect the desired information [24].

Functional capacity evaluations, such as all other tests performed in the field of rehabilitation, are generally planned according to the test and measurement standards established by the American Physical Therapy Association [32]. Functional capacity assessments are crucial to ensure reliable and valid results and to be safe and practical in practice [24, 30]. Reliability is stated as the most important factor that evaluations are standardized [24, 30]. Reliability studies of functional capacities for many different purposes have been accelerated after 1990, and clinicians have drawn attention to the importance of reliable assessment methods [33]. Reliability studies of newly produced evaluation methods continue at a rapid pace [33].

Lechner et al. [34] and Brouwer et al. [35] found that functional capacity evaluation protocols were reliable for people with low back pain and other musculoskeletal disorders. Lechner et al. evaluated 50 persons aged between 18 and 65 who had musculoskeletal discomfort and who spent at least 20 hours per week with the so-called Physical Work Performance Evaluation [34]. The reliability of interpersonal reliability when using the evaluation method of 11 physical therapists was found to be very high [34]. Gross and Battie [36] found that test–retest reliability of the results of functional capacity evaluation during lifting was high in people with low back pain. An evaluation system called 'Isernhagen Work System' was used in this study [36]. The authors state that when evaluating the operational definition, the safe and maximum performance detection is reliable when well explained to the evaluators [36].

Many types of validity were tested in the field of functional capacity assessments [30, 33]. Less validity studies were conducted compared to reliability studies [37]. The first study to question the validity of functional capacity assessment studies was conducted by Smith et al. [38]. In this study, 125 prisoners in prison were evaluated by 'Smith Functional Capacity Assessment Method', medical history was taken, and 'Patient Activity Questionnaire' was applied. According to these test results, the chances of returning to work were determined. One year after being released from prison, a questionnaire was sent to these persons, and their employment status was questioned. From the responses, it was determined that the results of the tests in the prison estimated the work situation to be 86%. Matheson et al. [39], who tested the predictive validity of functional capacity assessments, attempted to determine the return to work after 6 months without evaluating the individuals with chronic musculoskeletal system. In this study, a low lift was tested, and a 2% chance of returning to work for each added pound weight was found to increase by 2%. Lechner et al. [40] also tested the predictive validity of the 'Physical Business Performance Assessment', a functional capacity evaluation method, on 30 people with musculoskeletal dysfunction. As a result of this study, the results of functional capacity assessment were well validated in determining the chances of returning to work after vocational rehabilitation [40].

Compared to other assessments, functional capacity evaluations take longer [24, 30]. This can vary from a few hours to a few days, depending on the measurement protocol used [24, 30].

It is also stated that these evaluations are more suitable to be applied in the clinical environment instead of the business environment because they include equipment such as lifting units, weights and power measuring unit [30]. Because of these equipment, it is stated that the establishment of functional capacity evaluation units is almost as costly as the imaging methods at diagnostic centers [30].

The main components of functional capacity assessments can be summarized as data collection, physical assessment, physiological assessment and functional performance measures [24]. In the data collection section, file scans, interviews with people, or surveys are conducted [24]. Physical evaluations are performed to determine clinical findings related to the disease [24]. As a result of these findings, it is determined if there is inconvenience for physiological and functional evaluations to be done properly or if the person should be followed during evaluations [24, 30]. Physiological evaluations include sections such as assessment of muscle strength or cardiovascular endurance [24].

The business factors specified in the 'Job Titles Dictionary' (DOT) indicate both the physical requirements of the job and the capacity of the employee to fulfill those requirements [24]. These 20 physical requirements are used by rehabilitation specialists and business consultants to classify jobs [24, 26]. Functional performance assessments measure the physical requirements of this work [24, 26]. The lift capacity test is the most commonly used functional work measurement in the DOT [24]. However, it is stated that the measurement of lift capacity in different situations and in different positions is very important in terms of reliability of the test [24].

3. Ergonomic regulations at workplace

The study of ergonomics and work posture in workplaces has gained importance in recent years. Ergonomics is an interdisciplinary scientific discipline that scientifically examines and relates the relationship between people, the equipment and working environment they use to the field of application [41]. In order to harmonize the person, machine and work with each other in the best way, it examines the physiological, biological, anatomical and other specialties of the human being and enables the machine and work to be designed according to these characteristics [41]. This science helps to understand how human abilities and limitations are understood and how it can bring about performance in a safe, effective, comfortable and healthy way in relation to the environment [42, 43]. If a building is anthropologically, physiologically, sociologically and psychologically compatible, it must be able to perform daily activities [42, 44]. Effective and successful 'harmonization' guarantees high productivity, avoidance of disease and injury risk and increased satisfaction in the work [44]. In order to achieve these, technical and health teams must be in a successful cooperation [44].

Ergonomists should consider the special requests of the persons who will use the building during the construction, arrangement, or repair of a building, so that the space is useful, safe and effective [42]. Factors such as lighting, heat, noise, ventilation, cleanliness, humidity, as well as working hours and break times are examined in the field of ergonomics [11]. While arranging the environment of a disabled or elderly person, ergonomists find solutions by evaluating every field and activity [42]. Ergonomic problems that occur during the working life of people with physical disabilities should be solved with the participation of many disciplines. Ergonomics is a multidisciplinary approach which addresses many disciplines as engineers, physicians, psychologists, physiotherapists, ergotherapists, architects, home economists and other disciples who have knowledge about anatomy, biomechanics, psychology, physiology, engineering principles, anthropometry, and kinesiology and the ones who solve stress factors at home, school, and workplace [17, 45].

The main physical problems that may arise as a result of interaction between human, environment, and equipment are musculoskeletal diseases [41]. Work-related musculoskeletal disorders refer to musculoskeletal disorders that affect work environment and work performance significantly. Workplace risk factors are thought to develop work-related musculoskeletal disorders with personal characteristics and social factors [46]. Jobs with multiple risk factors or increased working at high-risk conditions will increase the likelihood of having a musculoskeletal system disorder [44]. Repeated hand tasks with heavy work, heavy lifting, pushing heavy objects, pulling or carrying, long sitting in poor posture, monotonous work, inadequate intermittent rests, vibration, or cooling are the main risk factors [41]. The level of risk generated is determined by the severity of exposure to the risks, frequency, duration, and strength capacity of the person to meet other job requirements [44].

Inadequate working postures in jobs that require intense labour force cause inefficiency as well as musculoskeletal discomfort [41, 44, 47]. One of the aims of the ergonomics is to improve worker postures and balance worker capabilities and work requirements, resulting in improved worker safety, health, and overall productivity of the system [41, 44, 47]. Workplace injuries cause a decrease in one's work capacity and production [41, 44, 47]. While these injuries cause discomfort, reduced work capacity, and production affect economics negatively [44]. Therefore, the role of preventive rehabilitation becomes increasingly important in preventing these injuries and having a healthy musculoskeletal system [44]. One of the mechanisms of injury that is resulted from many risk factors is muscle loading [43, 48]. In poor working posture, degenerative changes occur in the affected joints and in the connective tissue [43, 48]. Repetitive movements and inadequate rest periods cause discomfort caused by muscular loads together with degenerative changes resulting from poor and bad posture [43, 48]. Another mechanism of injury that occurs during exercise is muscle fatigue. Static and dynamic loading resulting in muscular work with maximum capacity leads to muscle fatigue [43, 48].

Points to consider when designing a workplace to avoid work injuries are listed below [49]:

1. When the person is working, he should provide a straight and face-to-face posture.
2. If the vision is required during a job, the required work points should be visible when the head and neck are upright or only when the head is tilted slightly forward.
3. All business activities should allow one to work with many different but equally healthy, safe postures without diminishing the capacity.
4. Work should be arranged in such a way that the person must be standing or sitting in position according to his wishes. While sitting, both feet should have equal load, and the foot supports must be adjusted accordingly.

5. When standing, both feet should be loaded equally, and the foot supports should be adjusted accordingly.

6. Work activities should be arranged such that the joint movements are in the middle of the range of motion. This is especially true for the head, neck, and upper limbs.

7. When muscle force is required for the work, the force applied should be along the relevant limb and should be performed by the contraction of the most suitable large muscles.

8. Work should not be performed at the heart level or above the heart level, especially when using force above the heart level. Even at the light work, the upper extremities need to be rested when work has to be done above the heart level.

9. If there is a continuous force application, arms or legs should be used without having to organize on the equipment.

10. Rest periods should be provided at all workloads including environmental load, information load, and length of work.

3.1. Ergonomics for persons with disabilities

Ergonomic arrangement of a workplace is done by making the work suitable for the person to be worked on. Although the employee is selected according to his/her ability according to the work to be done, it is very important that the place to work matches the physical and psychological characteristics of the employee [44, 45]. 'Appropriate Settlement' was first used in 1990 to prevent discrimination against the people with disabilities and to remove the barriers to employment [14]. This term includes [1] provision of assistive equipment necessary for the job to be done, [2] modification to make the business environment fully accessible, [3] arrangement of the workflow, and [4] provision of personal assistance when needed. Unreachable workstations constitute a physical barrier, and if the workspace is not modified, it will prevent the desired work [7, 14]. Some workplaces are affecting the physical condition negatively due to the work they have installed on the person, which can reduce the person's independence both at home and in daily life [1, 14]. The person may not be able to keep the job any longer and then may be forced to another job or not to work at all.

Providing the necessary tools to do the job is a step in removing the barriers at the workplace [14]. Easy access to computer technology, software that understands speech, ergonomic keyboards, and mouth-controlled mice are frequently used in many disability groups [14]. In fields where computer technology is not used, envelope folding machines, electrical staplers, telephone headsets, and similar equipment can be useful for productivity [14]. Another step in lifting the barriers is to organize the physical work environment both personally and in general [14]. Business areas should be well illuminated, crossing areas should be expanded, maneuvering areas should be separated, and entrances without stairs should be provided [14, 44]. The regulation of the workflow is also important in ensuring accessibility [14, 44]. It should be ensured that the energy of the person is activated by arranging activities that are not necessary for the business [14, 44]. For example, placing frequently used equipment in close proximity, or lowering shelves where heavy items are placed, prevents the occurrence of fatigue and walking difficulty [14]. In addition, to find the appropriate time to take a break without interruption and to change among employees in monotonous work are the steps that can be taken in order to streamline the workflow [14]. Some employees may need physical help despite all the arrangements [14]. Office design should be done in such a way that employees can help each other when needed or a place where an assistant can work if required [14].

Different studies done by Belgen et al. [50] and Çalık et al. [51] reported that the majority of people with disabilities work with high-risk posture and this creates risk of musculoskeletal problems [50, 51]. An employer who will hire a person with physical disabilities should follow a conscious attitude to what positions he or she will be employed and the places in which the person concerned will be interested. It is aimed to create the work to be done with the ergonomic arrangement to ensure the employee's harmony with the work environment [42, 44, 45, 50, 51]. This is only possible when anthropometric point of view, physiological point of view, psychological point of view, information point of view, and safety point of view are all considered [42, 44, 45]. Only when all these conditions are met, the person can perform all the necessary activities appropriately [42]. Conditions that are often neglected for people with disabilities are anthropometric, physiological, and psychological conditions [45].

3.2. Accessibility at work for people with disabilities

Accessibility means that a person with a disability can move around as he or she wants without any intermediary. Accessibility is the most important point that should be given importance in workplaces where people with disabilities are. Accessibility of the workplace is the independent completion of all phases between the door of the house and the start of work at the workplace. The barrier most frequently shown as an obstacle to work is a workstation that is inaccessible [7, 14].

The accessibility feature should also be considered parallel to the vertical area, also called the comfort zone. This area is the vertical field from the lowest level that a person can reach to the highest level that one can reach while standing. The limits set for the Turks in this regard are the upper reach limit of 115.6 mm (the small woman with the wheelchair) and the lowest reach limit of 665 mm (the long male using the seat handle) [44]. This area marks the location of many control buttons, such as power switches, door handles, sockets, and so on, which must be present at the workplace. Changes in this area in the business environment also prevent the disabled employee from being dependent to others [43, 45].

Optimum placement will not make anyone happy because the various places in the workplace can be used by people with many different characteristics. As a result, both horizontal and level of adjustability are always the best solutions. The height of the seat to be seated, the height of the counter, the height of the sinks, and the height of the cabinets to which the items of interest are to be placed must always be adjustable [14, 44, 52]. Özyörük and Kütük [52] reported that redesigning of working environment to increase work efficiency made positive changes and achievements were gained.

3.3. Ergonomic risk factors

Work-related factors that cause musculoskeletal disorders and accelerate discomfort are called ergonomic risk factors. These factors directly or indirectly affect the occurrence of discomfort. Ergonomic risk factors are examined under three main headings [41]. These are:

1. Physical factors
2. Environmental factors
3. Psychological factors

3.3.1. Physical factors

Repetition of the same movements during work, improper postures, static posture, excessive use of force, and squeeze are the physical dimensions of the ergonomic risks. Repetitions of the same or similar movements during work can cause pain and discomfort in the musculoskeletal system because the muscles are not given enough time to rest [41]. Natural postures are the safest and most convenient way to work. Non-natural postures force the physical limits of the body by putting pressure on the muscles and joints. The long standing of the worker in the same position limits the blood flow and makes the muscles tired and injured. The excessive force applied to the muscles causes the muscles to contract more than normal, causing the joints to overload and cause injuries. Compression of the soft tissue between a bone and a hard or sharp object reduces blood flow and nerve conduction, damaging tendon and tendon sheath [41].

3.3.2. Environmental factors

Noise, temperature, humidity and airflow, lighting, vibration, and chemicals are among the ergonomic risks. The organizer of the workplace should also pay attention to environmental factors. The obligation of the human body's limits, job requirements, and the characteristics of the equipment means to ignore the role of the environment.

The body of a working person may be exposed to certain environmental factors. Environmental interactions above the limits can cause different body parts, leading to cumulative trauma. The use of vibration absorbing equipment, the use of extreme cold or hot barriers or insulation clothing, the construction of barriers where there is airflow, and the introduction of a crusher on the computer screen for reflected light can reduce the environmental impacts of the body through simple, non-costly measures [41].

3.3.3. Psychological factors

Psychological risk factors include mental overload, psychosocial effects, social communication in the workplace, and organizational influences. It has been determined that these factors, which include all employees and employers, increase ergonomic risk and should therefore be considered [41, 44].

Many musculoskeletal system diseases that involve the abdomen, neck, upper extremity, and lower limbs in our country are accepted as occupational diseases in the law [41]. However, data on the frequency of these diseases, risk factors, workday loss, insurance indemnity, and cost are not available [41]. Work-related musculoskeletal diseases, which are among the most important problems of employees and which reduce work efficiency, and prevention of adverse effects of these diseases are possible with ergonomic education and initiatives [41, 53].

Employees, employers, and professionals and organizations dealing with occupational health should be informed about work-related musculoskeletal disorders and prevention, and community awareness should be established [41, 53–55]. Studies done with different groups of employees emphasize the importance of workplace assessment and health evaluations to be done actively, and continuous training should be provided for all workers [53–55].

3.4. Evaluation of ergonomic risk factors at workplace

It is important to assess risk in terms of health and safety, including the situation of employees who are likely to be affected by the risks present at the workplace [41]. Following these assessments, the protective measures to be taken and the protective equipment to be used can be determined [41]. Ergonomic analysis methods are used to evaluate the ergonomic risk factors in the study area. Ergonomic analysis is a mechanism used to facilitate the identification of existing problems in the field of work [12, 41, 56]. The work is carried out by systematically recording the effects of work on the person or the specific views of the work [56]. With these analyses, ergonomic defects and possible health hazards can be identified and subsequently eliminated. During the analysis, all factors considered for each individual situation, technical and personal factors, should be evaluated [56].

When choosing which of the many analysis methods available today is to be used, the objectives should be [43, 56]:

- Working environment, working place, working style, design of equipment.
- Prevention of work injuries, work-related disorders and diseases.
- Continuing and enhancing the ability of the disabled and elderly to work.
- Obtaining information for the prevention of occupational injury or illness.
- Evaluation of work and characteristics of the work related to health care and planning of research programs.

Assessment methods include checklists, workplace analysis observations of work postures and movements, and self-filled surveys [43, 56]. Checklists are an evaluation method that consists of many questions and examines various factors. The most commonly used checklist is the 'General Ergonomic Risk Analysis Checklist' prepared by the International Ergonomics Association [56, 57]. Workplace analysis determines workplace characteristics such as workplace, general physical activity, lifting, work postures and movements, accident risk, occupational satisfaction, difficulty in decision-making, work repetition, attention, air temperature, and noise. Work postures and movement analysis are needed to be done at work to make a more precise analysis of the problems caused by work postures and movements. Today, there are many observation methods. The most commonly used pole is the pencil-paper method based on visual observation. In recent years, photography, videotape, and computer systems have also been used frequently.

The Ovako Working Posture Analysis System (OWAS) and Rapid Upper Limb Assessment

(RULA) are commonly used methods for evaluation of easy and practical posture movements requiring direct observation. OWAS examines the upper extremity/shoulders, lower extremity, head, and load-lifting postures [56, 57], while RULA examines upper extremity working posture.

Author details

Beliz Belgen Kaygisiz

Address all correspondence to: bkaygisiz@eul.edu.tr

Faculty of Health Sciences, Department of Physiotherapy and Rehabilitation, European University of Lefke, Lefke, Turkey

References

[1] Pigini L, Andrich G, Liverani G, Bucciarelli P, Occhipinti E. Designing reasonable accommodation of the workplace: A new methodology based on risk assessment. Disability and Rehabilitation: Assistive Technology. 2010;**5**(3):184-198. DOI: 10.3109/17483100903488768

[2] Saunders SL, Nedelec B. What work means to people with work disability: A scoping review. Journal of Occupational Rehabilitation. 2014;**24**(1):100-110. DOI: 10.1007/s10926-013-9436-y

[3] Lindsay S, Cagliostro E, Albarico M, Mortaji N, Karon L. A systematic review of benefits of hiring people with disabilities. Journal of Occupational Rehabilitation. 2018:1-22. DOI: 10.1007/s10926-018-9756-z

[4] Erbahceci F, Kayıhan H, Uyanık M, Akçay T, Kırdı N. Ankara Mesleki Rehabilitasyon Merkezinde işe yönelik eğitim. Optimal Tıp Dergisi. 2000;**13**(3):57-63

[5] US Department of Justice. A guide to Disability Rights Laws. [Internet]. 2005. Available from: http://www.ada.gov/publicat.htm#Anchor-14210. [Accessed: Jan 30, 2018]

[6] Başbakanlık TC. Özürlüler İdaresi Başkanlığı. 4. Özürlüler Şurası. İstihdam. Ankara: Komisyon Raporları ve Genel Kurul Görüşmeleri; 2009

[7] Nevala N, Pehkonen I, Koskela I, Ruusuvuori J, Anttila H. Workplace accomodation among persons with disabilities. Journal of Occupational Rehabilitation. 2015;**25**(2):432-448. DOI: 10.1007/s10926-014-9548-z

[8] Wehmann PH, Revell G, Kregel J, Kreutzer JS. Supported employment: An alternative model for vocational rehabilitation of persons with severe neurologic psychiatric or physical disability. Archives of Physical Medicine and Rehabilitation. 1991;**72**:101-105

[9] Lyth JR. Disability management and functional capacity evaluations: A dynamic resource. Work. 2001;**16**:13-22

[10] Trombly CA. Chapter 21. Employment for the Physically Disabled. In: Occupational Therapy for Physically Disabled. 3rd ed. New York; 2000:441-451

[11] Holmes J. Introducing vocational rehabilitation. In: Vocational Rehabilitation. Great Britain, Blackwell Publishing Ltd; 2007

[12] Johnson KL, Brown PA, Knaster ES. Aging with disability in the workplace. Physical Medicine & Rehabilitation Clinics of North America. 2010;**21**:267-279

[13] Bureau of Labor Statistics. U.S Department of Labor.Persons with Disability: Barriers to Employment, Types of Assistance, and Other Labor-Related Issues. Bureau of Labor Statistics. U.S Department of Labor; 2012

[14] Zolna J, Sanford J, Sabata D, Goldthwaite J. Review of accommodation strategies in the workplace for persons with mobility and dexterity impairments: Application to criteria for universal design. Technology Disability. 2007;**19**:189-198

[15] Johnson KL, Yorkston KM, Klasner ER. The cost and benefits of employment: A qualitative study of experiences of persons with multiple sclerosis. Archives of Physical Medicine and Rehabilitation. 2004;**85**(2):201-209

[16] Yorkston KM, Johnson KL, Klasner ER. Getting the work done: A qualitative study of individuals with multiple sclerosis. Disability and Rehabilitation. 2003;**25**(8):369-379

[17] Kayıhan H. Mesleki Rehabilitasyon. Ankara: Hacettepe Üniversitesi Fizik Tedavi ve Rehabilitasyon Yüksekokulu; 2009

[18] Ercan S, Kayıhan H. Şizofreni Ve Mesleki Rehabilitasyon. Ergoterapi Ve Rehabilitasyon Dergisi. 2017;**5**:3, 278

[19] Akel S, Şahin S, Huri M. Kanser Tanılı Çocukların Meslek Tercihlerinin Belirlenmesi. Ergoterapi Ve Rehabilitasyon Dergisi. 2017;**5**(3):339

[20] World Helath Organisation [Internet]. Available from: http://www.who.int/disabilities/world_report/2011/report/en/ [Accessed: Jan 31, 2018]

[21] Escorpizo R, Finger ME, Glassel A, Gradinger F, Luckenkemper M, Cieza A. A systematic review of functioning in vocational rehabilitation using the international classification of functioning, disability and health. Journal of Occupational Rehabilitation. 2011;**21**(2):134-146. DOI: 10.1007/s10926-011-9290-8

[22] Homa DB. Using the international classification of functioning, disability and Helath (ICF) in job placement. Work. 2007;**29**:277-286

[23] Finger ME, Escorpizo R, Glassel A, Gmunder HP, Luckenkemper M, Chan C, Fritz J, Studer U, Ekholm J, Kostanjsek N, Stucki G, Cieza A. ICF core set for vocational rehabilitation: Results of an International Consensus Conference. Disability and Rehabilitation. 2012;**34**(5):429-438. DOI: 10.3109/09638288.2011.608145

[24] King PM, Tuckwell N, Barret TE. A critical review of functional capacity evaluations. Physical Therapy. 1998;**78**(8):852-866

[25] Gibson L, Strong J. Expert review of an approach to functional capacity evaluation. Work. 2002;**19**:231-242

[26] Gibson L. International Handbook of Occupational Therapy Interventions, Functional Capacity Evaluation: An Integrated Approach to Assessing Work Activity Limitations. Springer; 2009:497-505. DOI: 10.1007/978-0-387-75424-6_55

[27] Wind H, Gouttebarge V, Kuijer PPFM, Sluiter JK, Frings-Dresen MHW. Complementary value of functional capacity evaluation for physicians in assessing the physical work ability of workers with musculoskeletal disorders. International Archives of Occupational and Environmental Health. 2009;**82**:435-443. DOI: 10.1007/s00420-008-0361-x

[28] Kayıhan H. Özürlü Kişilerde Çalışma Kapasitesinin Değerlendirilmesi. Ankara: Hacettepe Universitesi; 2003 (Project No: 00001 401 001)

[29] Bhambhani Y, Esmail S, Brintnell S. The Baltimore therapeutic equipment work simulator: Biomechanical and physiological norms for three attachments in healthy men. American Journal of Occupational Therapy. 1994;**48**(1):19-25

[30] Gross DP. Measurement properties of performance-based assessment of functional capacity. Journal of Occupational Rehabilitation. 2004;**14**(3):165-174

[31] Cotton A, Schonstein E, Adams R. Use of functional capacity evaluations by rehabilitation providers in NSW. Work. 2006;**26**:287-295

[32] Task Force on Standarts for Tests and Measurements in Physical Therapy Practice. Standards for tests and measurements in physical therapy practice. Physical Therapy. 1991;**71**:589-622

[33] Innes E, Straker L. Reliability of work-related assessments. Work. 1999, 1999;**13**:107-124

[34] Lechner DE, Jackson JR, Roth DL, Straaton KV. Reliability and validity of a newly developed test of physical work performance. Journal of Occupational Medicine. 1994;**36**:997-1004

[35] Brouwer S, Reneman MF, Dijkstra PU, Groothoff JW. Test-retest reliability of the Isernhagen work systems functional capacity evaluation in patients with chronic low back pain. Journal of Occupational Rehabilitation. 2003;**13**:207-218

[36] Gross DP, Battie MC. Reliability of safe maximum lifting determinations of a functional capacity evaluation. Physical Therapy. 2002;**82**(4):364-371

[37] Innes E, Straker L. Validity of work-related assessments. Work. 1999;**13**:125-152

[38] Smith SL, Cunningham S, Weinberg R. The predictive validity of the functional capacities evaluation. American Journal of Occupational Therapy. 1986;**40**:564-567

[39] Matheson LN, Isernhagen SJ, Hart DL. Relationships among lifting ability, grip force, and return to work. Physical Therapy. 2002;**82**(3):249-256

[40] Lechner DE, Page JJ, Sheffield G. Predictive validity of a functional capacity evaluation: The physical work performance evaluation. Work. 2008;**31**:21-25

[41] T. C. Çalışma ve Sosyal Güvenlik Bakanlığı. İş Sağlığı ve Güvenliği Genel Müdürlüğü. İş Sağlığı ve Güvenliği Dergisi. Yükü Hafiflet. Özel Sayı. Mesleki Kas İskelet Sistemi Hastalıkları. 2007;**34**(7):6-9

[42] Ahasan R, Campbell D, Salmoni A, Lewko J. Ergonomics of living environment for the people with special needs. Journal of Physiological Anthropology. 2001;**20**(3):175-185

[43] Kayıhan H, Hazar G, Uyanık M, Düger T. Büro Çalışanlarında Çalışma Şartlarına Bağlı Ergonomik Risk Faktörlerinin Değerlendirilmesi. Vol. 570. Ankara: Milli Prodüktivite Merkezi Yayınları; 1995. pp. 369-376

[44] Jacobs K. Ergonomics for Therapists. 2nd ed. United States of America: Butterworth-Heinemann; 1999

[45] Uyanık M. Özürlüler İçin Verimli Çalışma. Seminar organized by "Hacettepe Üniversitesi Fizik Tedavi veRehabilitasyon Yüksekokulu ve Bedensel Engellileri Güçlendirme Vakfı", Ankara. 2002

[46] Armstrong TJ, Buckle P, Fine LJ, Hagberg M, Jonsson B, Kilbom A, Kuorinka IAA, Silverstein BA, Sjgaard G, Viikari-Juntura ERA. A conceptual model for wrok-related neck and upper-limb musculoskeletal disorders. Scandinavian Journal of Work Environment & Health. 1993;**19**:73-84

[47] Akay D, Dağdeviren M, Kurt M. Çalışma Duruşlarının Ergonomik Analizi. Gazi Üniversitesi, Mühendislik ve Mimarlık Fakültesi Dergisi. 2003;**18**(3):73-84

[48] Mc SCM, Glothlin JD. Occupational risk factors associated with soft tissue disorders of the shoulder: A review of recent investigations in the literature. Ergonomics. 1993; **36**(6):697-717

[49] Braddom RL. Chapter 16: Physical medicine and rehabilitation. In: Ergonomics. 2nd ed. United States of America: W.B. Saunders Company; 2000. pp. 435-459

[50] Belgen B, Uyanık M, Kayıhan H. Fiziksel Engelli Kişilerde Çalışma Kapasiteleri ile ilgili Ergonomik Risk Faktörlerinin Yaşam Kalitesine Etkisi. Ergoterapi ve Rehabilitasyon Dergisi. 2013;**1**(2):146-147

[51] Çalık BB, Çavlak U. Çalışan Engellilerde Ergonomik Risk Faktörleri Analizi. Ergoterapi ve Rehabilitasyon Dergisi. 2013;**1**(2):119

[52] Özyörük B, Kütük D. İş Ortamını Yeniden Düzenlemenin İş Verimliliğine Etkileri. Ergoterapi ve Rehabilitasyon Dergisi. 2014;**2**(2):73-81

[53] İlhan MN, Kurtcebe ZÖ, Koşar ED v L. Temizlik İşçilerinin Sosyodemografik Özellikleri ve Çalışma Koşulları ile İş Kazası ve Meslek Hastalığı Sıklığı. Fırat Üniversitesi Sağlık Bilimleri Dergisi. 2006;**20**(6):433-439

[54] Gülhan B, İlhan MN, Civil EF. Occupational accidents and affecting factors of metal industry in a factory in Ankara. Turkish Journal of Public Health. 2012;**10**(2):76-85

[55] Akal D, İlhan MN. Musculoskeletal system health complaints which is sourced from negative ergonomic work conditions in call center workers. Ergoterapi ve Rehabilitasyon Dergisi. 2017;**5**(1):2017, 27-2034

[56] Duger T, Uyanık M, Kayıhan H, Hazar G. Çalışma Yerinin Ergonomik Analizi. Vol. 570. Ankara: Milli Prodüktivite Merkezi Yayınları; 1995

[57] Pendelton HM, Schultz-Krohn W. Chapter 13. Work evaluation and work programs. In: Occupational Therapy, Practice Skills for Physical Dysfunction. 6th ed. 2006. pp. 264-295

10

Animal-Assisted Therapy in Occupational Therapy

Sedef Şahin, Barkın Kose and Meral Zarif

Abstract

Developing technology, rehabilitation services, and health definitions have brought about the use of different treatments as well as traditional treatments. Some of these methods are virtual reality, animal-assisted practices, and aqua therapy. Animal-assisted approaches are the therapeutic methods of eliminating and using the problems that an individual experiences in the physical, emotional, psychological, social, sensory, and environmental development areas by taking advantage of human and animal interaction. These methods consist of two basic chapters: animal-assisted activities (AAAs) and animal-assisted therapies (AATs). An interdisciplinary team is needed to implement the methods. This team is composed of personnel, such as occupational therapist (OT), physiotherapist, speech therapist, special education specialist, and a psychologist, who have been trained in this area. In recent years, these methods have been used to increase social interaction with physical structure and functions in neurodevelopmental disorders such as autism spectrum disorder and cerebral palsy. In addition, it is actively used in mental disorders such as depression and anxiety because an improvement is observed by providing the individual to feel safe. When participation is considered in the context of independence in daily life activities are very important, the use of animal-assisted in occupational therapy.

Keywords: animal-assisted, occupational therapy, rehabilitation

1. Introduction

Developing technology, rehabilitation services, and change in health definitions have brought about the use of different treatment methods as well as traditional treatments. Some of these methods are virtual reality, animal-assisted practices, and aqua therapy. Animal-assisted approaches are defined as using human and animal interaction in therapeutic methods to eliminate or decrease the problems that an individual experiences in the physical, psychological, and social environments. These methods consist of two basic topics, namely animal-assisted activities (AAA) and animal-assisted therapies (AAT). Both AAA and AAT can be implemented in an interdisciplinary team approach. Occupational therapists (OTs), physiotherapists, speech therapists, special education specialists, and psychologists are core elements of these approaches. In recent years, these methods have also been used to increase social interaction with physical structure and functions in neurodevelopmental disorders such as autism spectrum disorder and cerebral palsy in addition to mental health disorders such as depression and anxiety to increase the independence in daily life activities and social participation.

2. Overview of animal-assisted therapy

The American Veterinary Medical Association has been involved in human and animal interaction as psychological and physical functions between human beings and animals. In this interaction, they define individual's quality of life as a structure that contributes positively to their improvement [1]. Animal-assisted rehabilitation, the inclusion of animals that can interact with humans such as cats, dogs, and horses, has an active role in the rehabilitation process with the aim of achieving rehabilitation goals [2, 3]. When such approaches are incorporated into rehabilitation programs, the general condition of the individual and the treatment principle that the rehabilitation team has followed are taken into account [4, 5]. Animal-assisted rehabilitation approaches, rather than a stand-alone approach, are a strategic concept where multiple professionals work together to achieve interdisciplinary goals within a single goal [5]. This framework consists of three basic questions. The first question is "what are the benefits of the individual animal and therapeutic activities including animals?" The second question is "how to include the animal to the rehabilitation process?" The third question is "what are the most appropriate activities for the individual?" [1] Based on the answers of these questions, animal-supported approaches are grouped under two main headings: animal-assisted activities (AAA) and animal-assisted therapies (AAT). When therapeutic properties of AAA are investigated, it has been found that it helps to reduce the level of stress and anxiety and indirectly increasing the self-confidence and socializing. It is stated that AATs were predominantly used to support neurodevelopmental substructures of individuals and make a positive contribution to their well-being [6].

3. History of animal-assisted therapy

3.1. Animal souls and spiritual healing

Animals play an important role in the history of the disease with different ideas about disease and its treatments. However, the precise characteristics of these roles depend not only on the prevailing views of animals but also on supernatural or "scientific" belief systems in which they are buried. Probably, the oldest of these belief systems, often called "animism," includes the concept that all natural beings, as well as other natural objects and phenomena, are circulated by an invisible soul, spirit, or "essence," but with conscious bodybuilding, the carrier can act independently of the body when it dreams or is unconscious. In a typical animist worldview, all statements of illness or misfortune are the direct result of attacks by the other angry or evil spirits encountered during these periods of unconsciousness toward the spirit of the person or the "truth." In some cases, these spiritual attacks are thought to be reprisals. It is the result of moral accusation that the person intentionally or mistakenly does. On the other hand, a person can be the innocent victim of a malicious shaman or the attack of souls acting in the name of witches. Tips about the root of spiritual attacks are provided by the contents of dreams or images just before certain illnesses, injuries, or misfortunes [7–9]. Animist belief systems carry the characteristics of all communities that engage in hunting, and disturbing animal spirits among these communities are often seen as the most common source of malicious mental influences. Many hunters believe that the souls of hunted animals in the tribe have the ability to seek revenge as the ghosts of killed people. To avoid this accretion, all animals, whether dead or alive, are treated with great respect [10]. In other hunting and feeding cultures, there were more specific moral associations between people and the animals they hunted for food. For example, many Native American and Eurasian peoples believe in the concept of personal "protective spirits" [7, 11]. Between Ojibwa (Chippewa) and the Algonian neighbors, these spirits were known as *manito* and were often represented as spiritual representations of wild animals or figures of their ancestors. Live animals were regarded as "honorable servants" of their own *manitos*, and this kind of spirit apparently presided over and represented all the worldly members of their species. For this reason, the hunters made contradictory ceremonies after killing an animal, so that the "essence" would return to *manito* with a convenient explanation of how it was processed. According to Ojibwa worldview, *manito's* activities explained almost all conditions of everyday life. Every living thing, whether alive or dead, was equipped with spiritual powers and associated with any unfortunate *manito*, such as illness, injury, death, or hunting that resulted in failure or the lack of personalized intention of someone else [12]. It was believed that the protective spirits of the animals differed in power. The majority of insects and small animals, such as mice, rats, or squirrels, were referred to as not important species because there was the belief that these animals lacked the protective qualities. On the other hand, it was believed that animals such as the bear and eagle had good protective spirits and so they were considered valuable [7, 12].

3.2. Animals as socialization agents

The end of the seventeenth century which was called "Age of Enlightenment" brought some changes in the public perception of animals that are well documented by historians of the modern age [13, 14]. Among these changes, contrary to the pre-medieval and renaissance periods, sympathetic thoughts began to dominate attitudes toward animals and nature [15]. While perceptions of wildlife and threats to wildlife have diminished from prevalence, pet-feeding habits have expanded to aristocratic and middle-class communities living in newly founded cities. This change in animal-related attitudes and behaviors could at least partly reflect Europeans' migration from rural areas to the towns and cities, and the rapid spread of the human population. This rural migration made it possible for the population to be adapted to systems designed for growth [8, 14]. The reformers of the eighteenth century, deriving their authority from the works of John Calvin and Thomas Hobbes, thought that they could indirectly learns from the innate, unfavorable characteristics of children by using children's behavior to take care and control real animals [16]. Compassion and anxiety for the health of animals became one of the didactic themes of children's literature that lived in the eighteenth and nineteenth centuries; the main aim was to inspire the morality of the good and sex, respectively, especially in boys [17–19]. In the late eighteenth century, theories about the social effects on animal care were initiated in the treatment of mental illnesses. The best-documented studies took place in The York Retreat in England. The York Retreat used more innovative methods than the mental treatment methods used at that time. In this study, prisoners were encouraged to do handwriting, writing and reading books, and they were also allowed walking freely around the courtyards and gardens of the Retreat, where small pets were also part of the Retreat and prisoners could interact with them. In his description of the Retreat (1813, p. 96), Samuel Tuke, the founder's grandson, described how the internal courtyards of the Retreat were supplied "with a number of animals; such as rabbits, sea-gulls, hawks, and poultry. These creatures are generally very familiar with the patients: and it is believed they are not only the means of innocent pleasure; but that the interaction with the sometimes tends to awaken the social and benevolent feelings." In the nineteenth century, pets became an increasingly popular feature in the psychiatric departments of hospitals in the UK. For example, in a highly critical report on terrible conditions for patients in Bethlem Hospital in the 1830s, British Charity Commissioners proposed that the shelter of people with a mental problem is provided support for treatment of sheep, rabbits, apes or other domestic pets, they have also been described as social animals. Such recommendations are clearly taken seriously. According to a paper published in Illustrated London News of 1860, the regulations at Bethlem Hospital have been redesigned according to the stimulus [20]. It has been observed that animal companions have beneficial and therapeutic effects in the treatment of physical disorders. Florence Nightingale, for example, observed and wrote in Notes on Nursing (1880) that "a small pet is a particularly good friend, especially for the patient, long chronic cases" [21].

3.3. Psychotherapy and animals

Despite the success of animal-supported institutional care in scientific studies during the nineteenth century, with the development of evidence-based medicine in the early twentieth century, the use of animals in hospitals has declined dramatically [20]. For the next 50 years, animals were used in the context of zootomic illnesses, public health concerns, or psychoanalytic theories of the origin of mental illnesses. Sigmund Freud's ideas concerning the origins of neurosis tended to reiterate the Hobbesian idea of mankind's inherently beast-like nature [16]. According to Freud, infants and young children are in fact similar to animals, as long as they are governed by instinctual desires or could be influenced by organized basic biological functions such as nutrition, defecation, sexuality, and self-protection. Freud describes this basic and animal-like instinct of human nature as "identity." As children mature, their parents' behaviors will either cause too much impulsive behavior by reacting to the child's inner aggression or induce their sense of fear, guilt, and socialization. The suppression of these children under the consciousness of children ensures that their behavior in their daily lives is healthy. But they are like animals in their 30s. Freud refers to this as a bottled animal chart. It results in explosive situations where the individual cannot go out on regular outings [22]. Freud interpreted the recurrent animal images of his patients' dreams and "freethinking" as metaphorical means that hid the unacceptable thoughts and feelings of humans. "The Wild Beast" he argued, "It makes him happy that other dreams come true while the passionate spirits of the dreamer are afraid of himself" [23]. These crude thoughts and impulsions threaten the "ego" so deeply that they can be ignored in the dark corners of the consciousness in proportion to the capacity of the subconscious within the hours when at least one person is awake. According to Freud and his followers, the aim of psychoanalysis is to reveal these scary residents of the subconscious, to reveal them as they are in their true nature, and thus to neutralize them [24]. The notion of "id," Freud defines as the basic "animal" essence of human nature, contains more than a superficial resemblance to animistic and shamanic ideas about animal spirits and protective spirits, including bad thoughts/"evil self" or spiritual origins [24]. In the study on Carl Jung, especially his discussions of mythological archetypes in dreams and visions, and his concept of the "Collective Unconscious," this resemblance becomes more or less explicit [25]. It is also echoed in the writings of Boris Levinson, the founder of "pet-facilitated therapy." In his book *Pets and Human Development*, Levinson states that:

> *One of the chief reasons for man's present difficulties is his inability to come to terms with his inner self and to harmonize his culture with his membership in the world of nature. The rational man has become alienated from himself by refusing to face his irrational self, his own past as personified by animals* [26].

According to Levinson, the solution to this growing sense of alienation is through positive relationships with the animals, as if dogs, pets, and other domestic animals are within themselves. It is emphasized that this relationship has increased the quality of life by positively contributing to the solution of the problems experienced by the individual in the spiritual sense [27]. Levinson went one step further to the idea that Freud propagated and suggested symbolic patterning system of things where we fear to confront animals; in order to argue that their relationship with animals is an important part of human evolution and that it is now an integral part of our present psychological well-being [26].

3.4. Animals, social support, and relaxation

There has been considerable development in the theoretical substructure of animal-assisted approaches during the last 20 years and, at least in part, in response to the skepticism shown toward blood-based medicine. This substructure offers the basis for demonstration as a psycho-mental mediator by providing relief from relatively metaphysical-based thoughts about animals [24]. The primary catalyst for this change of emphasis was a single, groundbreaking study of 92 outpatients from a cardiac care unit who, statistically speaking, were found to live longer if they were pet owners [28]. This finding prompted a whole series of other health-related studies as well as stimulating a lot of discussion concerning the possible mechanism(s) responsible for the apparent salutary effects of pet ownership. Of these, at least two have stood the test of time. According to the first, animals are able to induce an immediate, physiologically de-arousing state of relaxation simply by attracting and holding our attention. According to the second, companion animals are capable of providing people with a form of stress-reducing or stress-buffering social support [29, 30]. Although the de-arousing effects of animal contact have been demonstrated by a considerable number of recent studies, little evidence exists at present that these effects are responsible for more than transient or short-term improvements in physiological parameters, such as heart rate and blood pressure. On the other hand, pets serving as a source of social support seem to provide a relatively high level of evidence for the longer-term benefits of animal companionship [31].Cobb has defined social support as "relationships that direct, to emphasize and give importance to, to describe that it is the pattern of mutual obligations." However, the newer authors have expressed it as "perceived social support" and "social networking" characteristics. The first represents a qualitative definition of the degree of satisfaction from the support that one receives from certain social relations; the second is a more quantitative measure involving the number, frequency, and propensity of the person's general social interactions [32]. However, the importance of social support to human well-being, which we wanted to describe, has been regarded as one of the top-down issues throughout history. Loneliness—lack of social support—has always been seen as a painful and distasteful phenomenon; since ancient times, societies have used single-cell imprisonment, exile, and social mobilization as methods of punishment. This, in fact, shows that loneliness is actually the basic punishment method. In addition, religious themes explain in detail the psychological effects of autobiographical, social isolation that homeland traitors and prisoners of war wrote. Many of them describe physical torture in a way that will emotionally, often sharply, up to the apex of gradual descent. This decrease in pain is associated with the onset of a serious indifference and hopelessness, which usually requires catatonic deprivation [29]. In the last 10–15 years, a comprehensive medical literature has emerged confirming that there is a strong and positive link between social support and improved human health and survival [33–35]. There is a great deal of social support in reducing the adverse effects of stress, which chronic life has brought. With the controversy still underestimating these effects, many authorities now accept the judgment that the main benefits arise from the buffering or healing capacities of long-term effects of supporting social relations [36]. Theoretically, this beneficial effect of social support should be applied to any positive social association. It has been observed that positive behaviors are exhibited within the two parties in relation to which one is loved or respected. Despite the increasing evidence for anthro-zoological research in the recent past, the idea that animal attendants contribute socially to human health, however, received very limited medical attention [8].

4. Animal-assisted therapy in occupational therapy

4.1. The role of animal-assisted approaches in rehabilitation

AAT is used as a therapeutic approach in rehabilitation. AAT approaches are being used all over the world in order to improve not only the emotional and psychosocial states but also the physical, sensory, and cognitive skills positively for individuals with various diseases or of different ages [37, 38]. Rehabilitation practices include holistic approaches, with divergence toward children, adolescents, adults, and elderly people.

It is known that there are many neurological, physiological, and genetic diseases seen in children, and the rehabilitation practices are widely used in these children [39]. In literature, AAT is commonly used in children with cerebral palsy, developmental neurological disorders, autism spectrum disorders, sensory processing disorders, degenerative neurological and muscle disorders that mainly focus on control of muscle tonus, mobility, and balance [40]. When the elderly and adult population rehabilitation applications are examined, it is seen that animal-assisted approaches are preferred in the treatment of diseases such as multiple sclerosis, head trauma, post-traumatic neurological conditions, Alzheimer Disease, dementia, anxiety, and depression [41–43]. These diseases can cause a reduction in postural symmetry and control, and deterioration in cognitive skills like attention, memory, and executive functions [37].

All of these patients with diseases, whether young or old, were psychologically affected, and their motivation decreased during rehabilitation. It is known that sensory, emotional, and physical characteristics of animals can be utilized to increase the level of motivation in rehabilitation. In fact, in most developed countries today, health-care providers employ animal-assisted therapy in a wide range of settings, including rehabilitation centers, acute care, psychiatric centers, and outpatient clinics. For example, doctors' consulting rooms have fish tanks in their waiting rooms to promote a sense of calm [44]. It is now well known that the presence of animals can induce relaxation, increase positive emotions, reduce resistance to treatment, and put patients' minds at ease.

Awareness of the advantages and disadvantages of the animals and species used by the professional practitioner team in rehabilitation practices involving many health disciplines involved in this area positively affect the effectiveness of rehabilitation [6]. At the same time, it also emphasizes the importance of knowing the animal's unique structure and instincts in these studies [6, 37]. Most studies and programs in AAT utilize animals such as livestocks, dolphins, dogs, cats, birds, hamsters, or horses [45]. All animals have certain advantages and disadvantages within themselves, so that the practitioner can make arrangements according to the individual and individual's needs.

4.1.1. Therapy with livestock

It is mentioned in the literature that all farm animals can be easily included in treatment approaches as long as they are checked by the veterinarian for good health and reliability. The benefits and difficulties of incorporating livestock into therapy approaches may vary according to the therapist's rehabilitation goal. These animals are preferred by the occupational therapists (OTs) in rehabilitation applications, in particular for those individuals who have difficulty in independent daily living skills, in terms of a large living space, and special need for care. There are also studies showing that AAT with livestock affects individuals' motor and cognitive functions positively [46, 47]. They are preferred by OTs because they can help improve their equilibrium, hand-eye coordination, executive function, and hand skills of individual.

4.1.2. Therapy with dolphin

AAT in individuals with both physical and cognitive impairment is a useful method for facilitating human interaction, stress reduction, relieving depression, and increasing motor and cognitive functions in therapeutic purposes. The dolphin is one of the most important animal species that provide them. There are two main reasons for choosing the dolphin in therapy session when compared to other species: the first is the dolphin's intelligence and learning style and the second is water as stress reduction [45]. On the other hand, there are also some difficulties or disadvantages to working with dolphins. Researchers suggest that the dolphin has some risks due to the fact that it is not a domestic animal, the results of evidence-based studies are very low, and treatment conditions come with very high costs [48].

Dolphin-assisted therapy is commonly used in people with head injuries, schizophrenia, cancer, or other chronic diseases for improving both gross and fine motor skills, developing sensory integration, and increasing communication skills. Nathanson et al. indicated that measurable improvement was observed in the functioning in children with autism spectrum disabilities when dolphin therapy was conducted 5 days per week for at least two weeks [49]. It is suggested that the dolphin should be used as a supportive therapy in the healing and motivational aspects as well as the positive aspects in human beings.

4.1.3. Therapy with dogs

One of the animals frequently used in therapy by professionals working in various fields is the dog to improve the physical, cognitive, functional, and social skills of individuals. The most important areas of use are autism spectrum disabilities in children and visually impaired individuals [50]. Many studies mentioned that the degree of independence in daily living activities improved when using dogs as a therapy companion [50, 51]. It is observed that dogs, one of the most important parts of AAT, interact better with people than other animals [6]. Dogs are highly preferred by experts because they are both AAA and AAT suitable for use in therapeutic approaches.

Dogs are often preferred for both children and adults in therapy because they are friendly, sympathetic, obedient, and playful. They are also used as a guide for the blind, as walking aids for physically challenged, and a hearing assistance for the deaf. Many studies have shown that dogs offer vital benefits in terms of reducing functional disability and facilitation of communication and interaction in humans [38, 52]. Therefore, it is important to remember that dogs can be used for animal-assisted approaches toward therapy, primarily for all ages and patients with diagnosis.

4.1.4. Therapy with cats

Cats can often help in both AAA and AAT like the dogs [53]. They are free spirited and can interact with humans and provide sensory and emotional support to individuals. Due to these characteristics, cats have shown that they especially affect individuals' well-being and quality of life positively [6]. It is known that they can be easily used in supplied everywhere as well as in the living space of the individual. However, it can be said that the most common disadvantage of using cats in therapy is their allergic furs [54]. It is therefore necessary that the therapist who applies the animal-assisted approach to patients has to understanding and know the patient's allergic conditions and chronic diseases.

Interest in AAT is increasing day by day in the literature. While it is generally believed that cats are widely used in AAT, we found no qualified studies that used a cat [37]. So, there is a need for OTs to investigate the disadvantages of utilizing a cat in the therapeutic approaches on patients with having a disability in daily life skills.

4.1.5. *Therapy with small animals*

Pets that are described as small pocket animals, feathers and furs of varying lengths, color, and characteristics that vary in appearance are categorized in this section. Small animals consist of fish, birds, hamsters, turtles, and rabbits, which can be found easily in the classrooms, offices, or schools rather than other large animals. OTs can benefit from the use of these animals in the development of activities in areas requiring community participation.

These animals often carry on with their lives as an ordinary part of the circle. But at this time, it is especially used in therapeutic approaches for both children and psychiatric patients in terms of learning to take responsibility for animals [43, 55]. These animals have a disadvantage in terms of the limited span of life (2–5 years) which can hamper rehabilitation process [56]. Although these animals are preferred in performing small tasks in AAA, the number of studies in the literature is inadequate.

4.1.6. *Therapy with horse*

Among animal-assisted approaches, horses are the most commonly used animals in therapeutic approaches toward patients [6]. When examining thousands of years of history, no matter how much the environmental conditions change, there has always been an intense relationship between societies and horses [57]. In the literature review on the therapeutic use of horses, the concept of AAT is under two headings: therapeutic riding and hippo-therapy. These concepts are named differently as both methods are different but basically with the same goal [58].

Although there is a belief that horses were tamed and ridden and used in the treatment of the human beings in B.C., there is no definite evidence on this subject [59]. Looking at history and the use of horses as therapeutic agents, horse riding was considered as a physically during exercise in the sixteenth and seventeenth centuries. This aspect was also observed during the 29 rehabilitation of war veterans after the World War II [58]. The use of horses for disabled people has been intensified since the middle of the twentieth century. The best example regarding this was the treatment process, which resulted in Lis Hartel, professional horse-rider, participating in the Olympics and winning a medal while losing lower extremity functions due to polio. After this excellent success, equestrian federations have been established in many developed countries, mainly in England, and AATs are being covered under universal health insurance [60].

Hippo-therapy, one of the commonly used methods of therapeutic intervention, is derived from the ancient Greek word "Hyppos." With this method, horses can be used to develop or rehabilitate the individual's physical, sensory, cognitive, and social functions through the use of horseback movements. Since 2010, American Hippo-therapy Association has created a conceptual framework that includes sensory integration, including dynamic systems theory and motor learning. This conceptual framework takes into account the natural rhythm or movement of the horse that can affect the participants' neurological, motor, vestibular, sensory, and functional considerations to achieve the intended goals or outcomes [61].

Choosing the appropriate horse for the therapy session helps the individual to meet the rehabilitation needs with the individual and the horse feeling more comfortable. The features of an ideal therapy horse are an average age of 10–12 years, an average height of 150–160 cm to help control horses and riders and side holders to about 45° tilt (the stepping stones will get harder as the angle of the bog is lowered), and being calm and gentile [6, 60]. The sessions with hippo therapy, which consist of meeting, warming, working, relaxation, and farewell, are planned by interdisciplinary professionals. Hippo-therapist, occupational therapist, physiotherapist, special education specialist, private horse instructors, and volunteers who have been educated about hippo therapy may be included in the rehabilitation sessions in menaj [61].

As a treatment strategy, hippo therapy may primarily be dependent on the theory of sensory integration because the movement of the horse provides a sensory experience for the rider. The role of therapists is to determine the amount of sensory stimulation and the input [61]. For example, walking slowly cannot be enough incentive to allow the rider to join a relative. On the other hand, brisk walking or jogging can increase the attention span. In addition, riding bareback can help the rider get the maximum possible proprioceptive input. As an alternative approach, stirrups (used with a saddle or backpack) can help proprioceptive input by gravity on the hard surface. Sans, Fortney, and Willenbring [71] argue about this approach of sensory integration as a rider. In addition, this internal drive can be further improved through the connection between the rider and the horse.

At a hippo-therapy session, the horse changes motion by an average of 2000 steps, which means that the rider is also taking 2000 strokes—about 2000 muscle contractions. It has been proved that the increased number of repetitions support motor learning. Therefore, the increase in the number of repetitions due to hippo therapy is the most important parameter supporting the development of static-dynamic balance, weight transfer, motor planning, and motor skill in the direction of the individual's motor learning principles [62]. During hippotherapy intervention, following the provision of a suitable position for the rider, the three planes are prepared in accordance with the principles of movement, rhythm, motor learning, and motivation. It has a positive effect on coordination, reaction time, sensory processing, respiratory control, motor planning, and postural control [6, 62]. This multifunctional approach helps to increase the positive effect of the therapy and success of the therapy.

4.1.7. Animal-assisted therapy and occupational therapy

Occupational therapy is a client-centered approach to these individuals in rehabilitation practices. The assessment and intervention of occupational therapy are aimed to improve the participation in their daily living activities more meaning and oriented [63]. Occupational therapists use a lot of approaches in their practice to improve quality of life and well-being in their patients. A range of target areas that can be addressed with the help of therapy animals are listed in the book for AAT interventions for OT: motor skills (gross and fine motor), neuro-musculoskeletal skills (range of motion, strength, balance), sensory functioning (tactile, visual, auditory), cognitive skills (orientation, attention, executive functions), weight bearing, communication skills (expression and acculturation language, cooperation), psychosocial skills (well-being, motivation), perception processing skills (body perception, depth perception, spatial relationships), and respiratory function (diaphragm force, positioning) [6, 64].

According to OTs' views and perceptions of evidence-based practice, AAT is one of the methods used in rehabilitation. Some researchers have investigated the impact of AAT on elderly participants who were diagnosed with psychiatric, physical, and developmental disabilities in long-term care settings [65]. Van Fleet and his colleagues describe an animal-supported occupational therapy as a learning process in which a professional therapist carries out a therapy session, using a dog, to facilitate the development of the skills needed by the child to have an independent function in self-help, playgrounds. A therapy dog may become part of the learning process when learning everyday tasks related to the animal [66]. OTs may add a wrist weight to gain strength from the weak arm or use a customized brush with a special handle to help the child hold the brush. Thus, the child becomes more motivated and excited to participate in the treatment. Thus, this method helps OTs, and the child can to reach the child's treatment goals more quickly and easily [67]. In another study, AAT was also applied on patients with post-traumatic stress disorder generally seen in personnel during military service; AAT was found to provide positive benefits. It was also observed that new gained in combat veterans learned new skills using trained dogs [68].

Dogs are a popular choice for many occupational therapists. OTs showed that treatment with dogs, which are often preferred for treatment, has improved social skills, motivation, having an interest in the environment, and self-awareness of children with autism spectrum who had behavioral problems [6]. A study performed on OTs found that senior citizens in a walking program at an assisted living facility walked further when with a dog than when they walked alone, indicating the potential value of pets in physical conditioning [69]. Due to the earlier studies mentioned, the OTs believed AAT impacted individuals through internal responses to the animal and thorough responses to the external environment. On the other hand, horses proved to be effective in treatment programs, especially for physically disabled people. Among the reasons for preferring the horse in these types of patients include; it can be said that walking on the horse can feel like as the walking accent, walking distance can be adjusted by the therapist or rider if necessary, and positive feeling can increase the motivation of the person [6, 70].

In almost all studies on AAT, animal interaction increased motivation of individuals:

- Those who refuse therapy may come to therapy sessions more often and easily when they know that animals are present.
- Interaction with animals raises morale of long-term care residents.
- People feel better socially people feel better about themselves the idea of ownership of animals and the responsibility for care given to them increases the daily devotion
- Sense, motor, perception, cognitive, and social skills improve.
- Participation in functioning and daily living activities are facilitated.

OT should focus on the use and participation of meaningful activities to improve the quality of life of an individual in AAT intervention. For these purposes, it is aimed to develop correct posture and walking pattern, mobility of the pelvis and hip region, head and trunk control, muscle tone and strength, sense regulation, social communication, self-confidence and empathy, motor and cognitive skills. It is thought that the ability of individuals to improve their skills, function, and quality of life can be improved by pet ownership, care of animals, and regular interaction during therapy.

The frequency of use of the AAT and AAA in the field of rehabilitation for the last 10 years has been rapidly increasing. Animal-supported approaches from different countries and disciplines showed positive effects on sensory, emotional, and cognitive functions, especially the physical structure and functions of individuals at different ages and diagnoses. OTs emphasize the effectiveness of this method in studies conducted in the field of occupational therapy. At the same time, we believe more qualitative and quantitative research and more detailed studies are still needed and OT's and OT intervention programs focusing on therapeutic use of animals in rehabilitation must continue.

Author details

Sedef Şahin*, Barkın Kose and Meral Zarif

*Address all correspondence to: sedefkarayazgan88@hotmail.com

Faculty of Health Sciences, Occupational Therapy Department, Hacettepe University, Ankara, Turkey

References

[1] Fine A, Mio J. The role of AAT in clinical practice: The importance of demonstrating empirically oriented psychotherapies. In: Handbook on Animal-Assisted Therapy: Theoretical Foundations and Guidelines for Practice. USA: Elseiver; 2010;**3**:563-578

[2] Cevizci S, Erginoz E, Baltas Z. Animal-assisted therapy for improving human health. TAF Preventive Medicine Bulletin. 2009;**8**(3):263-272

[3] Cevizci S, Sen HM, Güneş F, Karaahmet E. Animal assisted therapy and activities in alzheimer's disease. In: Understanding Alzheimer's Disease. Intech; 2013

[4] Cevizci S, Erginöz E, Baltaş Z. Ruh sağlığının iyileştirilmesinde destek bir tedavi yaklaşımı: Hayvan destekli tedavi. Nobel Med. 2009;**5**(1):4-9

[5] Frewin K, Gardiner B. New age or old sage? A review of equine assisted psychotherapy. Australian Journal of Counselling Psychology. 2005;**6**(2):13-17

[6] Fine AH. Animal-assisted therapy. In: Encyclopedia of Psychotherapy. USA: Elseiver; 2002;**1**:49-55

[7] Benedict R. The Concept of the Guardian Spirit in North America. USA: American Anthropological Association, Elseiver; 1923

[8] Serpell JA. Animal companions and human well-being: An historical exploration of the value of human—Animal relationships. In: Handbook on Animal-Assisted Therapy. 2nd ed. Philadelphia: Elsevier; 2006. pp. 3-19

[9] Noll R, Achterberg J, Bourguignon E, George L, Harner M, Honko L, et al. Mental imagery cultivation as a cultural phenomenon: The role of visions in shamanism [and comments and reply]. Current Anthropology. 1985;**26**(4):443-461

[10] Wenzel GW. Ningiqtuq: Resource sharing and generalized reciprocity in Clyde River, Nunavut. Arctic Anthropology. 1995:43-60

[11] Hultkrantz Å. On beliefs in non-shamanic guardian spirits among Saamis. Scripta Instituti Donneriani Aboensis. 1987;**12**:110-123

[12] Landes R. Ojibwa Religion and the Midéwiwin. USA: University of Wisconsin Press, Elseiver;1968

[13] Maehle A-H. Cruelty and kindness to the "brute creation: "stability and change in the ethics of the man-animal relationship, 1600-1850. In: Animals and Human Society: Changing Perspectives. USA: Elseiver; 1994. pp. 81-105

[14] Thomas K. Man and the Natural World: Changing Attitudes in England 1500-1800. UK: Penguin; 1991

[15] Salisbury JE. The Beast within: Animals in the Middle Ages. Philadelphia: Routledge; 2011

[16] Myers OG. Children and Animals: Social Development and our Connections to Other Species. Philadelphia: Westview Press; 1998

[17] Grier KC. Childhood socialization and companion animals: United States, 1820-1870. Society and Animals. 1999;**7**(2):95-120

[18] Toynbee JM. Animals in Roman Life and Art. Philadelphia: Johns Hopkins University Press; 1996

[19] Turner J. Reckoning with the Beast. Philadelphia. Johns Hopkins University, 1980

[20] Allderidge PH. A cat, surpassing in beauty, and other therapeutic animals. The Psychiatrist. 1991;**15**(12):759-762

[21] Nightingale F. Note on Nursing. Philadelphia: Simon and Schuster; 2013

[22] Shafton A. Dream Reader: Contemporary Approaches to the Understanding of Dreams. Philadelphia: SUNY Press; 1995

[23] Van de Castle RL. Our Dreaming Mind: Ballantine Books. USA: Elseiver; 1994

[24] Serpell JA. Creatures of the unconscious: Companion animals as mediators. In: Companion Animals and us: Exploring the Relationship between People and Pets. USA: Elseiver; 2000. pp. 108-124

[25] Gregory RL, Zangwill OL. The Oxford Companion to the Mind. Philadelphia: Oxford University Press; 1987

[26] Levinson BM. Pets and Human Development. USA: Elseiver; 1972

[27] Levinson BM, Mallon GP. Pet-Oriented Child Psychotherapy. Charles C. Philadelphia: Thomas Publisher; 1997

[28] Friedmann E, Katcher AH, Lynch JJ, Thomas SA. Animal companions and one-year survival of patients after discharge from a coronary care unit. Public Health Reports. 1980;**95**(4):307

[29] Kruger KA, Serpell JA. Animal-assisted interventions in mental health: Definitions and theoretical foundations. In: Handbook on Animal-Assisted Therapy. 3rd ed. Elsevier; 2010. pp. 33-48

[30] Siegel JM. Stressful life events and use of physician services among the elderly: The moderating role of pet ownership. Journal of Personality and Social Psychology. 1990;**58**(6):1081

[31] Cobb S. Social support as a moderator of life stress. Psychosomatic Medicine. 1976;**38**(5): 300-314

[32] Eriksen W. The role of social support in the pathogenesis of coronary heart disease. A literature review. Family Practice. 1994;**11**(2):201-209

[33] Esterling BA, Kiecolt-Glaser JK, Bodnar JC, Glaser R. Chronic stress, social support, and persistent alterations in the natural killer cell response to cytokines in older adults. Health Psychology. 1994;**13**(4):291

[34] House JS, Landis KR, Umberson D. Social relationships and health. Science. 1988; **241**(4865):540-545

[35] Sherbourne CD, Meredith LS, Rogers W, Ware JE. Social support and stressful life events: Age differences in their effects on health-related quality of life among the chronically ill. Quality of Life Research. 1992;**1**(4):235-246

[36] Ader R, Cohen N, Felten D. Psychoneuroimmunology: Interactions between the nervous system and the immune system. The Lancet. 1995;**345**(8942):99-103

[37] Chandler CK. Animal-Assisted Therapy in Counseling. Philadelphia: Taylor & Francis; 2017

[38] Barker SB, Pandurangi AK, Best AM. Effects of animal-assisted therapy on patients' anxiety, fear, and depression before ECT. The journal of ECT. 2003;**19**(1):38-44

[39] Katcher A, Wilkins GG. Animal-assisted therapy in the treatment of disruptive behavior disorders in children. In: The Environment and Mental Health: A Guide for Clinicians. USA: Elseiver; 1998. pp. 193-204

[40] Martin F, Farnum J. Animal-assisted therapy for children with pervasive developmental disorders. Western Journal of Nursing Research. 2002;**24**(6):657-670

[41] Filan SL, Llewellyn-Jones RH. Animal-assisted therapy for dementia: A review of the literature. International Psychogeriatrics. 2006;**18**(4):597-611

[42] Richeson NE. Effects of animal-assisted therapy on agitated behaviors and social interactions of older adults with dementia. American Journal of Alzheimer's Disease and Other Dementias. 2003;**18**(6):353-358

[43] Barker SB, Dawson KS. The effects of animal-assisted therapy on anxiety ratings of hospitalized psychiatric patients. Psychiatric Services. 1998;**49**(6):797-801

[44] Animal Assisted Therapy. Available from: https://www.allenmorecounseling.com/animal-assisted-therapy-tacoma/

[45] Nathanson DE, de Castro D, Friend H, McMahon M. Effectiveness of short-term dolphin-assisted therapy for children with severe disabilities. Anthrozoös. 1997;**10**(2-3):90-100

[46] Berget B, Ekeberg Ø, Braastad BO. Animal-assisted therapy with farm animals for persons with psychiatric disorders: Effects on self-efficacy, coping ability and quality of life, a randomized controlled trial. Clinical Practice & Epidemiology in Mental Health. 2008;**4**(1):9

[47] Berget B, Braastad BO. Animal-assisted therapy with farm animals for persons with psychiatric disorders. Annali dell'Istituto Superiore di Sanità. 2011;**47**:384-390

[48] Fiksdal BL, Houlihan D, Barnes AC. Dolphin-assisted therapy: Claims versus evidence. Autism research and treatment. 2012;**2012**

[49] Nathanson DE, de Faria S. Cognitive improvement of children in water with and without dolphins. Anthrozoös. 1993;**6**(1):17-29

[50] Weiss E, Greenberg G. Service dog selection tests: Effectiveness for dogs from animal shelters. Applied Animal Behaviour Science. 1997;**53**(4):297-308

[51] Svartberg K, Tapper I, Temrin H, Radesäter T, Thorman S. Consistency of personality traits in dogs. Animal Behaviour. 2005;**69**(2):283-291

[52] Nimer J, Lundahl B. Animal-assisted therapy: A meta-analysis. Anthrozoös. 2007; **20**(3):225-238

[53] Morrison ML. Health benefits of animal-assisted interventions. Complementary Health Practice Review. 2007;**12**(1):51-62

[54] Banks MR, Banks WA. The effects of animal-assisted therapy on loneliness in an elderly population in long-term care facilities. The Journals of Gerontology Series A: Biological Sciences and Medical Sciences. 2002;**57**(7):M428-M432

[55] Braun C, Stangler T, Narveson J, Pettingell S. Animal-assisted therapy as a pain relief intervention for children. Complementary Therapies in Clinical Practice. 2009;**15**(2):105-109

[56] Marcus DA, Bernstein CD, Constantin JM, Kunkel FA, Breuer P, Hanlon RB. Animal-assisted therapy at an outpatient pain management clinic. Pain Medicine. 2012;**13**(1):45-57

[57] Masini A. Equine-assisted psychotherapy in clinical practice. Journal of Psychosocial Nursing and Mental Health Services. 2010;**48**(10):30-34

[58] Lasa SM, Bocanegra NM, Alcaide RV, Arratibel MA, Donoso EV, Ferriero G. Animal assisted interventions in neurorehabilitation: A review of the most recent literature. Neurologia (English Edition). 2015;**30**(1):1-7

[59] Muñoz-Lasa S, Ferriero G, Valero R, Gomez-Muñiz F, Rabini A, Varela E. Effect of therapeutic horseback riding on balance and gait of people with multiple sclerosis. Giornale Italiano di Medicina del Lavoro ed Ergonomia. 2011;**33**(4):462-467

[60] Fry NE. Equine-Assisted Therapy: An Overview. Biotherapy-History, Principles and Practice: Springer; 2013. pp. 255-284

[61] American Hippotherapy Association. Available from: http://www.americanhippotherapyassociation.org/

[62] Zadnikar M, Kastrin A. Effects of hippotherapy and therapeutic horseback riding on postural control or balance in children with cerebral palsy: A meta-analysis. Developmental Medicine and Child Neurology. 2011;**53**(8):684-691

[63] Kielhofner G. Conceptual Foundations of Occupational Therapy Practice. FA Davis, Philadelphia. 2009

[64] Winkle M, Crowe TK, Hendrix I. Service dogs and people with physical disabilities partnerships: A systematic review. Occupational Therapy International. 2012;**19**(1):54-66

[65] Le Roux MC, Kemp R. Effect of a companion dog on depression and anxiety levels of elderly residents in a long-term care facility. Psychogeriatrics. 2009;**9**(1):23-26

[66] Van Fleet R, Fine AH, O'Callaghan D, Mackintosh T, Gimeno J. Application of animal-assisted interventions in professional settings: An overview of alternatives. In: Handbook on Animal-Assisted Therapy. 4th ed. Philadelphia: Elsevier; 2015. pp. 157-177

[67] Dimitrijević I. Animal-assisted therapy–a new trend in the treatment of children and adults. Psychiatria Danubina. 2009;**21**(2):236-241

[68] Alers EV, Simpson KM. Reclaiming identity through service to dogs in need. Canine Assisted Therapy In Military Medicine. 2012;72-83

[69] Herbert JH, Greene D. Effect of preference on distance walked by assisted living residents. Physical & Occupational Therapy In Geriatrics. 2001;**19**(4):1-15

[70] Velde BP, Cipriani J, Fisher G. Resident and therapist views of animal-assisted therapy: Implications for occupational therapy practice. Australian Occupational Therapy Journal. 2005;**52**(1):43-50

[71] Sams MJ, Fortney EV, Willenbring S. Occupational therapy incorporating animals for children with autism: A pilot investigation. American Journal of Occupational Therapy. 2006;**60**(3):268-274

11

New Flower Bed Design and Verification Supporting Horticultural Therapy Classes Based on Behavioral Observation

Meng-Cong Zheng

Abstract

Horticultural therapy improves the elderly's emotional and cognitive functions and also leads to their social participation and better overall health. We want to know about the problems of implementing horticultural therapy and how to improve it with the flower bed design. "House of Love" is a private nursing home in Taipei and had been the research base in this study. It was found that current horticultural classes heavily rely on teacher-centric and volunteer staff-assisted curricula, often not considering the specific physical and psychological needs the elderly usually face in classes. "Elderly Green" is a new design taking the requirements of horticultural classes in to consideration, providing for a maximum of flexibility under varying conditions by modulizing the flower bed. It allowed the elderly to do their gardening in a comfortable and less strenuous manner. "Elderly Green" is a centripetal flower bed design improved equally distributed care for each participant during class time and increased interaction among the elderly that reduces manpower needs.

Keywords: flower bed design, horticultural therapy, behavioral observation

1. Introduction

Taiwan has become an aging society. Even though many assisted living facilities are providing care services for the elderly, most of them do not want to move into nursing homes because the perceived lifestyle at these facilities is foreign to them. "Aging in place" is a concept that first originated from Northern Europe during the 1960s. The goal at the time was to care for the elderly with resources that are native to them so they could age in an environment that is familiar to their culture, which would give them the holistic care and independence that they deserve. On the contrary, some nursing homes limit the elderly's lifestyle choices and social functions, which may damage their mental health and self-respect resulting in deterioration of their body and mind [1]. The goal of "Aging in place" was to fulfill the native's needs with domestic goods and services, which would require community-like facilities to build a long-term care system. Most of the assisted living facilities today in Taiwan are based on community activities to promote interaction among the elderly. Healthcare-oriented facilities should be considered more when daily activities and movements become less convenient for the elders. Japanese welfare economist [2] proposed five basic measures to ensure that the elderly live a normal life: avoid taking quarantine measures; allow them to live in an environment with which they are familiar as much as possible; facilitate their social exchanges and mutual assistance; provide facilities and services to maintain quality of life when institutionalized care becomes necessary; and integrate social welfare, medical and health, and environmental maintenance policies to create a suitable living environment.

Sandberg indicated that 95% of the elderly in Hong Kong have one or more chronic diseases; however, only 5.5% require institutionalized care [3]. Although nursing homes can help the elderly who cannot live independently [1], institutionalized care entails a change in living environment, and consequently, disconnection from family and society as well as a reduction in physical activities and enhanced loneliness [4]. Another study found that the physical activity level of the nursing home-dwelling elderly is considerably lower than that of the community-dwelling elderly [5]. In addition to facing changes to their environment and mobility, the elderly who move into nursing homes must deal with changes in daily life routine, social network, and social support [6]. Moving into a nursing home means the discontinuation of a person's traditional lifestyle with which they are familiar. In addition, the elderly can sustain an enormous sense of loss caused by separation from families, neighbors, and friends [1, 7]. When the elderly face gradual decline in physical and mental status, what can be done to ensure they age stably is a question that requires an answer. The American Horticultural Therapy Association (AHTA) maintained that horticultural therapy can be applied to people of various ages, backgrounds, and abilities. It defined horticultural therapy as "engaging in gardening-related activities through the assistance of a trained therapist to complete a specific therapeutic goal." Horticultural therapy has four major types of benefits: intellectual, social, emotional, and physical [8–11].

Intellectual benefits: Through horticultural therapy, participants can acquire new skills and knowledge, increase their vocabulary and communication skills, have their curiosity aroused, improve observation, receive occupational and pre-occupational training, receive stimulation to their sensory organs [11–14], and obtain new learning opportunities [15].

Social benefits: A successful treatment should involve three types of interaction: between the therapist and the client, between clients, and between the client and nonclient [16]. Generally, these interactions mainly are aimed at socializing and collaborating; specifically, sharing gardening experiences facilitates creating meaningful interactions. Because group members have a common goal, interactions among them can be increased on the basis of mutual respect and support, as well as duty sharing. During the process of gardening, patients have the opportunity to connect with people other than their group members and share their own gardening results with external parties, thereby gaining the benefit of an enlarged interpersonal network [4, 11, 17].

Emotional benefits: Lewis and Mattson maintained that through gardening activities, people can experience serene satisfaction in the world of plants where no threats or discriminations exist, thereby alleviating their mental stress and fear [2]. Furthermore, when patients discern that they can work independently and have their own gardens, a sense of identification and belonging to the gardens emerge in them, and their self-respect is enhanced. When patients' confidence is elevated, their belligerent tendencies can be tempered and adjusted to socially acceptable behavioral models; in addition, their interests and passion for future life are triggered to satisfy their creative instinct [11]. Moreover, gardening activities can help patients develop an ideal self-image and continually develop work skills [12]. Because numerous factors in the living environment can affect people's emotions, a designed and selected environment can indeed quicken patients' emotional recovery [18–21]. For example, a successful therapeutic garden can reduce people's stress, even generating a sense of encouragement [22].

Physical benefits: In addition to mental benefits, gardening activities help wounded or physically disabled individuals to improve their coordination and effectively control their motor neurons through tasks such as carrying plants, sowing seeds, applying fertilizer, and watering plants [11].

For the elderly, gardening enables them to improve physical and mental health through a leisure activity. Therefore, an increasing number of the retired elderly have devoted themselves to gardening activities, and numerous elderly nursing and home care centers have introduced horticultural therapy. Research has shown that horticultural therapy can improve the elderly's arthritis symptoms, and it exerts positive effects on blood pressure and diet control [2]. Furthermore, gardening activities can increase regular physical activities that require physical and mental stability as well as high-level functional activities [23]. Gardening practices have the clear effects of enhancing muscle strength, fine motor skills, and balance; in particular, transplanting requires grasping and releasing with the thumb and index finger as well as muscle flexibility [23, 24]. Gardening activities boost enthusiasm and senses of responsibility and achievement. From selecting plants to their growth and eventual flowering, plants continually create hope for people. Furthermore, learning gardening skills enhances the elderly's curiosity. Therapeutic use of activity can help the geriatric individuals to improve their independence in daily life, and cognitive and motor skills [13, 21, 23]. The activity that will be used as a therapeutic agent can be determined according to the interests, activity preference, and the skills of the geriatrics [19, 25, 26]. Gardening can expand people's social networks by providing opportunities to socialize [27]; thus, gardening activities have positive effects on the community-dwelling elderly.

Brown administered a 5-week horticultural therapy course to 66 older residents in nursing homes [28], and found that compared with the control group, residents in the test group exhibited significantly greater improvements before and after receiving the horticultural therapy in several items on the activities of daily living (ADL) scale, namely physical ambulation, feeding, and toilet. Austin applied a 5-week horticultural therapy course to eight elderly people who lived by themselves, the results of which revealed that their fitness, ADL scores, and 6-min walk test results all improved significantly after the intervention [29]. In addition, Son administered a 5-week horticultural therapy to five community-dwelling elderly people, and found that during vegetable-planting activities, they could use adapted tools and aids to teach the elderly to adjust to appropriate joint movement angles, balance using suitable postures, and train gross and fine motor skills, eventually improving their physical activity and self-maintenance abilities [30]. Thelander introduced a 6-week outdoor gardening intervention to eight older residents with dementia at a frequency of three times a week, for 40–70 minutes per session [31]. The results indicated that landscape maintenance tasks such as watering, weeding, and fallen leaf picking significantly improved the residents' balance. Gigliotti and Jarrott compared the elderly participating in gardening activities with counterparts receiving conventional treatment, and found that those in the horticultural therapy group exhibited significantly higher levels of activity involvement and positive emotions [32]. Lee and Kim implemented a 4-week gardening intervention comprising selecting bean cultivars, sowing seeds, watering plants, touching the plants they had planted, cleaning and maintaining the planting environment, and harvesting, cutting, and washing the plants; their results indicated that these indoor gardening activities significantly reduced anxiety [33]. Austin determined that after receiving horticultural therapy, the elderly exhibited significantly lower levels of anxiety [29]. By touching the plants they had planted, cleaning and maintaining the planting environment, and harvesting, cutting, and cleaning the plants, the elderly were engaged in higher levels of physical activity, which in turn improved their cognitive functions [33]. In addition, Sempik, Aldridge, and Becker noted that gardening activities strengthened the elderly's sense of responsibility and increased the opportunities for decision-making, through which their degradation could be slowed and the group became consolidated because of sharpened social skills [34]. However, gardening activities remain inadequate in the elderly's nursing homes. Although lawns and gardens are common in nursing institutions, they are rarely designed according to user needs. SCUs in France conducted a survey from 1992 to 2007, determining that less than 82% of medical institutions had freely accessible outdoor space, and only 43% provided patients with access to this outdoor space; thus, gardens were not regarded as a part of health management. Nevertheless, compared with conventional treatments that require hospitalization, horticultural therapy is generally more accessible to patients and easier to adapt to; furthermore, the costs are cheaper than other types of therapy. Despite gardening activities being widely recognized as a positive therapy, substantial efforts are still required to popularize this therapy in public care systems. Engaging in gardening activities typically requires the elderly to bend or squat. When planting is conducted in a standing posture, people in a wheelchair have difficulty participating because square tables have limited availability. Therefore, defining design conditions that support the elderly's participation in gardening activities is paramount. Research has shown that the first condition to be considered in horticultural equipment design is to lower the participants' physical burden. When the elderly are allowed to engage in the activities by themselves, their opportunities for mutual communication increased; however, their exchanges and communications reduced when a facilitator joined [35]. Circle theory in the field of environmental psychology maintains that using a round table enables people to see each other. However, results of one experiment revealed that simple concentric tables could not satisfy the requirements of wheelchair users and others with diversified physical conditions [36]. Even so, designers may still experiment with other shapes that have the effect of a circle to determine which table shape facilitates the interaction of people with varying physical conditions in a variety of venues. Horticultural therapy courses stimulate emotions, boost activity levels, reduce stress and fear through human-to-plant interactions, increase muscle relaxation, and promote confidence and knowledge. These courses promote user's sense of responsibility and self-fulfillment through plant care, which also enhances cognitive capabilities. Group activities in planting and sharing experiences create community opportunities and respect among each other. There is a connection between social participation and environment recognition of the elderly [37, 38]. Besides, there is also a strong correlation between the elderly's ability to successfully interact with society and the quality of their facilities and surroundings. Their comfort with the surrounding environment and perception of the social interactions significantly aid their social ability [39]. Horticulture courses are crucial in planning regarding retirement and assisted-living facilities. Many studies showed mind-body health improvements among the elderly who partake in horticulture classes. However, implementing horticulture courses through assisted care and planning in these facilities are not enough. We need to consider an elder's activity level, physical ability, and health condition in gardening classes to implement communication and activity in their curriculum.

This study investigates facilities that have implemented horticulture classes in their treatment. Through interviews and behavioral observation to find out the problems and conditions associated with horticulture classes, also understand the different types of gardening, facility deployment, and gardening treatment details and execution. This study also focuses on the duration of these classes to understand the effectiveness of horticulture classes that will be helpful for future class design and planning.

2. Method

"House of Love" is a private nursing home and a research base established in 1923, for the elderly, people with no assistance, the sick, and the homeless. "House of Love" is also awarded for excellence by the Ministry of Home Affairs and Taipei City Hall. "House of Love" is the best long-term care center in Taipei that focuses on treatment of the body and mind (**Figure 1**). This study implemented records of long-term behavioral observation in "House of Love" with a focus on cases who participated in these horticulture classes, the

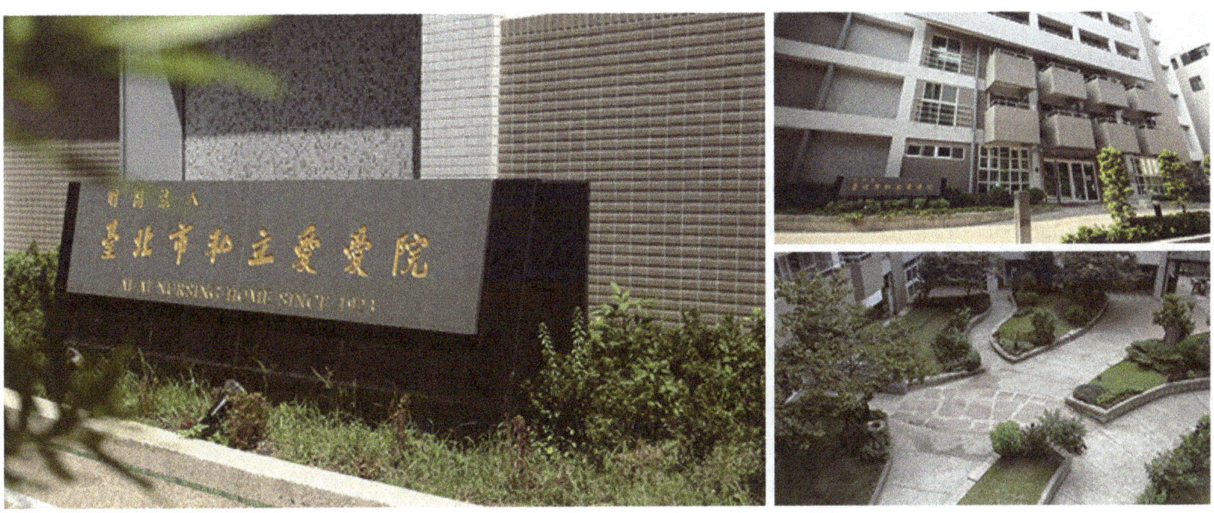

Figure 1. Private nursing home "House of Love".

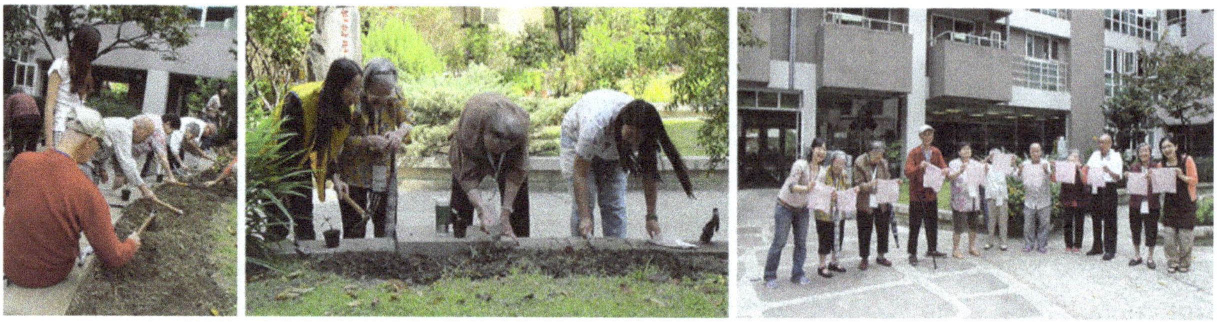

Figure 2. Observation one, class one (control group).

interaction between them, their problems in grading, and studies of these classes. Behavioral observation and post-occupancy evaluation were used in this study. Behavioral observation is referred to as sequential action marking; this method is a type of continuous observation-recording, and its objective is to record the relationship between time and actions. This study adopted behavioral observation to record the process of the elderly's engagement in gardening activities. Post-occupancy evaluation was adopted to evaluate user evaluations after experiencing the design. Weaknesses in the proposed design could be determined from users' behaviors and reactions, and corresponding design strategies could be developed.

This study was carried out in three sections. The first section focuses on observation of elders who participated in horticulture classes. We implemented behavioral observations in the three classes as below:

1. Observation of class one (control group) (**Figure 2**)

   Class location: flower beds with sitting areas.

   Elder group: the elderly with dementia and ambulatory.

   Class participation: nine elders, one teacher, one social worker, and three volunteers

2. Observation one, class two (control group) (**Figure 3**)

   Class location: operating area.

   Elder group: the elderly in wheelchair and ambulatory.

   Class participation: total of 13 elders. Nine in wheelchair and four ambulatory, one teacher, one social worker, and seven volunteers

3. Observation one, class three (control group) (**Figure 4**)

   Class location: low floral display area in the back of the garden.

   Elder group: the elderly on lower treatment.

   Class participation: total of eight elders, one teacher, one social worker, and 10 volunteers.

The investigation was conducted using behavioral observation. The gardening course was implemented in the Garden of Fragrance in the House of Love. Classes for the control group were documented faithfully in their entirety with videos and photographs. The collected files

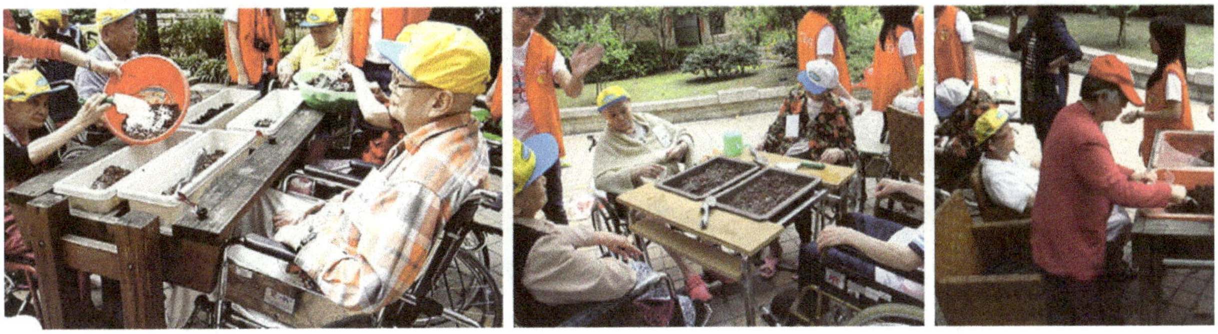

Figure 3. Observation one, class two (control group).

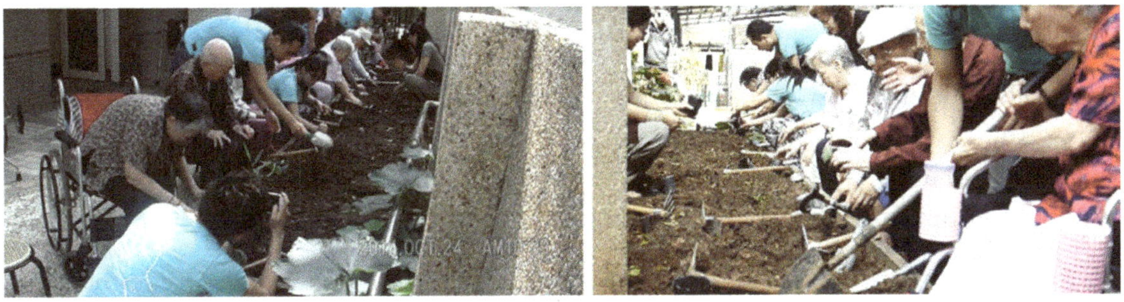

Figure 4. Observation one, class three (control group).

were coded and divided into four categories: class-related objects, classroom interactions, the elderly's upper extremity activities, and the elderly's lower extremity activities.

Section 2 focuses on how we make a design proposal of gardening tools and then new design proposal will put into section three which uses behavioral observation again in another horticultural therapy class to see its effect.

4. Observation of new class (test group)

    Class location: side exit of the main building in the plaza.

    Elder group: currently in wheelchair.

    Class participation: five elders, one teacher, no social workers, and no volunteer.

This study is based on behavioral observation and post-occupancy evaluation. We hope the result would combine gardening therapy and class design in an amicable environment for elders.

3. Results

The observation results indicated that classes two and three involved longer durations of activities conducted in a sitting posture. Compared with a standing posture, engaging the elderly during the classes in a sitting posture led to more satisfactory evaluations from the teacher in the postclass interviews. Both the teacher and social workers expressed that adopting a sitting posture effectively prevented the elderly from developing exhaustion or muscle pain, whereas

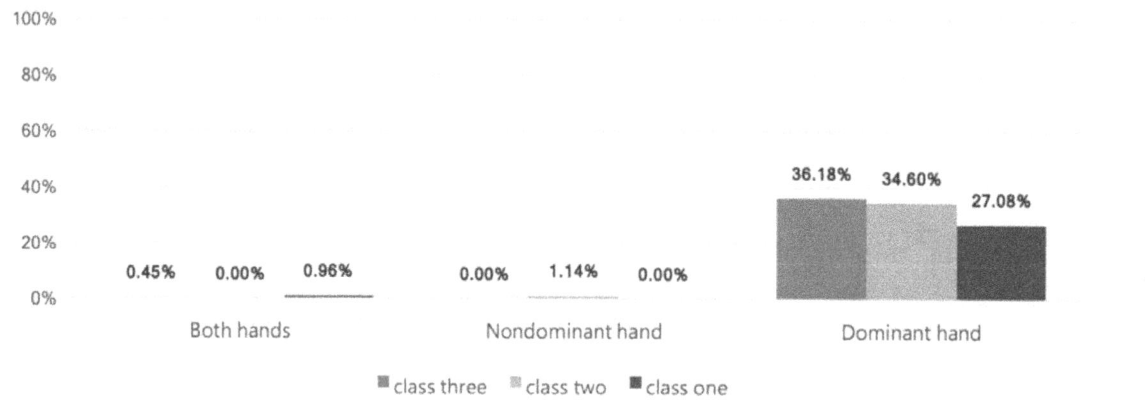

Figure 5. Behavior of tool use.

adopting a standing posture could result in these symptoms. In addition, **Figure 5** reveals considerable difference between the dominant and nondominant hand in the rate of tool use, indicating that the elderly did not use their two hands in turn for equal lengths of time. Even when engaged in bare hand operations, the elderly spent significantly longer on average operating with their dominant hand than with their nondominant hand or both hands.

There are more elders staring into space and resting behavior in class two. Even though class two has a longer duration, there is no increase in time between the interaction of plants and elders. Furthermore, elders in class two have at the highest, a 39.47% increase in time duration to observe others (**Figure 6**). The observation reveals that the unequal attention from instructors causes the unattended elders to look around at other elders in boredom.

The instructor in three horticulture classes pointed out that sedentary positions are more suitable for elders in gardening activities that prevent fatigue from stooping or repetitive movements. Only class two has three gardening platforms, providing more assistance during gardening. The operating platforms make it easier for elders to reach, which makes it a more suitable platform for elders to use. On the contrary, there is a high discrepancy between dominant and nondominant hand users in gardening work in class two. Moreover, observations of the three classes reveal that elders who use tools use their dominant hand 32.62% of the time more than their nondominant hand. Elders who use their bare hands use their dominant hand 17.31% of the time more than their nondominant hand. It is one point where the platform design can improve. We also know that elders more frequently use tools than bare hands to work with soil

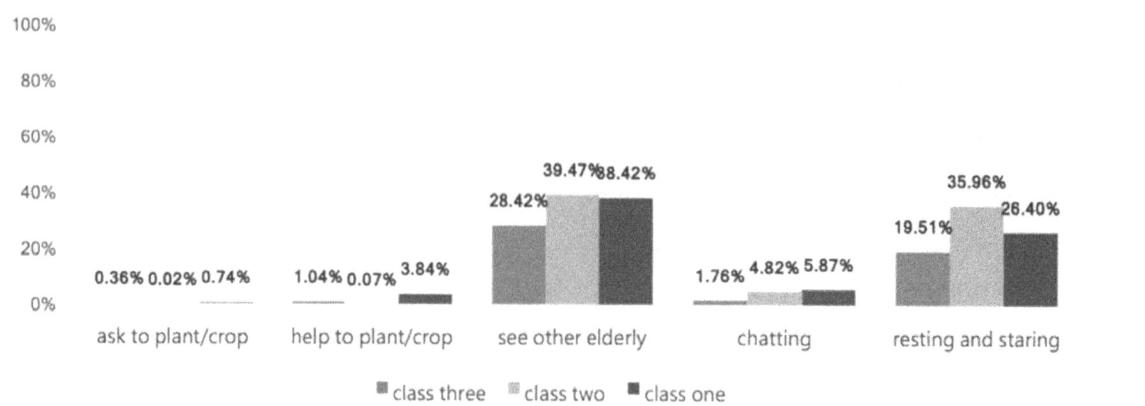

Figure 6. Intensity of elder interaction in horticulture class.

and plants based on observation. This study also focuses on the design proposals of how users place gardening tools, to give an effect of horticulture activities.

Moreover, staring into space and resting behavior are the highest in class two. When instructors are unavailable to attend to an elder, this elder ends up staring into space because he/she is confused about next steps. Observations in class two also reveal that instructors, volunteers, and social workers on average spend the most time assisting elders. The purpose of these horticulture classes is for elders to achieve therapeutic effect through finishing class experiments on their own. Over-guidance from instructors or volunteers could decrease the opportunity for elders to work on their own. One of the 13 elders in class two had less attendance. Finally, the flower platform from class two with nine elders in the wheelchair, compared to the fixed flower beds at the center of the plaza, is associated with higher mobility which can easily accompany with other classes. Therefore, we should consider the different physical condition of elders and use the mobile floral platform as a base, as a template for future gardening design.

3.1. Horticultural flower bed design concerns and conditions

Three most common problems occurred in gardening work among the elders during the first observation:

1. Bad posture: inadequate tools encourage poor posture in elders, which offsets the therapeutic benefits of the classes. The tools they used affected many postures in classes.
2. Lack of interaction of classes: horticulture classes stimulate interactions between the elderly and also reduce the aging of body function. Staring-into-space and resting behaviors take up a large percentage of class interaction based on our observations. Sharing and helping interactions among elders should be a critical design criterion for a flower bed.
3. Uneven care among elders: many staff, other than the instructor, need to focus on the situation of all elders also, which increases the burden on them. Therefore, most of these horticultural classes arrange volunteers to help. However, an oversupply of volunteers will cause uneven care among the elders, and reduce their independence to work in gardening activities. A goal of flower bed design should be taken into account the volunteer-to-elder ratio and save manpower.

3.2. Concept drafts

Horticultural therapy courses were conducted in groups. Most flower beds available on the market could be used by multiple users. However, this study aimed to develop a flower bed featuring sufficient personal space and the ability to support multiple users, thereby enhancing a sense of exclusiveness in the users. From the starting point of user space, modularized separable designs were developed to meet the aforementioned requirements (**Figure 7**).

Eventually, a hexagonal design was adopted. A set of flower beds comprising six pieces was created and modularized. The advantage of hexagon-based modularization was that the comprising pieces could be assembled into various shapes in response to varying class requirements. During the design process, the researchers considered the possibility of future production and designed the flower beds to be self-assembly pieces for the convenience of those purchasing and using the products. Hence, all components were made from planks and

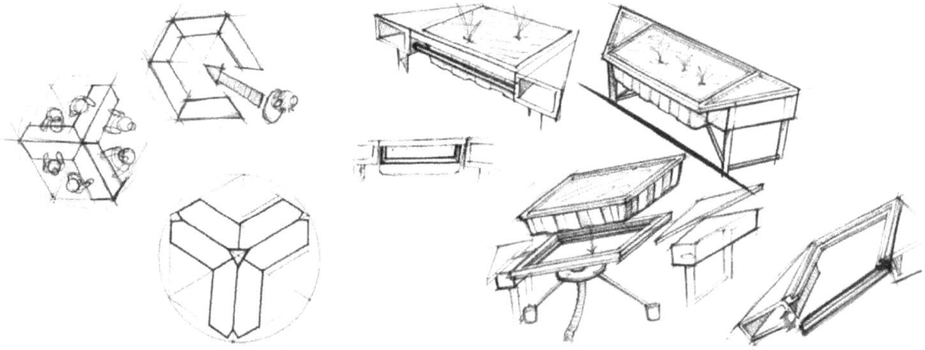

Figure 7. Development of design concepts.

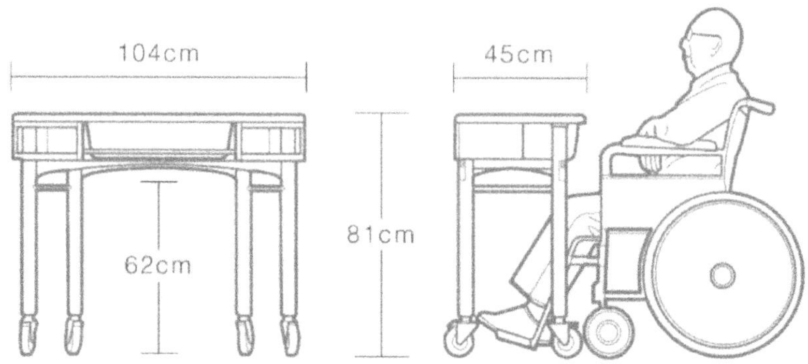

Figure 8. Flower bed dimensions.

tubes. To meet the requirements of various older users, the use of height of an ordinary elderly in the sitting and standing postures as well as that of the elderly in wheelchairs were considered. A 1:1 model was produced by measuring available wheelchairs on the market to obtain the most appropriate dimensions (**Figure 8**): 104 cm (l) × 45 cm (w) × 81 cm (h). Furthermore, the height under the table was set to 62 cm, to be compatible with the knee height of most the elderly in a sitting posture, and to allow wheelchairs to enter and exit easily.

In a satisfactory drainage system, flower bed design should be considered. The drainage system was first placed at the center of the table; however, experimental results indicated that the drainage effect was poor. Subsequently, a pipeless drainage system was designed, in which table beams were used as water channels to guide water to be discharged through table legs. With a pipeless design, water pipes or water pot damage caused by prolonged use could be prevented, and the space under the table could be effectively minimized to allow the elderly to enter and exit more easily. The soil pot that was readily available was Model-600 sealed pot, which could be used once it was pierced along the directions of the water channels, and furthermore, it could be replaced conveniently. Previous observations have suggested that approximately 15 items should be used in each gardening course session, including hoes, shovels, potted plants, and the elderly's personal belongings. Considering users' need for storage, operating platforms and drawers were added to both sides of the newly designed flower bed. The operating platforms were designed to be inclined surfaces with water drainage holes to facilitate water discharge. In addition, a round hole was designed on the top to place 5–7″ potted plants or hoes and shovels. Moreover, most of the elderly would hold on to the chair or the flower bed when standing or sitting. Therefore, iron bars were installed to surround the operating platform with raised edges for the elderly to hold on to. Multiple methods of flower bed arrangement were simulated to ensure the design was compatible with multiple course requirements. In addition to facilitating teaching, the operating platform served as a display platform after class to enhance the elderly's sense of connection with the plants they had planted. We have designed a new wooden flower bed based on all of the conditions and concerns on the sizing and interaction design factors. The flower bed is a trapezoidal desk, which allows everyone to gather around in a circle. We hope it is more convenient for the instructor to communicate with the elderly than before.

In addition, top pulleys were adopted for the casters, which featured a stamp-and-press switch to stop slippage, enable the flower beds to be arranged in class, and prevent flower bed movement when the elderly hold them for support. Because horticultural therapy classes are often implemented outdoors, all flower beds were finished with wood oils that were extracted from plants and exhibited UV-resistant and water-proof features. Subsequently, simple loading and drainage tests were conducted. A sealed pot containing approximately 30 liters of water was used in the loading test, and the results indicated that the flower bed remains stable both under normal use conditions and violent shaking. Furthermore, the drainage system was proved to be effective in leading the water to drain through the framework-turned-channels under the sealed pot to the sides of table legs to be discharged.

4. Discussions

This discussion takes the new design of the flower desk into the curriculum. The test group has a total of five participants, including four women, one man, where three of them are in wheelchairs. They sit equidistant from the teacher in a circle. The five new flower desks are arranged radially, with an opening for the instructor to freely walk in and out of it.

In the test group during the horticulture class, the elderly used the dominant hand 26.30% of the time, nondominant hand 17.58% and both hands 12.32% of the time (**Figure 9**). The test group has a much higher usage of hands in all three categories compared to the control group, especially in the nondominant hand category. The test group uses bare hands 56.21% of the class, which is much higher than the control group of 25.28%. Previous observations revealed that inappropriate flower bed dimensions can lead to a forward-leaning sitting posture. When the table top was too low, or when the elderly could not approach the flower bed with ease from their chair, they could not make effective use of the work table. However, the newly designed flower bed "Elder Green" may effectively prevent bad posture in its users. As a result, this new flower bed design stimulates both hand usage and balance in the elderly. From flipping soil to digging a hole to placing a seed to burying soil, all elders fulfilled the hand movement goals. It could be the design of "Elder Green" that allow elders to feel more intimate toward the product.

The total time that the test group spent using their dominant hands was 26.32% for tool use and 26.30% for bare hand operations. In contrast, time spent in the control group was 34.60%

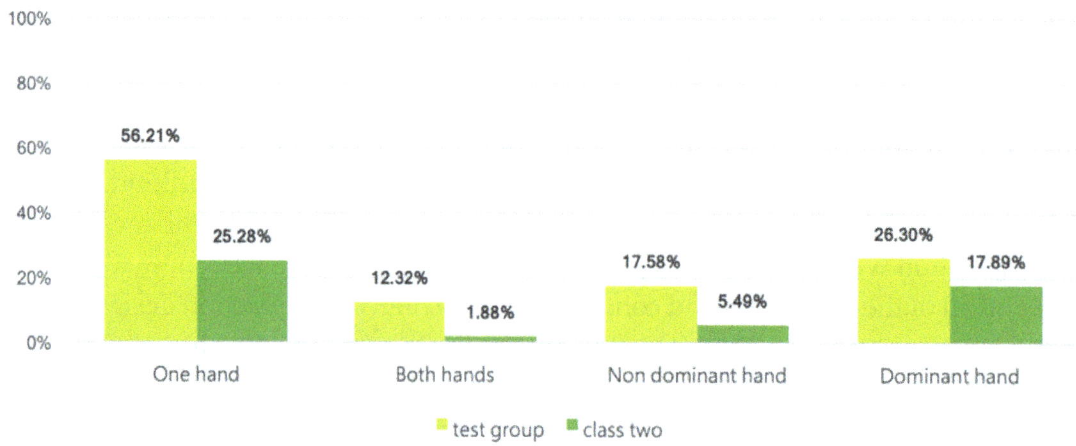

Figure 9. Average percentage of time working with bare hands.

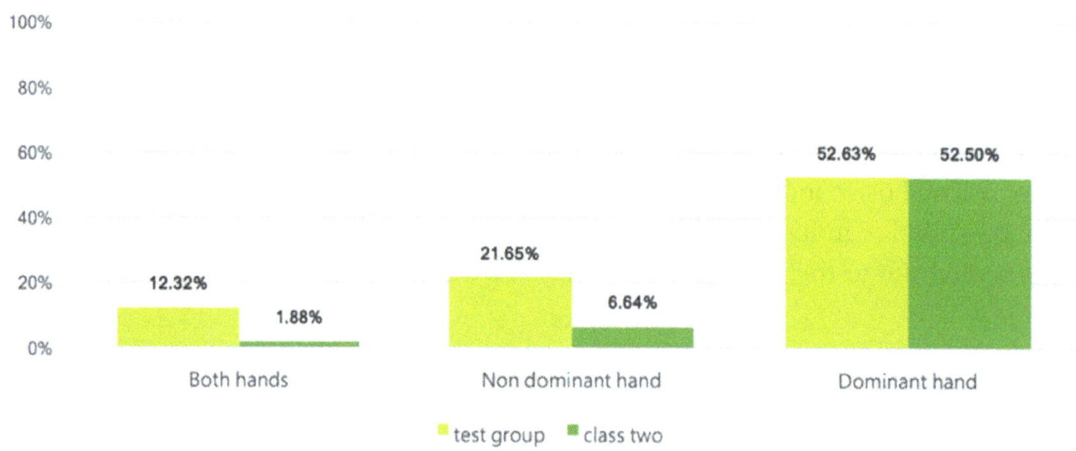

Figure 10. Average percentage of time working with tool-assisted and bare hands.

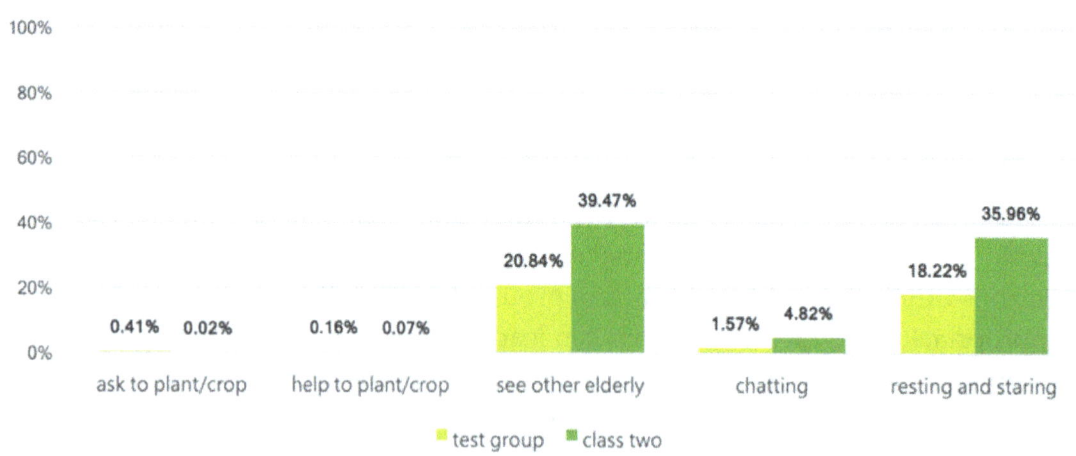

Figure 11. Interaction of the elders in class in percentage.

for tool use and 17.89% for bare hand operations (**Figure 10**). The results indicated that the elderly in the test group were involved in tool-assisted and bare hand operations more evenly. In addition, compared with the control group, the elderly in the test group had considerably higher percentages of dominant hand use and both hand use in terms of total time. Therefore, the newly designed flower bed was proved effective at enhancing the elderly's willingness to use the nondominant hand and both hands, thereby encouraging balanced exercise in both hands and enhancing the positive effects of horticultural therapy.

The percentage of time in the test group where the elderly spent staring into space or resting is 18.22%. It is significantly lower than that of the control group at 35.96% (**Figure 11**). The elders in the test group spent a lot more time on planting activities and less time being idle. We also observed that the elderly immersed in their tasks that were under only one instructor's supervision. This means that "Elder Green" causes participants to be more interested in the whole class.

4.1. A comparison between pre- and post-design behavior, factoring in the number of elders

The control group of class two has a total of 13 participants, accompanied by nine volunteers and one teacher (**Figure 12**). Based on the new and unique design function of the flower bed with professional garden therapist advisory, the user base of "Elder Green" is set at five, accompanied by one instructor.

4.2. A comparison of caregiving to elders between the pre- and post-design

The percentage of time where an elder gets verbal instruction in class is 7.19%, physical instruction is 6.46%, and the average time where instructor demonstrates for an elder is 57.4 s, 1.97% of class time (**Figure 13**). Compared to class two, volunteer demonstrations have decreased.

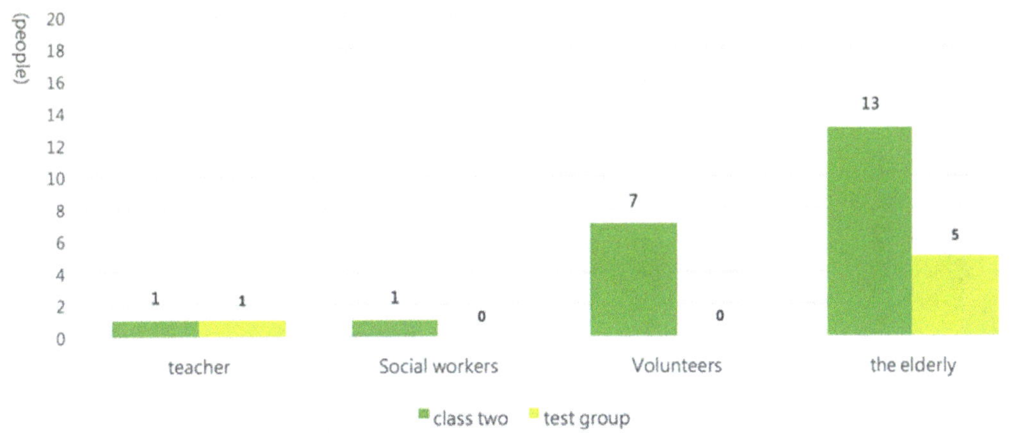

Figure 12. The relationship between the number of instructors and elders.

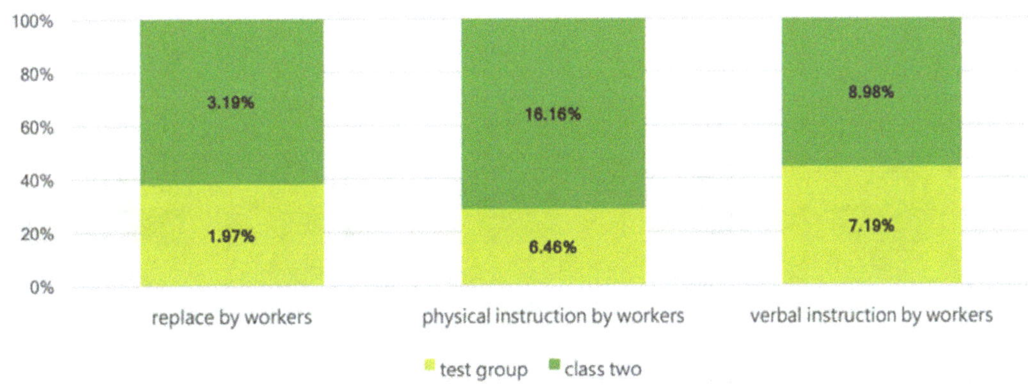

Figure 13. The percentage of time when an elder receives care.

Also, the elderly in the test group are much more enthusiastic about the curriculum, which reduces any distraction from other volunteers. The new design makes the elderly to get the therapeutic effect when working independently as same as the goal of horticultural classes. Implementation of "Elder Green" in the new curriculum will have positive effect on horticultural activities.

4.3. Comparison of pre- and post-design, factoring workers to elder interaction

The attention on all the elderly residents was unequal even though there were 13 elders and 9 volunteers in the control group of class two (**Figure 14**). On the contrary, there is only one instructor for every five elders, the elders of test group have more even guidance and care from one instructor (**Figure 15**). The test group had a much better experience than the control group in increased mental stimulation and physical exercise. This reveals how the instructor-centric class mode of "Elder Green" works. "Elder Green" helps the elders with fewer instructors and volunteers, conducting a quality fulfilling class more than creating a balance of instruction to each student.

In the test group, the elderly achieved higher amounts of exercise in a more balanced manner. The percentage of time involved in bare hand operations was higher than that spent on tool use. During the classes, the horticultural therapist encouraged the elderly to touch the soil often with their hands, and even smell the soil to increase tactile and olfactory sensory stimulation. Because

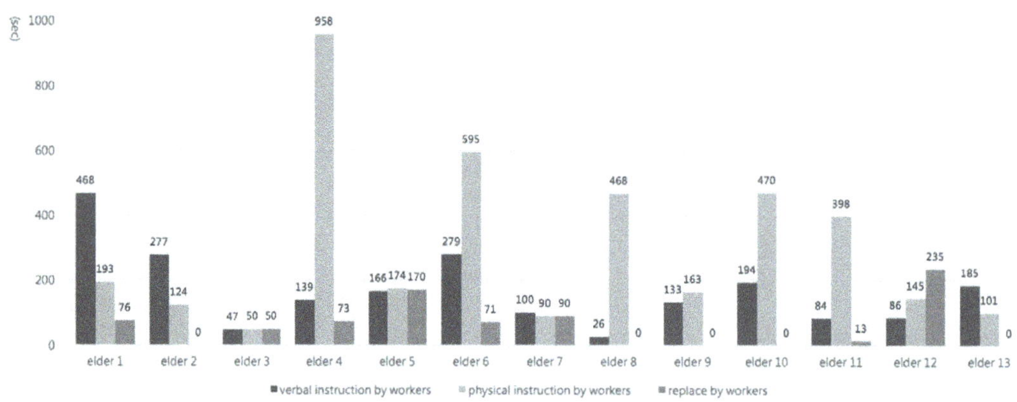

Figure 14. Relationship of class two (control group) between workers and elders.

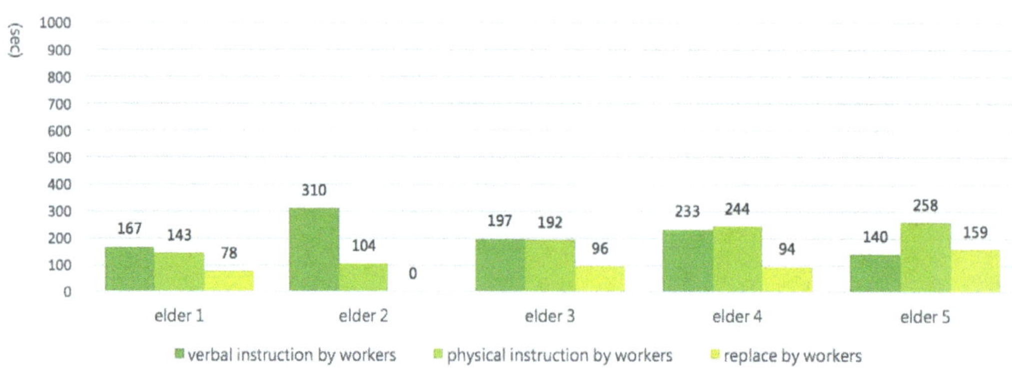

Figure 15. Relationship of the test group between workers and elders.

the dimensions of Elder Green were more suitable for the elderly, and because it featured individual operating platforms, the elderly could engage in planting more easily, which enhanced their willingness to use bare hands. In addition to encouraging the elderly to use both hands evenly, Elder Green enabled the horticultural therapist to provide equal attention to each older adult because of its radial arrangement when in teaching mode. Moreover, the arrangement elevated the elderly's perceived respect from others during the activities. The results indicated that idle time for the elderly in the test group decreased and mutual assistance increased. Again, this showed that higher enthusiasm in the elderly promotes the effects of horticultural therapy. Overall, this teaching style can enable institutions to provide quality gardening courses with less manpower.

5. Conclusions

The horticultural therapist can stand at the center of the radial flower beds to interact with the elderly during gardening courses. This study adopted universal design; both the elderly who were wheelchair users and nonwheelchair users could sit by the side of the flower bed. The flower bed was primarily made of wood, the pattern and color of which conveyed comfort and warmth to the elderly. After completing the gardening course, the flower bed naturally became a display shelf showcasing the planting results (**Figure 16**). The Elder Green flower bed helped every older adult focus on the course contents. It mitigated the problem of forward-leaning sitting postures commonly observed in users of existing products by improving flower bed dimensions; moreover, even the elderly in wheelchairs could approach the flower bed at a proper distance to effectively use the work table and reach the depth of the flower bed at ease, rendering gardening activities easier. In previous observations, marked differences were observed between the percentage of time the elderly spent using their dominant hand and using their nondominant hand. However, with the Elder Green flower bed, the elderly' physical activity conducted with both hands holding objects was substantially elevated, and they used their nondominant hand more frequently to accomplish the movements required in the class instead of simply using the same hand repetitively. Therefore, the Elder Green flower bed created more opportunities for physical activity among the elderly by effectively guiding them in spreading their strength to both hands (**Figure 17**).

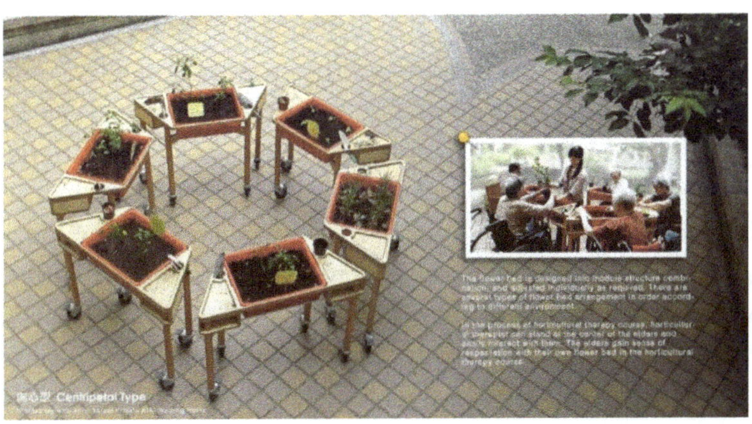

Figure 16. Different type of "Elder Green" arrangements.

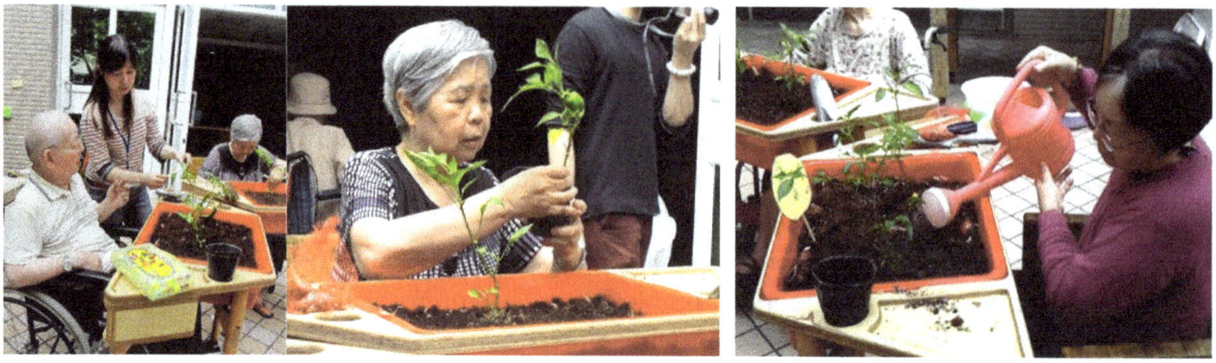

Figure 17. Actual situations of the elderly holding objects, using tools, and interactions between them and the teacher.

Observations on the bare hand operations of the elderly using Elder Green revealed notable increases in the average time of dominant hand, nondominant hand, and both hand usage compared with those observed with conventional methods. This finding indicated that the elderly became more active in bare hand operations, which enabled them to receive more comprehensive hand motor training. The individual seat attached to each Elder Green flower bed provided each participating older adult with an exclusive operating platform, enhancing their subsequent willingness to care for the plant and generating a sense of connection with the plant. In addition, this study noted that after Elder Green was introduced, the elderly were more enthusiastically involved in the tasks assigned by the teacher in class, which reduced distraction caused by boredom. Overall, the combination of a tight class tempo and concentrated movements rendered the gardening course fruitful; moreover, after Elder Green was adopted, the elderly spent more time helping each other. This indicated that the new teaching method inspired by Elder Green encourages mutual assistance and collaboration in a group of the elderly, and can adequately achieve the effects that horticultural therapy is expected to exert on the elderly. Using this method, the elderly have greater opportunities to complete gardening operations independently during horticultural therapy. Although the five elderly participants in the test group were only cared for by a horticulture teacher, the course proceeded successfully and they received relatively equal attention. This method allows organizing a quality horticultural therapy course with less manpower, and is likely to promote the willingness of related institutions to organize such courses. The flower bed of "Elder Green" allows soil depth of at least 15 cm. The height of the space under the desk is set at 62 cm which is a one-size-fits-all for elders of different heights and wheelchair users. The specification for the different basin choices are available in the market which makes future replacements easier (**Figure 13**). Users can arrange "Elder Green" in different forms according to the number of participants and the purpose of the horticulture class. Users also arrange flower beds in different shapes as the number of desks increase. "Elder Green" desks are mostly made out of wood. The protective wooden oil creates a warm and moist feeling when touching the wooden desk. Users can place the tools such as a hoe, shovel, plant, etc. on top of the desk or in the built-in drawer, which allows an elder to work seamlessly. Besides, an elder can use the desk of "Elder Green" as a hand-holder when sitting down or standing up for class. The installed wheel can make moving arrangements easier on the desk, and wheel lock also prevents the flower basin from shifting around.

The "Elder Green" flower beds have the potential to improve in many aspects. Studies support that individuals with cancer and chronic disease also benefit from therapeutic use of activities such as gardening, which helps the individual in terms of strengthening his/her bonds with life [19, 21]. Thus, different types of wooden patterns and the color of the flower basin are examples of customization which can meet the different requirements by design. Also, how different horticultural class curriculums combined with different medical aids are worthy of investigation for the future.

Author details

Meng-Cong Zheng

Address all correspondence to: zmcdesign@gmail.com

Department of Industrial Design, National Taipei University of Technology, Taiwan

References

[1] Kamp D. Design considerations for the development of therapeutic gardens. Journal of Therapeutic Horticulture. 1996;**8**:6-10

[2] Lee Y, Kim S. Effects of indoor gardening on sleep, agitation, and cognition in dementia patients—A pilot study. International Journal of Geriatric Psychiatry. 2008;**23**(5):485-489

[3] Relf D. Human issues in horticulture. Horti Technology. 1992;**2**(Suppl. 2):159-171

[4] Brown VM, Allen AC, Dwozan M, Mercer I, Warren K. Indoor gardening the elderly: Effects on socialization, activities of daily living, and loneliness. Journal of Gerontological Nursing. 2004;**30**(10):34-42

[5] Kavanaugh JS, Musiak TA. Selecting design services for therapeutic landscapes. Journal of Therapeutic Horticulture. 1993;**7**:19-22

[6] Gigliottic CM, Jarrott SE. Effect of horticultural therapy on engagement and affect. Canadian Journal on Aging. 2005;**24**(4):367-377

[7] Mami M. Japanese Society for the Promotion of Welfare (53). Japan: Broadcast Publishing Association; 1984

[8] AHTA. About Horticultural Therapy. [Internet]. Seattle, WA: American Horticultural Therapy Association; 2005. Available from: http://www.ahta.org

[9] Azar JA, Conroy T. The development of an empirical instrument designed to measure the effects of horticultural therapy. Journal of Therapeutic Horticulture. 1989;**4**:21-28

[10] Eckerling M. Guidelines for designing healing gardens. Journal of Therapeutic Horticulture. 1996;**8**:21-25

[11] Huri M, Kayıhan H. Investigation of relationship between independence in activities of daily living and cognitive function variables in geriatric individuals. Ergoterapi ve Rehabilitasyon Dergisi. 2014;**2**(1):1-10

[12] Airhart DL, Willis T, Westrick P. Horticultural training for adolescent special education students. Journal of Therapeutic Horticulture. 1987;**2**:17-22

[13] Reed J, Roskell Payton V. Challenging 'the institution'. Journal of Psychiatric and Mental Health Nursing. 1996;**3**:274-277

[14] Sinem S, Ayla G, Serkan P, Meral H, Babak Kashefi M, Gülfer K. Mine UYANIK7 relationship between activity. Environment and Life Satisfaction in Older Adults Ergoterapi ve Rehabilitasyon Dergisi. 2016;**4**(2):89-96

[15] McGuire DL. Implementing horticultural therapy into a geriatric long-term care facility. In: Wells SE, editor. Horticultural Therapy and the Older Adult Population. New York: The Haworth Press; 1997. pp. 107-139

[16] Meral H, Emre H, Hülya K. Determination of activity preferences and effects of occupational therapy on activity profile and participation of patients with metastatic prostate cancer. Ergoterapi ve Rehabilitasyon Dergisi. 2013;**1**(2):1-10

[17] D'Amico PD, Sommer J. Promoting and maintaining mobility in the homebound elderly client. In: Zang S, Allemer JA, editors. Home Care of the Elderly. Philadelphia: Lippincott; 1999

[18] Brownson RC, Baker EA, Housemann RA, Brennan LK, Bacak SJ. Environmental and Policy Determinants of Physical Activity in the United States. American Journal of Public Health 91. December 1, 2001;(12):1995-2003

[19] Johnson RA. The meaning of relocation among elderly religious sisters. Western Journal of Nursing Research. 1996;**18**:172-185

[20] Jancey JM, Clarke A, Howat P, Maycock B, et al. Perceptions of physical activity by the elderly: A qualitative study. Health Education Journal. 2009;**68**(3):196-206

[21] Onur A, Berkan T, Mine U. Occupational therapy for elderly people book chapter In: Meral H, editor. Occupational Therapy-Occupation Focused Holistic Practice in Rehabilitation. ISBN 978-953-51-3322-3, Print ISBN 978-953-51-3321-6

[22] Dobbs GS, Relf PD. Enclave employment of disabled individuals in a university grounds maintenance department: A case study. Journal of Therapeutic Horticulture. 1991;**6**:38-49

[23] Ayşe G, Serkan P, Bilgehan T, Hülya K, Mine U. Impact of activity preferences on cognitive skills and life satisfaction in elderly. Ergoterapi ve Rehabilitasyon Dergisi. 2016;**4**(1):1-14

[24] Lewis JF, Mattson RH. Gardening may reduce blood pressure of elderly people: Activity suggestions and models for intervention. Journal of Therapeutic Horticulture. 1988;**3**:25-38

[25] Parsons AB, Relf PD. The need for organized information of horticulture projects which involve the disabled population in developing countries. Journal of Therapeutic Horticulture. 1989;**4**:3-9

[26] Sempik J, Aldridge J, Becker S. Social and Therapeutic Horticulture: Evidence and Messages from Research. Reading: Thrive and Loughborough: CCFR; 2003

[27] Lee YK, Lee TF, Woo J. Predictors of satisfaction among cognitively intact nursing home residents in Hong Kong. Research in Nursing & Health. 2005;**28**(Suppl. 5):376-378

[28] Barnes M. Designing for emotional restoration: Understanding environmental cues. Journal of Therapeutic Horticulture. 1996;**8**:11-14

[29] Austin E, Johnston Y, Morgan LL. Community gardening in a senior center: A therapeutic intervention to improve the health of older adults. Therapeutic Recreation Journal. 2006;**40**(1):48-57

[30] Relf D. Putting the consumer in horticulture. PPGA News Feb. 1990:4-5

[31] Schleien S, Rynders J, Musonen T, Heyne L, Kaase S. Teaching horticulture skills to adults with autism: A replicated case study. Journal of Therapeutic Horticulture. 1991;**6**:21-37

[32] Flagler J. Correctional youth and the green industry. Journal of Therapeutic Horticulture. 1993;**7**:49-55

[33] Lassey WR, Lassey ML. Quality of Life for Older People: An International Perspective. New Jersey: Prentice Hall; 2001

[34] Relf D. Dynamics of horticulture therapy. Journal of Rehabilitation. 1981;**42**:147-150

[35] Tadao S. Community Planter, Annual design review of Japanese Society for the Science of Design. 2013;**18**(18):54-59

[36] Relf D. Horticulture: A therapeutic tool. Journal of Rehabilitation. 1972;**39**(1):27-29

[37] Bunn DE. Group cohesiveness is enhanced as children engage in plant stimulated discovery activities. Journal of Therapeutic Horticulture. 1986;**1**:37-43

[38] Huri M, Huri E, Kayihan H, Altuntas O. Effects of occupational therapy on quality of life of patients with metastatic prostate cancer: A randomized controlled study. Saudi Medical Journal. 2015;**36**(8):954-961. DOI: 10.15537/smj.2015.8.11461

[39] Bowling A. Research Methods in Health: Investigating Health and Health Services. McGraw-Hill Education, UK: Open University Press; 2007

Permissions

All chapters in this book were first published in OTTCUA, by InTech Open; hereby published with permission under the Creative Commons Attribution License or equivalent. Every chapter published in this book has been scrutinized by our experts. Their significance has been extensively debated. The topics covered herein carry significant findings which will fuel the growth of the discipline. They may even be implemented as practical applications or may be referred to as a beginning point for another development.

The contributors of this book come from diverse backgrounds, making this book a truly international effort. This book will bring forth new frontiers with its revolutionizing research information and detailed analysis of the nascent developments around the world.

We would like to thank all the contributing authors for lending their expertise to make the book truly unique. They have played a crucial role in the development of this book. Without their invaluable contributions this book wouldn't have been possible. They have made vital efforts to compile up to date information on the varied aspects of this subject to make this book a valuable addition to the collection of many professionals and students.

This book was conceptualized with the vision of imparting up-to-date information and advanced data in this field. To ensure the same, a matchless editorial board was set up. Every individual on the board went through rigorous rounds of assessment to prove their worth. After which they invested a large part of their time researching and compiling the most relevant data for our readers.

The editorial board has been involved in producing this book since its inception. They have spent rigorous hours researching and exploring the diverse topics which have resulted in the successful publishing of this book. They have passed on their knowledge of decades through this book. To expedite this challenging task, the publisher supported the team at every step. A small team of assistant editors was also appointed to further simplify the editing procedure and attain best results for the readers.

Apart from the editorial board, the designing team has also invested a significant amount of their time in understanding the subject and creating the most relevant covers. They scrutinized every image to scout for the most suitable representation of the subject and create an appropriate cover for the book.

The publishing team has been an ardent support to the editorial, designing and production team. Their endless efforts to recruit the best for this project, has resulted in the accomplishment of this book. They are a veteran in the field of academics and their pool of knowledge is as vast as their experience in printing. Their expertise and guidance has proved useful at every step. Their uncompromising quality standards have made this book an exceptional effort. Their encouragement from time to time has been an inspiration for everyone.

The publisher and the editorial board hope that this book will prove to be a valuable piece of knowledge for researchers, students, practitioners and scholars across the globe.

List of Contributors

S. Doria, F. Irtelli, R. Sanlorenzo and F. Durbano
Department of Psychiatry and Neuroscience, "Fatebenefratelli e Oftalmico" Hospital, Milano, Italy

Joaquim G. Machado-Neto
São Paulo State University, Jaboticabal, Brazil

Grethel León-Mejía
Laboratory of Molecular Radiobiology, Center of Biotechnology, Postgraduate Program in Cell and Molecular Biology (PPGBCM), Federal University of Rio Grande do Sul (UFRGS), Porto Alegre, Rio Grande do Sul, Brazil
Simon Bolivar University, Faculty of Basic Sciences, Unit of Research, Development and Innovation in Genetics and Molecular Biology, Barranquilla, Colombia

Milton Quintana Sosa
Simon Bolivar University, Faculty of Basic Sciences, Unit of Research, Development and Innovation in Genetics and Molecular Biology, Barranquilla, Colombia

Paula Rohr
Laboratory of Celular and Molecular Biology, Academic Unit of Health Sciences, Universidade do Extremo Sul Catarinense (UNESC) - Criciúma SC), Brazil

Katia Kvitko
Postgraduate Program in Genetics and Molecular Biology (PPGBM), Federal University of Rio Grande do Sul (UFRGS) Porto Alegre, Rio Grande do Sul, Brazil

João Antonio Pêgas Henriques
Laboratory of Molecular Radiobiology, Center of Biotechnology, Postgraduate Program in Cell and Molecular Biology (PPGBCM), Federal University of Rio Grande do Sul (UFRGS), Porto Alegre, Rio Grande do Sul, Brazil
Laboratory of Molecular Radiobiology, Center of Biotechnology, Federal University of Rio Grande do Sul (UFRGS) Porto Alegre, Rio Grande do Sul, Brazil

Juliana da Silva
Laboratory of Genetic Toxicology, Postgraduate Program in Molecular and Cell Biology Applied to Health (PPGBioSaúde), Lutheran University of Brazil (ULBRA), Canoas, Rio Grande do Sul, Brazil

Meral Huri, Burcu Semin Akel and Sedef Şahin
Hacettepe University, Faculty of Health Sciences, Department of Occupational Therapy, Ankara, Turkey

Ayse Numanoğlu Akbas
Department of Physical Therapy and Rehabilitation, Abant İzzet Baysal University, Bolu, Turkey

Bryan M. Gee and Theodore W. Peterson
Idaho State University, Pocatello, ID, USA

Amy Nwora
D'Youville College, Buffalo, NY, USA

Gokcen Akyurek
Department of Occupational Therapy, Faculty of Health Science, Hacettepe University, Ankara, Turkey

Esma Ozkan and Sümeyye Belhan
Department of Occupational Therapy, Faculty of Health Sciences, Sağlık Bilimleri University, Istanbul, Turkey

Mahmut Yaran
Department of Therapy and Rehabilitation, Havza Vocational School, Ondokuz Mayıs University, Samsun, Turkey

Meral Zarif
Department of Occupational Therapy, Faculty of Health Sciences, Hacettepe University, Ankara, Turkey

Beliz Belgen Kaygisiz
Faculty of Health Sciences, Department of Physiotherapy and Rehabilitation, European University of Lefke, Lefke, Turkey

Sedef Şahin, Barkın Kose and Meral Zarif
Faculty of Health Sciences, Occupational Therapy Department, Hacettepe University, Ankara, Turkey

Meng-Cong Zheng
Department of Industrial Design, National Taipei University of Technology, Taiwan

Index

www.ingramcontent.com/pod-product-compliance
Lightning Source LLC
LaVergne TN
LVHW060557210926
848485LV00005B/1332
* 9 7 8 1 6 3 9 8 9 3 9 1 1 *